About *Your Body, Your Yoga*

Your Body, Your Yoga **is a fascinating, provocative, and sci-entifically-informed look at the inner workings of the body as it affects the practice of asana.** Bernie Clark challenges much dogma in the modern postural yoga world, including a few heretofore sacrosanct principles of alignment, to demon-strate that a healthy and effective yoga practice should be adapted to each individual's unique needs, abilities and anat-omy. Required reading for yoga teachers and yoga therapists, and highly recommended for avid practitioners.
—*Timothy McCall, MD, author of* Yoga As Medicine, **USA**

An exceptionally well-informed and interesting way of approaching the human enterprise of doing yoga. Full of beautiful and stimulating pictures and analogies, awakening a deep thirst to know more and think more yet.
—*Loren M. Fishman, MD, BPhil (Oxon.)* **USA**

Your Body, Your Yoga **is an essential book for all serious yoga practitioners.** Through skillful marshaling of evidence, Bernie Clark decisively illustrates the importance of individ-uality in yoga practice.
—*Norman Blair, yoga teacher, author and trainer,* **United Kingdom**

This book will revolutionize the practicing and teaching of yoga. It is going to be the next yoga bible! It is an incredible treasure, and it will help everybody to truly understand the essence of physical yoga practice.
—*Stefanie Arend, author of* Yin Yoga, Detox Yoga, *and* Fascia Massage, **Germany**

Teachers will benefit greatly from understanding all that this book has to offer, and advancing students will enjoy and benefit all the more because of it. Bernie Clark's book is a ter-rific contribution to the field of yoga, which until recently has been overly "posture-centric." Bernie gives a readable, clear account of individual differences—how to recognize them, their consequences for asana practice, and how to sense when you are going too far. There is a wealth of information on the deeper mechanics of muscles and fascia, and an extensive treatment of the specifics of the joints.
—*Doug Keller, author of* Yoga As Therapy *and associate profes-sor in the Maryland University of Integrative Health Master's Degree Program in Yoga Therapy,* **USA**

Instant Classic: Bernie Clark has done a tremendous service in producing this book. It is as thorough in its scope as it is excellent in its content. He has systematically accounted for an-atomical variation. I feel indebted to Bernie and Paul Grilley for promoting an anatomically functional approach to yoga.
—*Gil Hedley, Ph.D., Director, Integral Anatomy Productions, LLC,* **USA**

Finally, a book that dares to combine yoga with state-of-the art critical thinking and scientific reflection! To my knowledge, the most accurate and anatomically knowledgeable book in this field. I knew that Bernie Clark would contribute something remarkable. But this book goes way beyond even the highest expectations. A truly groundbreaking contribution to the field of science-inspired yoga.
—*Professor Robert Schleip, PhD, Ulm University,* **Germany**

A must-read for yoga teachers and practitioners. This book will reframe the way you think about body movements.
—*Jo Phee, senior yoga teacher trainer,* **Singapore**

This is an instant classic. *Your Body, Your Yoga* demystifies and reveals the limitations in one's yoga practice in a very clear and in-depth manner.
—*Sebastian and Murielle, senior yoga teacher trainers,* **Indonesia**

I am so amazed: *Your Body, Your Yoga* **is more than a great book**—it is like participating in a training at home. I could not stop myself from finishing it.
—*Devrim Akkaya, senior yoga teacher trainer,* **Turkey**

This is a brilliant book. It is an absolutely essential research resource for anyone who teaches, hopes to teach, or wants to practice the asana component of yoga in a safe, therapeutic, and effective way. Bernie Clark's thesis that we are not all the same and therefore there are no universal alignment princi-ples that work for everyone is a huge contribution to today's yoga literature. I couldn't agree more. It is hard to believe that anyone would say this about a book on anatomy, physiology and human movement, but once I started reading, I was so excited I couldn't put it down! —*Beryl Bender Birch, author of 4 books on yoga and the founder/director of* The Hard & The Soft Yoga Institute *and* The Give Back Yoga Foundation, **USA**

YOUR BODY YOUR YOGA

116°

82°

BERNIE CLARK

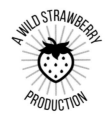

A WILD STRAWBERRY PRODUCTION

This book is dedicated to Paul Grilley,
whom I am proud to call my teacher and my friend.
This truly is his book.

All rights reserved. Copyright © 2016 by Bernie Clark. No part of this book may be reproduced or transmitted in any form or by any means whatsoever, including graphic, electronic, or mechanical, including photocopying, recording, taping, or by any information storage or retrieval system, without permission from the publisher. Inquiries should be addressed to:

Wild Strawberry Productions
1906 West 11th Avenue,
Vancouver, B.C.
Canada V6J 2C6
Website: www.YourBodyYourYoga.com

Editor: Dania Sheldon

Cover and interior design by Alex Hennig

Illustrations by Morgan Jeske unless otherwise indicated

First edition: 2016

Printed in the U.S.A.

ISBN 978-0-9687665-3-8 (pbk.)

MEDICAL DISCLAIMER

The contents of this book are intended for general information only and not as specific medical advice. Please check in with your health-care provider before following any suggestions found herein. The guidance given in this book is not meant to replace medical advice and should be used only as a supplement if you are under the care of a health-care professional. When you are not sure of any aspect of the practice, or feel unwell, seek medical advice.

Acknowledgements

It takes a village to raise a child, and a similar amount of loving kindness, attention and intention to create a book like this one. I would like to acknowledge the village of people who helped inspire and create this book, beginning with Paul Grilley. Paul had the original genius to recognize the importance of human variation in yoga and of compression in limiting our range of motion. His dedication to educating yoga students and teachers through his classes, courses and DVDs changed the way I taught and practiced yoga asanas. It was because of Paul that I learned to stop trying to destroy my knees by forcing myself into hip-opening postures. I have now humbly accepted that Lotus pose (Padmasana) will never be a close personal friend. Paul, from the bottom of my heart and the heart of my knees, thank you!

Along with my gratitude for the enthusiasm and support provided by Paul and his wife and fellow yogi, Suzee, I would like to thank the students of the September 2013 Yin Yoga Teacher Training, conducted by Paul and Suzee at Land of Medicine Buddha, in Soquel, California, for sharing their stories, body shapes, proportions, and enthusiasm for this project. To Douglas, Dace, Danielle, Debby, Amanda, Stephanie, Sebastian, Murielle, Leslie, Helga, Karin, Maheshwara, Rich, Perry and all the others who shared those 16 days together, my heartfelt thanks.

My gratitude extends also to the reviewers who gave of their time and knowledge to look over the early and later drafts of my work: Dr. Chelsea Barry, Dr. Robin Armstrong and especially Katrina Sovio, thank you so much for keeping my thinking clear and my writing readable and relevant. To Dr. Sammy Chan for his invaluable research assistance, my great appreciation. A special thanks goes to Professor Stuart McGill for his reviews, thoughts and encouragement.

Of course, words alone fail to convey concepts completely, and I turned to Morgan Jeske time and again to help illustrate my ideas. Many thanks for your patience and your pen in creating and revising the drawings for this book. Speaking of illustrations, my thanks also go to OpenStax College for their commitment to providing free education to all, including free anatomical drawings for educators to use. And, once more, my thanks to Paul Grilley—this time for freely making his "bone photos" available to everyone via his website, for his reviews of the work in progress, and for our many Skype calls discussing the intricate points of skeletal anatomy and its implications for our yoga practice.

Thanks also to Dania Sheldon for her patient editing, the many reviews and many profitable suggestions. And thanks to Alex Hennig for coming up with the design concept for the book, laying it out in such an attractive and accessible way, and creating the graphic design of the cover. What makes a book fully usable is the index: my thanks to Pilar Wyman for once again creating such a comprehensive one.

Throughout my journey to create this book, I have often been absent, both physically and mentally, from my home and home life. I would like to thank my partner, Nathalie Keiller, for her patience and support, and for being there to let me bounce off half-formed ideas.

Finally, my thanks to all my students who have helped me shape these ideas over the years and test them out on so many varied bodies.

How to Read this Book

The human body and the human experience of our body are complex, vast and varied. It will never be possible to reduce the full range of variation and its implications for our yoga practice into one book. But scientists have a methodology for addressing vast questions: break them down into smaller bits. Much is lost in such a reductionist approach to reality, but the process has its merits, which is why it is so commonly applied. We will also use a reductionist approach, beginning by segmenting our investigation into several volumes, presented in a number of books. Book One, this book, consists of Volumes 1 and 2.

Volume 1: What Stops Me? will investigate the nature of our tissues and how they contribute to a reduced range of motion. We will introduce and quantify the vital concepts of human variation, the value of stress and our tissues' need for stress, the sources of tension and compression, and the contributions that different kinds of tissues make to tension. We will learn that what gives rise to tension in our tissues is much more than simply short, tight muscles. Through this realization, we will understand that we need to go beyond simply stretching our muscles to gain our optimal health and range of motion.

Volume 2: The Lower Body will put what we learned in Volume 1 into the specific context of our joints. We will investigate the major joint segments that play a role in our yoga practice in the lower body (hips, knees, ankles and feet.) We will look at their anatomical structures and what can restrain movement. We will answer the "What stops me?" question in relation to the lower body.

First, we will look at the *form* of the joint segments, including their architectures, bones, joint capsules, ligaments, fascia and muscles. We will also investigate the ranges of variation in the tissues comprising the joint, focusing mainly on the variations in the bones. This section will appeal to those teachers who are really interested in anatomy, and not just from a yoga perspective. Many yoga students may choose to skip the *form* section and move straight to the second section, where we will examine the *function* of the joint segment and the implications of this functionality for our

yoga practice. In this second investigation, we will look at the sources of tension that can limit movement, and at how human variations can affect the possible movements and individuals' ultimate ranges of motion. We will also look at the implications of these factors for selected yoga postures.

Volumes 3 and 4 in the next book will continue to investigate the rest of the body in the same manner as we do for the lower body: the axial body (from the sacrum to the cervical spine) and the upper body (shoulders, arms, wrists and hands.)

Volume 5 will look at the other aspects of human variation not yet addressed: those of individual proportions of the body, and the reality of the asymmetries that we all have. The frequency and consequences of these asymmetries will be investigated, along with their implications for our yoga practice.

Sidebars and Appendices. Selected materials and interesting topics are broken out into sidebars and appendices. In these instances, more detail can be offered than is desirable in the general stream of investigation. For the student who loves lots of details, sidebars called "It's Complicated" will dive more deeply into certain topics. Longer investigations of these complex topics will be placed in the appendices at the end of each volume. Most students, however, can skip any of the sidebars that begin with "It's Complicated." For yoga teachers, there are sidebars called "Notes to the Teacher." And for virtually everybody, there are sidebars called "It's Important"; these will contain information that is a little bit off the main topic but nonetheless important to any student of yoga.

An Apology to Purists

Our intention is to help educate yoga students and teachers on the reality of human variation and its impact on range of motion. We are not attempting to offer any original research, and we are not addressing an academic audience. Where practical, we offer citations for studies, claims and statistics in the endnotes. In the process of illustrating sometimes complex topics, we have taken certain liberties with strict academic diligence. For this, we beg your indulgence. For example, we do not always choose the conventional nomenclature. Likewise, when we make a claim that a certain movement results in an angular displacement of 110°, we will not always show how we derived that figure. There are a lot of detailed calculations that are not shared with the reader, because to do so would clutter the text and not add value or clarity. We have chosen to err on the side of accuracy over precision: due to the nature of human variation, approximate figures are precise enough, as long as they are accurate. Except where specifically noted, we have not used the most extreme examples of human variations, but rather have opted for the range of variations most likely to show up in 95% of the students attending a yoga class (those falling within two standard deviations of the norm, which means one person in 20 will fall outside the illustrated range). Even here, we are using an approximation: two standard deviations in a normal distribution includes 95.45% of the population and excludes 4.55%. We will round these amounts, so that we can simply say 19 people out of 20, or one person out of 20, even though that may not be mathematically precise. We have opted for simplicity over thoroughness, but not at the expense of accuracy or truthfulness. If, in this process, we offend your sensibilities, we beg your understanding.

Bernie Clark
Vancouver
December 2015

Contents

VOLUME 2: The Lower Body: The Consequences of Human Variation and the Sources of Tension and Compression

Sidebars

IT'S IMPORTANT

IT'S COMPLICATED

NOTE TO TEACHERS

FOREWORD
The History of Teaching Alignment in America

Assuming that everyone is the same makes the teaching of yoga simpler but, unfortunately, not safer. We are *not* all the same: just as you would be ill advised to take someone else's prescription drugs, or drive while wearing someone else's glasses, an alignment cue that works well for one yoga student may be quite harmful to you. Where did this emphasis on universal alignment cues come from? Paul Grilley explains:

When did the "rules of alignment" in yoga classes become ubiquitous? Rules of alignment became both rigid and pervasive with the rise of yoga teacher training (TT) programs. Teacher training programs were rare until the late 1980s and early 1990s. There were some yoga studios in Los Angeles and San Francisco, but their bread and butter were daily and weekly classes, not TT programs.

Before the rise of TT programs, yoga teachers trained by showing up regularly at classes and then being asked to substitute for the regular instructor; eventually, they started teaching regularly. There were no formal training programs. In fact, the people who opened and ran these studios had very little formal training themselves. Yoga culture then was like surfing culture is now: people learned from others, practiced on their own and occasionally practiced in groups. Most "studios" were people's living rooms.

Yoga benefitted from the birth of the modern fitness culture, just as did other forms of exercise such as body building, jogging, dance classes and aerobics. Body building and running are not conducive to group class participation, but dance and aerobics classes were born in the group environment. Yoga classes began to model themselves after dance classes, and the modern "yoga class" was born. People practicing on their own became less common.

Just prior to the fitness boom, yoga was a small niche of hippie/Hindu yogis whose practices focused on calmness and stillness. Yoga might not have benefitted from the fitness explosion had it not been for the Ashtanga/Vinyasa yoga of Pattabhi Jois. This style of yoga was hot, sweaty and similar in feel to aerobics classes. Vinyasa styles of yoga eventually became as popular as aerobics, while the gentle hippie yoga of the previous years was nearly forgotten.

Thanks to Ashtanga/Vinyasa, yoga exploded, and there were not enough teachers or studios to keep up with the demand. Yoga TT programs were created to meet this need. There wasn't time to cultivate teachers in the old-fashioned way of "show up regularly, then substitute teach, then teach"; teachers needed to be mass-produced in 200-hour chunks of time. None of this was a cynical manipulation—it was motivated by a genuinely felt need.

But how to produce a teacher in 200 hours? The education had to be systematized to be time efficient, and students needed to be assessed unambiguously. Both needs were met by creating manuals with strict and memorizable "rules of alignment" on how postures should be taught.

Continuing along for many years before the yoga boom was a TT program that was not patterned after the "show up regularly, then substitute teach, then teach" model. This was the Iyengar School of Yoga in India, and its branches in the USA, particularly in San Francisco. In fact, *Yoga Journal* started life as a journal of the Iyengar School in San Francisco.

Iyengar teachers prided themselves on having exact rules of alignment; in this very significant way, they stood out from other styles of yoga and from yoga TT programs. Mr. Iyengar had already developed many "levels" of certification. This is important because the manual first used by Yoga Works in Los Angeles was written by Iyengar and other alignment devotees.

Yoga Works developed the most successful TT program in the hot-bed of the booming yoga business: Los Angeles. Yoga Works has since then expanded to many studios in LA and across the USA, and they have actively exported their TT program to as far away as Asia.

But it isn't just Iyengar Yoga or Yoga Works that have sought to standardize the rules of alignment: every style of yoga that seeks rapid expansion does the same. Bikram yoga turns out cookie-cutter teachers by the hundreds, and their "training" is largely the strict memorization of a script of alignment instructions. Anusara yoga used to bill itself as "the fastest growing style of yoga in the world!" and its rules of alignment have been described as "Iyengar with spirals." And almost monthly, someone trademarks their "brand" of yoga, which is essentially trademarking their alignment rules.

Alignment is not a "Western corruption" of yoga tradition. Mr. Iyengar is an Indian from an Indian tradition. But there are many Indian schools of yoga without rigid alignment, and Pattabhi Jois's Ashtanga yoga is one of them. There are also Western schools of yoga that are not alignment rigid, such as Kripalu yoga. So, alignment rigidity is not Eastern or Western or universal, it is a consequence of TT programs trying to make it simpler to mass-produce teachers.

Any time an art is constrained to mass production, it will be simplified, codified and rigidified. This is true in yoga, in dance, in the martial arts and in religion. Simpler is easier to teach and absorb, but it also leads to inaccurate generalizations and intolerance of individuality.

Yet it must be said that the impulse to embrace rigid rules of alignment is not motivated only by TT necessities. It is one part of human nature to codify and rigidify, just as it is another part of human nature to break with tradition and create something new. We cannot teach effectively without some generalizations, but we haven't reached maturity until we have outgrown generalizations and can competently focus on the unique needs of every student in every pose. This is not an impossible dream—it just takes more time than a TT program can afford. The onus of continuing growth is on each and every yoga teacher. This is the only way a teacher can reach his or her full potential.

Swami Vivekananda addressed this issue in the field of religion: "It is good to be born in a church; it is bad to die in one."

Paul Grilley, September 2015

VOLUME 1
What Stops Me?

Sources of Tension and Compression

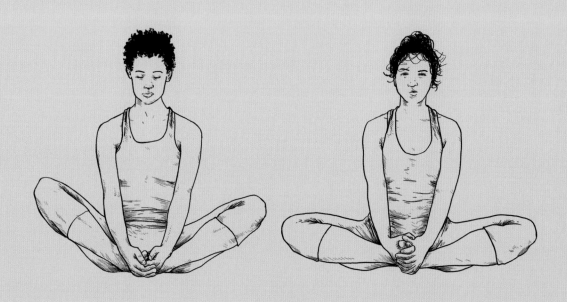

Intentions

You are unique. That is nothing new, but the implications of this short statement are vast. You are unique and therefore, what works for you, what suits your body (your biology) will be different from what works for other people. Your history (your biography) is also uniquely yours. When you consider both your biology and your biography—the raw materials that made you and the forces that shaped you—it is not surprising to find that your needs differ considerably from everyone else's. Your eye glasses prescription, your shoe size, the position of your driver's seat in your car, which hand you use to write or throw, the way your lips curl when you smile, the curve of your spine and the arches of your feet—all these little and grand variations make you uniquely and undeniably you.

So why do we default to a belief that we are all the same on the inside? Why do we believe that there is one and only one way to do a yoga posture, that there is one "right" way for every body? Why do we believe that alignment cues are universal and that all people should move their bodies in the same way?

The first intention of this book is to help you understand your uniqueness and what it means for your yoga practice. However, this realization goes far beyond yoga. As you come to understand your uniqueness, many things in your life may shift. What diet works best for you, how much rest you need, how much exercise and which type is most beneficial, which medicines and therapeutic interventions will prove beneficial, all these and more will become worthy of assessing. The fact that something worked for a friend or a family member (or a complete stranger) does not mean that it will work for you. It might, but you are not them, so maybe it won't. How can you know?

When we apply this overriding intention to the investigation of yoga, we quickly come to a question that will be repeated numerous times in this volume: "What stops me?" Sometimes we will simply abbreviate it to "WSM?". Due to your uniqueness, what stops you may be totally different from what stops your yoga teacher; or, if you are a yoga

teacher, what stops your students may be very different from what stops you.

The second intention of this book, and of this volume in particular, is to help you answer your WSM? question. Modern Hatha yoga instruction looks for the physical answer in the musculature of the body: invariably, the answer will be couched in terms of short, tight, restricting muscles. Wonderful drawings and computer-generated graphics have been created to show which muscles are the culprits and how to work these muscles to keep going deeper and further in our postural work. The psychologist Abraham Maslow once noted that if all you have is a hammer, then everything starts to look like a nail. If your theory of yoga revolves only around the muscles, then the solution for every problem will be to address the muscles. However, as we journey through Volume 1, the answer to the WSM? question will broaden considerably. We will discover two main contributors to physical restrictions: tension and compression. We will also discover that these are complex categories.

Many books do an excellent job of describing the role of muscles in various yoga postures. It is not our intention to duplicate such work, so we will not spend much time describing which muscles articulate which limbs and which muscles resist movement; we will cover these in a generalized, overview fashion. For the reader who wants to learn more about the muscles, one highly recommended resource is Leslie Kaminoff's *Yoga Anatomy*. We will spend even less time describing the pervasive effects of our fascia and its contribution to tensile resistance. This is not to imply that fascia is unimportant—it is very important. Fascial restrictions can contribute far more to restrictions in our range of movements than short, tight muscles ever will. This topic is simply beyond our scope of investigation and requires a detailed book all on its own. Fortunately, such a book already exists: Thomas Myers's *Anatomy Trains*. Serious students of anatomy are also advised to pick up a good university-level anatomy textbook, such as Thieme's *Atlas of Anatomy*.

This book aims to make you aware of your uniqueness within the vast range of human variation, to explain the principles of tension and compression, to raise and answer the question "What stops me?" and to help you realize what all this means for your yoga practice: Your Body —> Your Yoga! This book was written for *you*, about *you*, and to help *you* get to know yourself much better. I hope you enjoy and benefit from it.

Postscript: Science is ever-changing, which is both its blessing and its curse: the scientific models and theories that we believe to be true today may turn out to be not so true in a few years. Stay open, stay humble, keep learning. The theories and facts shared in this book may well change, but what can remain constant is the intention—finding *your* yoga. To do this, trust your *experience* over any theory or dogma.

CHAPTER 1
You Are Unique—So Is Your Yoga

You are unique! These three words imply something amazing. In the whole universe, there is no one like you. You are not "average" and you are not "normal"—no one is actually average, normal or regular. You may share a few similar traits with other people: you may wear a medium-sized shirt like millions of others; your shoe size may be the same as your sibling's; you are made up of identically shaped protons, neutrons and electrons, as is everyone you know. But when you examine the whole of who you are, the ways these particular parts come together to form a "you," you are totally and indisputably unique.

Consider what this means: if you are totally unique, then what you need to be healthy and whole will be very different from what someone else needs. Roger Williams, scientist, author and discoverer of vitamin B5, coined the term "biochemical individuality" to express how vastly different all humans are from each other.[1] It is this variation that makes all the difference when we look at what keeps us healthy and what causes us to become sick and suffer disease. The nature of human variation has been largely ignored in both medicine and the fitness world (including the yoga industry), an error that Williams and others have tried to correct. The 18th-century physician Parry of Bath said, "[It is] more important to know what sort of patient has a disease, than to know what sort of disease has a patient."[2] We can paraphrase this in relation to yoga as: "It is more important to know what sort of student can do a pose, than to know what sort of pose is doing the student." In advising how to train an elite athlete, Stuart McGill, a medical researcher of lower back disorders, notes, "Each person has different proportions of body segment lengths, muscle insertion lengths, muscle to tendon length ratios, nerve conductance velocities, intrinsic tissue tolerances, etc. . . . Imposing a stereotyped 'ideal' technique will often prevent an athlete from reaching their full potential."[3] Figures 1.1 and 1.2 give simple illustrations of how our uniqueness will affect our yoga postures.

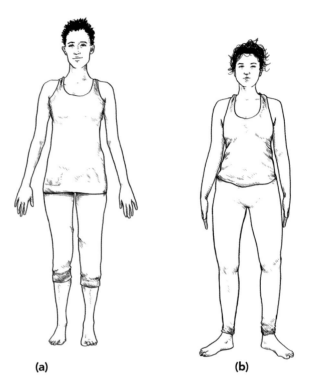

(a)   **(b)**

FIGURE 1.1 The woman on the right (b) has a distinct varus of the legs, causing her bowlegged appearance, and her hips are quite externally rotated, causing her feet to point outwards. The lady on the left (a) is slightly internally rotated in the hips, and her legs are straighter.

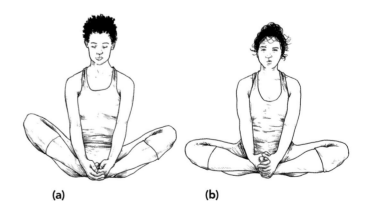

(a)   **(b)**

FIGURE 1.2 The variations in the shapes of our legs affect not only our appearance but also our ability to do yoga postures. Student (b) finds it easier than student (a) to get her knees to the floor in Butterfly Pose (Baddhakonasana).

Just as no one else has your dental pattern, no one else has your bone structure, your spine or your hips. Why think, then, that what someone else can do, you should be able to do, too? Or why think that because someone else can't do something, you also will fail? There are things you can do right now, there are things that you will be able to do in time, and there are things that you will never be able to do. This is not a critique of your abilities or a reflection of your personality or some flaw that needs to be fixed—this is simply the reality of your existence. A five-foot-tall ballerina will never play right tackle for the Seattle Seahawks, and the right tackle for the Seahawks will never win an Olympic gold medal for figure skating. This does not mean that the ballerina is flawed or the right tackle is lazy. A snowflake, in all its beautiful uniqueness, will never be a galaxy of stars. Why would it ever try to be something it cannot be? Better to be a great snowflake. We need to understand our uniqueness and our natural limitations.

Think of the ways we can be measured: height, weight, age, education, income level, family size, city of upbringing, blood pressure, heart rate, the length of our arms relative to our spine, the degree to which our feet point outwards, the amount of curvature in our legs… The list can go on and on. In any one of these categories, you might fall within the "average range"—you may indeed be an average height and maybe even an average weight, but when you add in the parameters of your blood chemistry, personality, diet, lifestyle, job, body shape, birthdate[4] and so on, you move far away from being an average person. No one is average (see It's Complicated: Averages and norms, on page 7). This means that whatever works for an "average person" (who does not actually exist) may not work for you.

To quote Roger Williams again: "[P]ractically every human being is a deviate in some respects."[5] There is no normal and no abnormal. There is only you in all your uniqueness, and this uniqueness will determine what, of all life's offerings, is available for you to partake in, and what you should, with wisdom, leave on the plate.

The Range of Human Variations

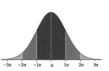

Where is your appendix? Most people who have studied anatomy will point to their lower right abdominal area. But as figure 1.6 illustrates, that is only where the appendix is located "on average." This is where an appendix is normally, but are you "normal"? Imagine you are suffering an acute attack of pain in your upper left abdomen. Your friends rush you to hospital, where a new intern comes to your aid. His first instincts are that you are suffering from appendicitis, but then he realizes that your pain is nowhere near your appendix, or at least where he thinks your appendix is supposed to be. He puts you on painkillers and sends you home instead of ordering the life-saving operation you need. Not good![11] *(continued on page 8)*

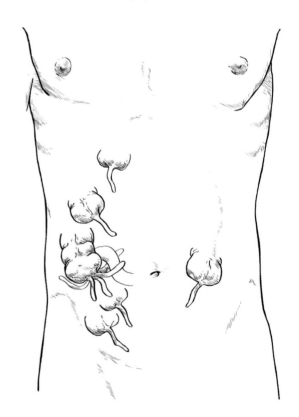

FIGURE 1.6 Where is your appendix? Here are a few of the observed locations.[12]

IT'S COMPLICATED: Averages and norms

"Statistics mean never having to say you're certain."

Average, also known as *mean*, is obtained by adding up all values in a range of measurements and dividing by the number of samples.

Median is the middle value of a range of measurements, where half the values are above the median and half are below it.

Mode is the most commonly occurring value.

Imagine you were invited to arrange the entertainment for a boy's birthday party. Being an intelligent person, you ask, "What will be the average age of the people at the party?" You are told 18. Great. Now you know how to prepare. You find some fantastic games that will challenge and stimulate 18-year-old boys, some killer videos with loud rock music and sexy women, and you think you are all set. You arrive at the party to discover 10 moms who are 30 years old and 10 boys who are six years old. The average age—18! We determine the average age by adding up the ages of everyone at the party and dividing by the number of people. The simple average (mean) is 18. (However, in this bi-model distribution, the modes are six and 30.) Unfortunately, no one at the party is able to enjoy the entertainment you arranged, because you pegged your thinking to the average. No one at that party is average. It is dangerous to think only of averages.

Scientists and medical researchers use a concept called *the norm* to measure human variation. They consider people inside the norm *normal* and apply this term to 95% of the population. People outside the norm—the remaining 5%—are considered, by definition, *abnormal*. If you are a teacher of a yoga class with 20 students, this means that on average, one student will be abnormal in some respect. But it is not that simple.

Human variation can be mapped out in what is called a bell curve (see figure 1.3). For a given characteristic, people will fall somewhere along this distribution curve. Towards the middle of the curve you find more people; 68% of people fall within a range called one standard deviation (denoted by the Greek letter sigma, σ), and 95% are within 2σ. Anyone outside 2σ is considered abnormal. (This doesn't mean that they are bad, just that they are very unusual.) Within the range of 2σ is the norm, as mathematicians define the term.

You may well be within the norm for height and weight, but are you in the norm for both height and weight together? When we consider two factors at the same time, we may end up with a multi-normal distribution. For example, consider gender and height. What is the normal height for someone? Well, that depends on different factors (see figure 1.4). What is normal for a woman is not necessarily normal for a man. We see also that the range of human variation is not constant; there is a wider range of heights for men than for women.[6]

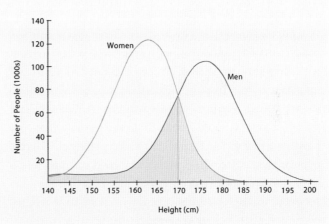

FIGURE 1.4 A multi-normal distribution, showing the distribution of height versus gender.

If we start to add in other factors, such as age, weight, blood pressure and fasting blood glucose, we find fewer and fewer people in the norm. Now consider yet more factors, like our genetic makeup. No two people have exactly the same DNA, not even identical twins![7] So, if no two people are exactly alike, how can we say what is normal, or average? Treating everyone as if they are all the same runs a grave risk of mistreating everyone. Treating every yoga student identically also runs a big risk of harming some students while under-challenging others.

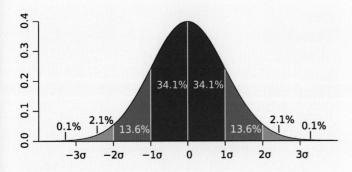

FIGURE 1.3 A bell curve graphically depicts a normal distribution; people generally fall within the curve, with many people close to the norm and fewer people further away from the norm.

Now imagine attending a yoga class where the teacher believes everyone can, eventually, do Lotus Pose (Padmasana). Maybe not today, but with diligence, practice and a firm guiding hand, with the right Lululemon pants and the best Himalayan incense, the teacher can show you how to get into this challenging cross-legged posture. He notes that every student who has stayed with his program long enough has managed to do this. What if you have never been able to sit cross-legged comfortably? Your knees are always up by your ears when you sit on the floor, but you are game. You try—you ignore the little tweaky feelings in your knees until one day, the pain escalates into a burning fire that won't stop even after the class is over. You have torn your medial meniscus and are no closer to doing Lotus Pose than when you started yoga. The teacher has been ignoring the reality of your uniqueness. Due to the shape of your pelvis and femurs, you will never be able to do Lotus Pose, and trying to get there is destroying your knees.

Yoga is a self-selecting practice. Those who have the correctly shaped bones to be able to do certain postures keep working and progressing. They stretch out all the tensile resistance that prevents achieving their maximum range of motion, and they get to their desire positions. However, those whose bones are not shaped so optimally, who are not stopped by tension but rather have reached compression, where the bones are hitting each other, will never be able to do the pose. They quit in frustration, convinced that some deep personality flaw is preventing their progress, a delusion secretly shared by some teachers.

IT'S IMPORTANT: Beware of studies

As a popular saying goes: studies have shown that people will believe anything you say as long as you begin your statement with "Studies have shown." A fact is defined as a piece of information, or a truth verifiable from experience or observation.[8] When scientists give us a fact, we naturally believe them—it saves us from having to do the research that they have done. But please, do not believe every study cited in the popular press. Often these studies are brand new, and that is what makes them newsworthy, but they have not yet been subjected to vigorous review and duplication. Time will tell whether the results bear up under further scrutiny.

As one example, the graphic shown in figure 1.5 displays the number of studies that have found that what we eat may both contribute to cancer and prevent cancer.[9] How can this be the case? It depends upon the design of the study, the particular people who participated in the study, the quality of the research and researchers, and many other factors. One solitary study is not sufficient to make an overall claim of causation. Plus, not all studies are equivalent in quality and scope, and not all participants have the same genetic and biographical backgrounds. Only repetition and time will uncover the true situation, and that truth may be that we cannot generalize about the effects of a given food on every body. Biological science is not nearly as exact as we would like it to be. Take everything you read with a grain of salt, even if studies have shown that salt intake may increase your risk of cancer.

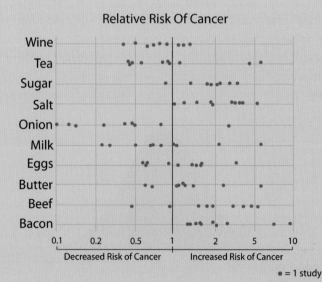

FIGURE 1.5 Single studies can create an incorrect perception of reality.[10] It takes multiple studies, repeated with differing populations, to understand causality.

Examples of Human Variations

Scientists love to and need to make generalizations. They draw a line through a myriad of points on a graph and say that this line represents reality, but it does not. It is a generalization. These generalizations are useful, but they miss an important part of the story. Consider the statistic that claims that the human thigh bone (femur) neck-shaft angle is 126°.[13] Figure 1.7 shows two femurs, and neither one has this average angle. Indeed, one study determined that the average femoral neck-shaft angle varies considerably across cultures. The North American average for urban people of European heritage is closer to 134°.[14]

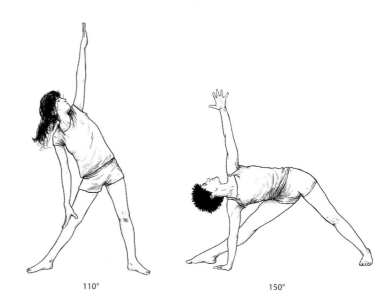

110°   150°

FIGURE 1.8 Our ability to abduct in Triangle Pose is determined in part by the femoral neck angle. The student on the left has a femoral neck-shaft angle of only 110°, while the student on the right has an angle of 150°.

Medical researchers term anyone who has a femoral neck-shaft angle of 120° or less *coxa vara* and those with an angle greater than 135° *coxa valga*. People with *coxa vara* or *coxa valga* are considered deviants; they are not "normal." But an extensive study of femoral neck-shaft angles shows that many people are above or below this range; indeed, "normal individuals are found from around 110° to almost 150°."[15]

Genetics will play a role in this ultimate angle, but genetics alone is not the whole story. When we are babies, the neck angle is around 150°.[16] As we mature and begin to stand, then walk, stress is placed upon the hip socket and the neck of the femur; over the years, this stress lessens the angle. The more active we are as children, the greater the remodeling of this bone.[17] By the time we enter puberty, the angle of the neck of the femur to the shaft of the femur reaches a value that will remain virtually unchanged throughout our adult life (see figure 1.9). But what is that final angle? This depends upon a number of factors, which are described in It's Complicated: Femoral neck-shaft-angle variations, on page 10.

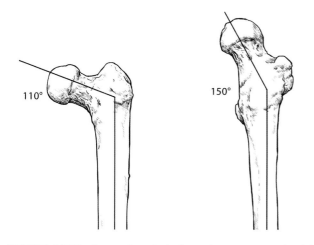

110°   150°

FIGURE 1.7 The femoral neck-shaft angle varies considerably.

What does this mean for us in our yoga practice? A teacher who is not aware of human variations is not risking your life, as might a doctor who is not aware of variations in the location of the appendix, but a yoga teacher's ignorance can still lead to problems. The neck angle of the femur (and the shape of the pelvis) dictates the ultimate range of motion in abduction (moving the legs apart.) Triangle Pose (Trikonasana), for example, requires an ability to abduct the legs, but once the tensile resistance to abduction has been worked through, the range of motion available is determined in part by the angle of the neck of the femur. The two students who own the femurs shown in figure 1.7 will not look the same in Triangle Pose (see figure 1.8) because of their bones, not because of their dedication or desire.

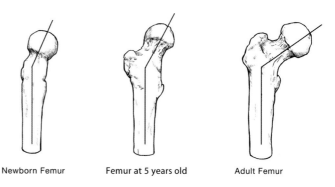

Newborn Femur   Femur at 5 years old   Adult Femur

FIGURE 1.9 The femoral neck angle varies as we mature.[18]

THE MYRIAD WAYS OF HUMAN VARIATION

Paul Grilley, a yoga teacher who has studied in depth the consequences of anatomical variation in individual yoga practices, emphasizes uniqueness by having his students recite the following mantra:

> *I'm the only one.*
> *There is something wrong with me.*
> *I must be inadequate in some way.*
> *Shanti, Shanti, Om...*

We all think that we are the only ones who cannot do a particular pose. And when we can't, we believe that there is, indeed, "something wrong" with ourselves. Understanding the reality of human variation, of your uniqueness, helps to sweep away these delusions. You are not the only one who cannot do a particular posture! You are unique, and that uniqueness is what makes the difference between what "everyone" seems to be able to do and what you can do. There is no pose in yoga that everybody can do, and no one can do every pose.

Barry Anson, a well-known medical scientist, doctor and professor, noted the frustration of medical students who dearly want a standard model to follow. "The student's attachment to the concept of an archetypal plan in the fabric of the human body is perennial and persistent. Frequently he is annoyed by departure from the standard."[19] Arguably, yoga students and yoga teachers have the same desire: it would sure be nice if every person's body was the same and if we all looked like the drawings in the anatomy books or the plastic skeleton hanging in the corner of an anatomy classroom. But we aren't and we don't.

As Roger Williams explains: "Variations encompass all structures, brain, nerves, muscles, tendons, bones, blood, organ weights, endocrine gland weights, etc. . . . These structures often vary tremendously from one individual to another."[20] He also points out that "human anatomists have been aware of variations for many generations but . . . for pedagogical reasons they have concentrated on the 'norm' and have shown little or no concern for the possible significance of the ever-present variations."[21]

IT'S COMPLICATED: Femoral neck-shaft-angle variations

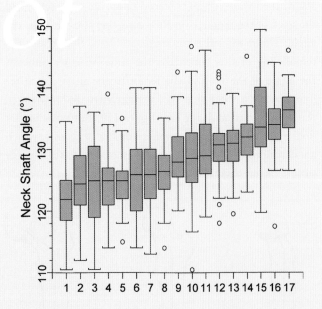

Different human populations have always had different femoral neck-shaft angles, depending upon their predominant activities. While modern North Americans living in an urban setting have an angle of around ~134°,[22] farmers, hunter-gatherers, and people who were very active as youngsters can average closer to 120°.[23] The range is what is most interesting. Note the variations shown in figure 1.10, from 110° to 150°—quite significant! The shaded areas range from 118° to 140°, and this too is significant because the shaded areas show a two-quartile range in the population, which means that 50% of the people studied are within that shaded range—and, of course, 50% are outside of it. So, this wide range of variation is very likely to show up in an average yoga classroom, meaning not everyone will be able to reach their hands to their ankles in Triangle Pose (Trikonasana)—ever!

FIGURE 1.10 The range of femoral neck angles by population types. The numbers along the bottom axis represent different population types, from #1 = South Africans to #17 = modern Chinese. Modern North-East Americans of European descent are shown in #15; they range from 118° to 150°, with 50% of the population being between 130° and 140°.[24]

Again, we find the same tendencies in the yoga world. It is inconvenient to describe all the ways our students are unique and easier to assume that the anatomy book assigned to help the student learn which muscles are worked in each yoga pose is the reality for every student. Unfortunately, it isn't. In addition, what stops us from obtaining the aesthetically pleasing shape in the majority of movements is compression, not tension. We will look at these two key concepts when we investigate the important question: "What stops me?"

I will be citing many studies that show great ranges of variation in the shape and size of our bones, joints, muscles and so forth. The key point is not what *one* particular study finds but that *all* studies show that ranges in human variation exist, are often wide, and are often quite significant. My point in citing studies is not to claim that any one of them represents "the truth" of how the human body is but to illustrate the ever-present range of variability in our bodies. Please do not focus on a particular statistic or measurement, or even on a particular range of values. The key is that ranges exist. We will use the reality of ranges to guide us when we look at the implications of human variation for our yoga practice.

Throughout Volume 1, I will offer examples of human variation. The intention of these snippets is to remind you that we are all unique and that this truth will eventually come to inform everything you try to do.

IT'S IMPORTANT: Who is flying the airplane?

In the Kalama Sutta, the good people of Kalama ask the Buddha whom to believe, as they are confused by the abundance of gurus, monks and teachers claiming to know the truth and dismissing anyone else's teachings. The Buddha advises them to take as truth only what they can verify for themselves. A person should not be believed simply because he seems learned, has a long white beard, is teaching from an ancient book, has a fancy title or a certificate from a prestigious university, or has written a book. The only method is to evaluate the doctrine personally to see whether it works, whether it diminishes suffering. If it doesn't, then drop it. The Buddha was both a rationalist and an empiricist.

Bruce Lipton, a professor of genetics, speaker and author of the book *The Biology of Belief*, once asked: "What is the difference between your doctor and an airplane pilot?" Before delivering the punch line, he pointed out that a pilot, by law, has to go through a large checklist of items before he can taxi the plane away from the airport terminal. Your doctor likewise is expected to go over a standard list of questions and procedures when you come to see her, but since she has only about 10 minutes allocated to your visit, there isn't time to actually do the full job. What's the real difference between the doctor and the pilot? "The pilot is on the plane with you." This bears repeating: **The pilot is *on* the plane with you!**

Lipton's comment is not meant to disparage doctors, and it also applies to dentists, accountants, lawyers and yoga teachers. You may be surrounded by bright, educated and well-intentioned people, but you are the one flying your own plane. Experts can be part of your advisory council, but you have to take the final responsibility for your life, for your health, for your yoga practice.

Don't take anything a yoga teacher tells you as gospel: check it out. The teacher's advice is no doubt well intentioned, but you are flying your plane. If the advice doesn't suit you, don't follow it. You are unique. Your teacher will never know you as well as you know yourself. Her advice is guidance, but it is not a commandment from God! How will you know whether the advice doesn't work for you? As the Buddha suggested, consider it, try it, but pay attention: pain is often a great signal that something isn't right. If it isn't right for you, ask for options. Theory is great, but never ignore your experience simply because it is at odds with someone's theory or philosophy.

You do not attend a yoga class for the teacher's benefit: she is there for your benefit. If she is not benefitting you, find another teacher who will.

CHAPTER 2
What Stops Me?

Along with realizing our uniqueness, it is also important to comprehend where our challenges lie. The Serenity Prayer expresses this understanding:

> *God, grant me the serenity to accept the things I cannot change,*
> *The courage to change the things I can,*
> *And the wisdom to know the difference.*[58]

The wisdom to know the difference is the goal of our journey. To understand what is possible for us, to have the courage to grow to the limits available to us, and to recognize and honor our limitations when we meet them—that is the wisdom we seek. This gives rise to an important question, one that we will benefit from asking any time life presents us with a challenge or high drama: "What stops me?" We will look at this predominately from a physical perspective, but please be aware that what is stopping you may have no physical component at all—it may be psychological or emotional. (For more on these obstructions, please read It's Important: Playing your edge, on page 15.)

Physically, we reach our edge when one of two things occurs: our tissues can stretch no further, or our body is hitting itself. We will use the term *tension* for the former: tension arises when the body's tissues can elongate no more, and further movement is therefore restricted. This tension can be found in our muscles but also in our fascia, ligaments and joint capsules. A common example of tension occurs for many people in their hamstrings. If your hamstrings are short and tight, when you try to come into a seated or standing forward bend with straight legs, you feel the tension in the back of your legs. The tension in your hamstrings restricts your range of motion (see figure 1.12a).

The second reason we may be unable to progress further is *compression*. This occurs when one part of the body comes into contact with another part and further movement in that direction is therefore not possible. There are several kinds and causes of compression. The first we will call *soft* compression—what occurs when flesh comes into contact with other flesh. A good example is presented in figure, 1.12b where the flesh of our chest hits the flesh our legs. The

second we will call *medium*—what arises when our bones compress our flesh. An example is when the bone of your pelvis (technically called the ASIS, or anterior superior iliac spine) compresses into the flesh of your thigh in a lunge posture. The third kind we will call *hard*; this is the unyielding compression of a bone hitting another bone.

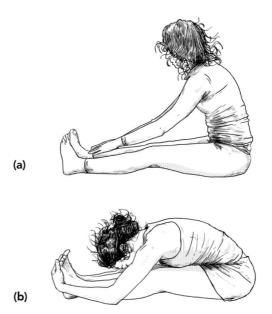

(a)

(b)

FIGURE 1.12 Tension (a) and compression (b) limit our range of movement. Tension is felt in the direction away from the movement, indicated in (a) by the shading along the hamstrings. Compression is felt in the direction of movement, indicated by the shading along the chest and thighs in (b).

From a technical point of view, there are several kinds of stress that we can apply to our tissues, and each form of stress has a limit. However, for our purposes, it is sufficient to look only at tension and compression. (For a complete discussion on the five kinds of stress we can create in our yoga practice, see Appendix A: The Forms of Stress.)

The stress of tension and compression can be arranged in a spectrum that starts with the weakest form of tensile resistance to movement and moves all the way to the finality of bone-on-bone compression. I call this the *WSM? spectrum*

"DIFFERENCES AREN'T DEFICITS," said Theodosius Dobzhansky, a population geneticist.[25] There are many ways we are different, and that is okay. Sometimes the differences have consequences, and sometimes they don't. The differences may become a problem when we either ignore or deny them. They are real, and that is normal.

(see figure 1.11). We can view our yoga practice as moving us from the far left of the *WSM? spectrum* to the far right, at which point the game stops. But for many people, the progress is not so linear. Our biography dictates how fast we move along this spectrum, but our biology may reorder the major stopping points. For example, due to your unique anatomical biology, you may not be able to stretch out your tensile resistance in one particular posture, because your hard edge is so close: you get stopped before you even get started.

In general, beginners to yoga will find that tension restricts their range of motion. In time, the tension will diminish. At some point, however, the student will find her restrictions are no longer due to tension—she will reach points of compression. An exception may arise when the tension occurs in joint capsules: capsular ligaments provide restraining tension that may greatly limit the range of motion in that joint. This tension may not disappear over time and may be the ultimate limit to how far she can go. A good example is the capsular ligaments of the hip joint that prevent extension beyond 30°. Our intention in yoga practice is not to become hypermobile in the joints; thus, we accept the tensile limitations presented by our joint capsules and do not try to stretch them further.

Unlike tensions, the points of restriction caused by compression will not change with further practice. When compression arises, you will have reached a fundamental limit to your range of motion—for *that* posture in *that* direction. It is important to acknowledge this point. Once you have reached compression, you cannot go further, but sometimes you can go around. In the example of the yogini who is doing a deep-seated forward fold in figure 1.12b, she cannot go any further because her upper body is contacting her lower body. She has reached a point of compression. However, if she abducts (spreads) her legs apart, as shown in figure 1.13a, she can go around this compression and continue her

journey, continue to work through tension, until the next point of compression is reached—in this case, the floor! She can't go further because her chest is hitting the floor. We could allow her to go further either by digging a pit beneath her or by building her a platform: we could put blocks under her sitting bones and calves and lift her higher (see figure 1.13b). Now she could continue her journey until, finally, at some point, some part of her body would hit another part of her body, and this would be a point of final compression. Ultimately, after you have stretched out your tissues as much as you can, you will reach the end of your progress for that posture. To try to go further now may be dangerous, and injuries often happen to students who try to push through compression. (See It's Important: Injuries caused by yoga, on page 17.)

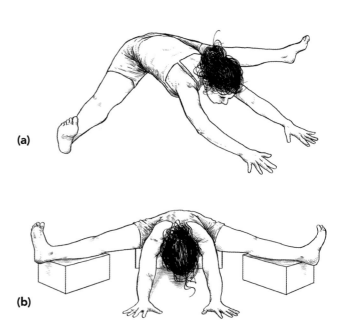

(a)

(b)

FIGURE 1.13 The points of compression experienced in a seated forward fold may be gotten around temporarily, but eventually, compression is the ultimate edge beyond which we cannot go.

These two concepts of tension and compression will resurface many times in our investigation of the body and will dictate what movements are available to us. While the concepts are simple, their manifestations are varied.

TENSILE RESISTANCE				COMPRESSION		
Surface Tensions	Myofascial Meridians	Muscles & Tendons	Ligaments & Joint Capsules	SOFT: flesh on flesh	MEDIUM: bone on flesh	HARD: bone on bone

FIGURE 1.11 The WSM? spectrum.

IT'S IMPORTANT: Playing your edge

There are valid reasons for fearing your edge—danger lurks there. But so does growth. If fear prevents you from playing your edge, that same fear is preventing you from learning, from progressing, from developing your full potential, including full health. A special teacher can show you how to play your edge and when to go past your edge. This requires trust—of your teacher and of yourself.

In yoga, the edge is the cliff of challenge and change. It may be high, it may be scary, but it is necessary. There are many kinds of edges. There is the physical edge, beyond which injury awaits. There is the emotional edge, beyond which both tears and laughter blossom. There is also the psychological edge, beyond which psychosis may erupt. And there is the spiritual edge, beyond which freedom is found. Edges are where something is about to happen—sometimes for ill and sometimes for good.

THE PHYSICAL EDGE

The body is always talking to us, if we listen. In our physical yoga practice, we are encouraged to approach the edge, which is the limit of tolerance of the tissues to the mechanical stresses being applied through the postures. Going beyond our tissues' tolerance invites damage. The body speaks, warning us of impending injuries by sending us little "tweaks." These small signals of pain or discomfort are important, and we ignore them at our peril, for little tweaks become big tweaks that suddenly turn into structural failure and long-lasting injury. The body needs challenges to stay strong and healthy. Too little stress and the tissues atrophy. However, too much stress and the tissues degenerate. If we fear our edge, we will default to a situation of too little, and that is unfortunate. If we ignore our edge, we will ignorantly go over the cliff and fall into damage and decay.

Playing the physical edge requires both intention and attention: the intention to be whole and healthy, and attention to the body's signals and sensations. In a yoga pose, we come to the point of challenge, our first edge, but then we back off a little. That first approach is a brief look over the cliff, to see what danger lurks below if we push too far. But our body is adaptable, and our edges are living things: they change, if we respect them. Once we have approached the edge, checked it out, then backed off a little bit—not so far

that there is no challenge at all, but enough so the edge is still in sight—the body relaxes. When the body fully trusts, it opens; the edge recedes, inviting you to follow. In time (and it can be a very short time or a very long time—you will only know by paying attention), the edge moves, and you may safely approach it once more, repeating the cycle of approach, observation, slight withdrawal and patience, awaiting the next movement.

Your physical edge is not reached by worrying about your alignment or engaging in physical contortion; your edge is reached by paying attention to sensation. How you look is irrelevant. How you feel is key. Based on your feelings, you adapt, you adjust, you advance and you retreat. Alignment cues can guide you, but they are never the ends, just one means of finding your edge.

Under certain special circumstances, your guide may push you beyond your physical edge. This may be beneficial in the right circumstances but not in a classroom filled with many other students. A physical therapist who knows you and your body well, a health-care specialist who has taken the time to understand you, a healer who is working with you one-on-one: these guides may take you beyond, because sometimes to heal, one must become injured again. Scar tissue is an incomplete response to damage; to get to the place of total healing, a therapist may have to push you past your comfort zone to break down the scars. Prolotherapy and other techniques, like scarring cartilage, can restimulate the body's repair mechanism and allow full healing to proceed. At times like these, we need to be pushed.

THE EMOTIONAL EDGE

Our body responds to emotions in observable ways,[59] and our emotions respond to our body. When we experience strong emotions, our body reacts: we may feel flushed, tight, hot, butterflies in the stomach, and a host of other sensations. But when we move our body, as we do in our yoga practice, we may also trigger emotional responses. There is a circular flow between the body and the heart/mind, well understood by Chinese Daoists and Indian yogis. Cause and effect—a favorite Western conceptual map—is linear, but look beyond this to the circularity of effect —> cause —> effect —> cause.

Our emotions cause bodily responses, and our body's movements cause emotional responses.

As we have physical edges beyond which we risk tearing open the tissues of the body, so too we have emotional edges beyond which we risk tearing open the heart. If the edge is pushed too fast and too hard, an emotional opening may become an emotional injury.

Pay attention! If you can't go deeper in a posture, you may have reached an emotional edge; you may well be able to physically go deeper, but your heart knows that to go deeper may trigger an emotional crisis that you are not yet ready to face. Play this edge, too—approach it, but then back off a little. Wait. In time, your heart may soften and invite you to come closer. Your emotional edge may move, and it may once more be safe to look over the precipice.

Never force the edge. That said, at times we need to be pushed over the emotional edge, and a dedicated guide may then be very helpful. When fear prevents our opening, when we are afraid to love or afraid to be angry, we avoid the edges. When our teacher knows us better than we know ourselves and pushes us over the emotional edge, the fear is shattered and our hearts are free: to love, to be angry, to express the emotions we have repressed. The shock and joy of this sudden freedom from fear is expressed in joyous tears and uncontrolled laughter. We fly.

THE PSYCHOLOGICAL EDGE

The mystic swims in waters where the psychotic drowns.[60] It is not surprising that, along with physical and emotional edges, we all have our psychological edges, beyond which there is an opening to the deep psyche—a shadowy, frightening view from which our ego recoils. It is rarer in our yoga practices to approach these edges, but it does happen. If one is not prepared, a leap off this edge can lead to psychosis. The ego will not willingly go there, and a sign that this edge is close is a strong physical and emotional signal: a visceral sense of danger, of fear, a compulsion to withdraw. The edge

is the place where our concepts change and we enter an alternate state of consciousness. The familiar is lost and the unfamiliar assaults us. We have gone too far.

Listen to that inner voice warning you that the edge is not to be passed. Back off again. Play the edge and view the abyss, but there is no need to dive in. Stay safe, stay grounded, and allow understanding to dawn slowly.

The shamans of primal cultures were guided through their childhood psychosis by elders who had gone before them. In modern times, the psychoses of childhood and early adulthood are disrupted through chemical treatments: the journey interrupted. An experienced guide and the necessary push are not to be found in a yoga classroom. Unless you are being taught yoga privately by an experienced psychotherapist, continue to play this edge respectfully.

THE SPIRITUAL EDGE

Each edge that we have visited holds potential danger and reward. This also applies to the final edge, the biggest edge of your life: the spiritual. Beyond this edge is freedom, but not as we imagine it in the West. This is not a freedom to *do* what we want. It is a freedom *from* want: no more wanting … anything! Are you ready for that? Probably not; few are. Such a vast freedom will affect the social fabric of your life. You will see friends and family in the same way you see everyone else. That sounds scary, but think of it this way: you will see everyone else the same way you see friends and family. There will be no attachments, and there will be no detachments. Boundaries will cease to exist.

Depending upon the spiritual map you have chosen to follow and the guide who chose you, your journey may take you to a beatific sight or to a full absorption in the divine. There will be no self and other: the ultimate boundary that your ego used to define itself will be lost. "Tat tvam asi," said the sage: "You are it!" As you fly over the edge, you will see that there is only one reality, and you are already in it.

Enjoy your edge, then enjoy your flight.

PAIN: We all have different abilities to feel pain, due to the number of pain receptors we possess. Fewer pain receptors can lead to longer life; this throws the whole bad idea of "no pain, no gain" right out the window! People with chronic pain die younger. Studies with mice have shown that blocking a gene that activates pain receptors allows mice to not only live longer but also stay healthier longer. We need some pain receptors so that we are aware when we damage our bodies, but too many, or suffering too much pain, has a cost.[54]

IT'S IMPORTANT: Injuries caused by yoga

Beginners starting their yoga practice are often quite stiff—so stiff, in fact, that many claim they are far too stiff to do yoga. This is akin to saying one is too dirty to have a shower, or too sick to see a doctor.[61] We do yoga *because* we are stiff! But we don't do yoga to become injured. Yet many advanced, experienced yoga students and teachers are injured through their yoga practice, whereas the beginning students are not. Why?

For most beginners, tension is restricting their range of motion. Over the years of their yoga practice, these yogis will work through their resistance and increase their range of motion until tension is no longer preventing further progress; only compression stops them now. The student has reached the limit of what her body will allow. This is a dangerous time! For the past several years, she has become more and more open and she has fallen in love with her yoga practice. Now, if she can continue the progression for a few more years, she will be able to touch her head to her butt in deep backbends and bring both feet behind her head in Dwipadasirsasana (as shown in figure 1.14). That day may never come for you, because once you have reached compression, which is dictated by the structure of your bones, more yoga will not open you up any further. Trying to go past the point of final compression is inviting injury, not further progress.

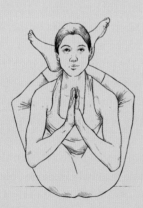

FIGURE 1.14 Dwipadasirsasana. Most people will be unable to achieve this position due to compression in their hip socket or tension in the capsular ligaments, not because of tension in their muscles.

Imagine that you are working towards a deep backbend, like the Wheel Pose (Urdvadhanurasana). Each day, you do 108 drop-backs from standing into the Wheel (see figure 1.15). If tension is restricting you from going further, you are feeling the stress of this posture along the front side of the body, but if you have worked through that tension until you have reached compression—the vertebrae of your spine hitting each other—then you are not going to go any further. You will not be able to create a deeper Wheel or grab your ankles. Tension along the front of the body helps to prevent the deep dynamic stress on the spine, but once you have worked through all that tensile resistance, the bones now start to hit each other, and degeneration (also called osteoarthritis) sets in. One of the reasons we are taught to engage our muscles in Hatha yoga classes is to prevent the dynamic stresses of the poses from damaging our joints and cartilage. (A safer way to stress the joints—and they do need stress to stay healthy—is to apply a static, lingering stress. This is the principle behind the practice known as yin yoga.)

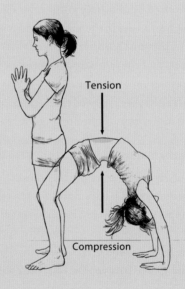

Tension

Compression

FIGURE 1.15 Dropping back into the Wheel (Urdvadhanurasana). To protect the spine, students are taught to engage their core muscles so that the tension of the tissues takes the stress of the pose, preventing dynamic compression of the joints of the spine.

Beginners do not have to worry nearly as much about damaging their joints as experienced students do. Beginners have a high degree of tension that prevents the dynamic stress of the poses from reaching the joints. Experienced student who ignore the sensations of compression and keep trying to gain a greater range of motion than their body will allow are the ones who run the risk of injuring themselves.

Tension

I gave the definition of tension as the resistance of our tissues to being stretched, which restricts further movement, then presented the example of the hamstrings being too tight to allow further flexion of the hips. However, this implies that tension is purely muscular. Tension may arise in a variety of tissues, though, not only in our muscles. Tension can be found in our muscles, tendons, skin, ligaments and the fascia that envelops and invests all of our tissues. A study[62] found four main contributors to tension in the midrange of a joint's movement:

- Skin: 2%
- Muscles: 41%
- Tendons: 10%
- Joint capsule: 47%

A progression from minimal tension to significant tension is reflected in the study's findings and in our *WSM? spectrum*. The *WSM? spectrum* shows that tension can arise minimally in the skin (which I am referring to as surface tension), then more significantly within the superficial fascia and deeper fascia, and in the muscles and tendons. After these tensile restrictions have been worked through, tension in the ligaments and the joint capsule becomes the governing cause of restriction to motion.

The study cited above showed that tightness in the muscles is not the major factor in limiting our range of motion: the joint capsule has a greater effect on our mobility than the muscles. As we reach the end range of our movement, the muscles have even less effect on further movement; now the connective tissues are fully responsible for tensile resistance. Missing from this study, however, are many other factors that also contribute to limitations in our mobility, such as restrictions between fascial boundaries. Often what keeps us stiff and tight are adhesions between the otherwise sliding surfaces of the body. Scar tissue is a common example of such adhesions. When an injury results in scar tissue forming between the normally sliding surfaces of our muscle fibers, we grow tighter and less able to move. This form of tension is not removed by lengthening our muscles because it is not shortness

FACES: Our faces contain more variability than any other part of the body. The greatest variation occurs in the triangular region formed by the eyes and the mouth. Humans have a relatively poor sense of smell, so we have to rely instead upon visual cues and our enormous brains to recognize other individuals. Our faces evolved their wide range of unique appearances to help us keep track of each other.[27]

in the muscles or the joint capsule that is stopping us now, but a contraction or stuckness in one area of our fascial network. Another cause of fascial tension is contracture of the fascia itself. The fascia may shrink, causing tension, which again restricts our natural mobility.

Tension is felt in the side opposite from the movement. For example, in the seated forward fold posture we looked at in figure 1.12a, the tensile resistance to going forward is felt in the *back* of the body (in the hamstrings). When tension restricts movement, it shows up in the opposite direction of the movement. This is important—training is required to help us recognize when tension is stopping us. Once we realize that tension will always arise in the opposite direction from which we are trying to move, we are able to pay attention to and discern when tension has arisen. Remember that tension can be changed, over time, with diligent practice. If what is stopping us is not tension, then we have reached compression, and our journey will require different strategies: either going around that point of compression or humbly accepting that we have reached our ultimate limit.

Compression

We have defined compression to be when one part of the body comes into contact with another part of the body, making further movement impossible. A trivial but illustrative example is the elbow joint: extend your arm out to the side, then investigate why you can't move your forearm further away from your shoulder. What is happening at your elbow joint to restrict further movement? The answer will probably be compression, as shown in figure 1.16a: your ulna is hitting the humerus and can't go any further. Mysteriously, for many people flexing the arm is also stopped by bone-on-bone compression (see figure 1.16b): in this case, the coronoid process of the ulna is coming into contact with the humerus. We can define this form of compression, where the bones impinge upon each other, as *hard* compression. It has a firm, solid, final feel.

Bone hitting bone is one example of compression, but it can arise in other ways. Notice again the yogini in figure 1.12b, who is folding her chest onto her thighs. This is a flesh-on-flesh form of compression rather than a bone-on-bone one. We are calling this *soft* compression. It has a soft, spongy or bouncy feeling to it. Yoga is not going to change this: she has reached a fundamental limit in how far she can fold in that pose and in that direction. In her case, it is possible to go around the points of soft compression. But there is no going around the elbow's points of compression. Wisdom suggests that she not try and instead accept this as a limitation of her body.

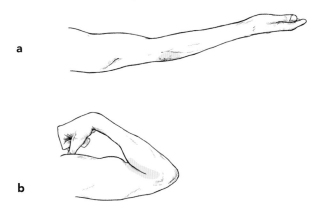

a

b

FIGURE 1.16 Hard compression. Bone-on-bone compression has a hard and final feel to it.

A third form of compression occurs when bone hits flesh. We are calling this *medium* compression. It has a pinching, uncomfortable feeling to it. An example of this often occurs for many students when they flex their hips. Due to the shape of their pelvis and the size of their thighs, the pelvis hits the thigh. This point of compression often shows up in poses like Child's Pose (Balasana) and low lunges (Anjaneyasana), or any time the thighs are drawn towards the chest. Fortunately, in this case there is an easy option for going around the point of compression: students can simply abduct the leg a bit (or a lot). This abduction allows the pelvis to go inside the thigh, and the point of compression is bypassed, allowing greater movement. Unfortunately, this option is often not offered to the student, because her teacher believes that "proper alignment" dictates the legs must be together in Child's Pose, or that the front knee must always point straight ahead in lunges. This emphasis on alignment over function causes more harm than good (and is dangerous enough to warrant a discussion of its own—please see page 22, Functional Yoga versus Aesthetic Yoga).

Compression has a very different feel than tension, and it occurs in a very different area. As mentioned, tension is felt in the direction *away* from the movement; compression is felt in the direction *of* the movement. Again, consider the yogini doing the seated forward fold in figure 1.12b who has pressed her chest into her legs. She has reached compression: she is moving forward, so compression is felt in the *front* of the body—where her chest hits her thighs.

Sensing Tension and Compression

The concepts of tension and compression are simple. During our yoga practice, it will often be very obvious what is stopping us. However, there will also be many places, deep and subtle, where we will not be so sure what is stopping us from going further. For example, in the hip sockets, tension may arise due to tightness of the ligaments wrapping the joint capsule. Or our movement may be stopped by compression of the neck of the thigh bone (the femur) against the rim of the hip socket (the acetabulum). Which is it? How can we know?

One of the greatest gifts a yoga teacher can give to her students is the ability to pay attention: to find for themselves the answer to WSM? To know whether what we are experiencing in this area is due to tension or compression requires great focus, concentration and attention. That is something we will develop over time. We can start by noticing what is stopping us in simpler situations. To develop this skill, continually ask yourself: "What stops me?" and determine whether it is tension or compression. Once you know the answer to that question, next try to figure out what *type* of tension (tension in the muscles, the ligaments, the fascia?) or what *type* of compression (soft, medium or hard?) is stopping you.

There are several clues that you can look for to help you answer WSM? When compression has been reached, there will still be some sensation of tension. To remove all the sensations of tension, we would have to stretch out the area where the tension arises, but by definition, once you have reached compression you cannot go any further, so whatever tension is still there will remain. This means that while you may be stopped due to compression, there will still be some feelings of tension as well. However, when you are stopped solely due to tension, there generally is little or no sensation of compression yet.

Table 1.1 shows correlations between the possible sources of resistance and the sensations that may arise. This table is not a definitive list, as everyone is different; use it as a

EYES: Retinal scans and iris scan are routinely used in security systems around the world to identify individuals. These work because everyone's eyes are different: even your left eye is different from your right eye. The differences are due to variations in the patterns of blood vessels supplying the retinas, and the ridges and furrows found in the muscles, ligaments and capillaries of the iris.[32]

guideline that you can adapt and modify to determine what sensations arise when *you* reach these edges. The intention of the table is to help guide your awareness and develop a level of sensitivity so that you can answer for yourself: WSM?

Pain does not belong in our yoga practice, but many students do not know whether the sensations they are experiencing are truly painful or not. If you experience the sensations listed in the pain column, it is a good idea to back away from that edge. Pain does have a place in physical therapy, and in the enlightened hands of a qualified therapist, pain can be a useful tool—to break through scar tissue for example. But most yoga teachers are not trained physical therapists, and a yoga class with 20 or more students is not the venue for seeking personalized therapy. If you are experiencing the sensations of pain listed, slowly back away from the edge.

NOTE TO TEACHERS: When students can't go further

You cannot tell by *looking* at a student what is stopping her from going further. You have to *ask her* what she is experiencing. Unless and until you have developed X-ray vision, don't assume that a student is not going deeper in a pose because she is (i) not listening to you, (ii) lazy or (iii) simply tight and needs to stretch her muscles more. Most of the time, students *are* listening to you, they *are* trying to do what you've asked, but they are stuck. Determine what is stopping her. Ask: "What are you feeling?" Then, based on what she says, give the appropriate direction. Remember, the most appropriate direction may be to back off! The student may have reached an edge beyond which it is not safe for her to go (see It's Important: Playing your edge, on pages 15–16). Ultimately, the greatest gift you can give any student is the ability to determine for herself what is stopping her, for then, she can be the one to determine the most skillful course of action.

If you have a student who responds to "What are you feeling?" with a shrug and a blank expression, if she doesn't know what she is feeling, then guide her awareness. Use some of the adjectives in Table 1.2 to help her know what to look for. Explain the differences between tension and compression. Tension is usually quite obvious, and if tension is stopping her, she will notice it and point to that area. If compression is the culprit, then you may need to point this out to her. Point to the targeted area of the pose and ask whether she is feeling anything there. If she is not feeling the pose where you would like her to feel it, try to figure out what is stopping her. Point to the common compression points and ask whether she is feeling anything there. If this is where she is being stopped, offer her options for going around those points. If she has reached her ultimate depth in the pose and there is no going around it, you have two options:

1) **Let her linger.** Sometimes there is great value in staying at a point of compression. Many tissues benefit from staying under compression. (See It's Important: The value of compression, on page 30.) Compression is not bad! *Painful* compression is not good, but painful tension is not good either. Pain is not good, at least not in a normal yoga classroom setting. There may be times when a therapist has to work through painful areas in order to break through scar tissue or other adhesions, but unless you are a trained therapist, don't subject your yoga students to pain.

2) **Give her another pose that targets the same area that you want her to touch.** A different pose may be able to reach this area without hitting the same points of compression. This is one of the benefits in the richness of Hatha yoga: there is an abundance of postures. If one pose cannot get to the target area, there are probably several other poses that can. Experiment, but also suggest to the student that she experiment, too—by moving slightly, she may find a path to the sensation you want her to experience. These slight movements or adjustments may take her out of the aesthetically pleasing alignment you originally asked for, but they will put her into a functional alignment, where she actually benefits from the pose. And that *is* the point, after all.

TABLE 1.1 The sensations arising in a posture can give us a clue as to the cause of resistance to further movement.

WSM? SPECTRUM	RESISTANCE SENSATION	PAIN
Surface Tensions	• Spread out • Mild • Stretchy or tugging	• Like a mild burn • Localized • Tolerable
Myofascial Meridian	• Spread out—multiple areas sensed at once • Linear or rope-like • Tugging or pulling • Dull	• Scratchy • Swirly • Circling • Achy
Muscles & Tendons	• Localized • Tugging • Tightness • Follows the shape of the muscle • Broad • Flat • Muscle: sensation found in the belly of the muscle • Tendon: sensation found in the attachments closer to the bone	• Sharp • Burning
Ligaments & Joint Capsule	• Stuckness • Deep • Mysterious (vague)	• Radiating • Sparkly • Electrical • Zingers (shooting)
Soft Compression	• Soft • Squishy • Bouncy • Spread out over a large area	
Medium Compression	• Stuck or blocked • Impinging • Localized	• Pinching • Uncomfortable
Hard Compression	• Stuck • Hard • Heavy • Very localized	• Dull • Achy[63] • Boring • Risky

A final point regarding pain: it is valuable to pay attention to pain not only while you are in the pose, but also as you come out of the pose, or even over the next day or two. Delayed onset of pain may be due to some things that you were doing in your practice that were not healthy. Whenever you feel pain, it is worthwhile to investigate the cause. If you can correlate it to what you were doing in your yoga practice, you have the option to skillfully modify your practice.

Part of your yoga practice is building your ability to attend, to be present, to notice what is happening. It can be helpful to have an idea of what to look for, to help us sharpen our perception. Table 1.2 offers several adjectives that we can use when trying to describe our sensations. It may be helpful as well to physically trace your sensation: use your fingertips to outline where you feel the sensation, and lightly draw on top of it.[64] This will guide your awareness and help you to deepen your attention. Several sensations are unique to tension, while others are more often indicative of compression. While everyone's experience is unique, you may find that the sensations shown in colour in the table are more typical of compression than tension. (Please be aware that these sensations may arise from other causes beyond yoga stresses, such as inflammation or other pathologies.)

Functional Yoga versus Aesthetic Yoga

There are two main reasons to do a yoga practice: to become healthier or to master postures. If your goal is the former, you will be more successful if you adopt a functional approach to your practice, which means you focus on the intention of the postures rather than their appearance. If your intention is to look good—perhaps you are a dancer or a gymnast, and looking good is essential to your profession—an aesthetic approach may be required. If you wish to follow a functional approach, however, there are three keys to adopt in your yoga practice ethic:

OUR WATER CONTENT: You have probably heard that we are 60% water. That is an average—the range of values is quite broad and differs significantly by gender. One study found that in a group of 18 men and 11 women, the water content varied from 46% to 70%.[26] The average for the men was 62%, but the average for the women was only 52%! This gender variation is due in part to the fact that fat contains less water than other tissues, and women have more fatty deposits than men.

TABLE 1.2 There is a wide range of qualities of sensations that we can look for. (Sensations shown in red are more typical of compression than tension.)

DESCRIPTORS OF SENSATION	
Location	• Deep or superficial • Spread out • Concentrated/localized • Amorphous • Wandering • Moving up or down
Shape	• Broad • Flat • Ropy • Strap-like • Cord-like • Linear • Dotted line • Dashed line • Interrupted line/jumping • Circular
Pressure	• Light • Heavy • Crushing
Intensity	• Hard • Medium • Mild • Soft
Duration/pulsations	• Constant • Throbbing • Intermittent
Temperature	• Cool • Warm • Hot • Burning
Resistance	• Sticky • Stuck • Leathery • Taffy • Elastic • Pulling • Tugging • Stretching
Other qualities (may indicate pain):	• Vague • Sharp • Dull • Stabbing • Achy • Piercing • Radiating • Activity related

1. Know the targeted area you are trying to affect.

2. Determine what you are feeling in the targeted area while you are in the posture.

3. If you are not feeling the pose in the targeted area, change what you are doing and find a position that creates the intended sensations.

A targeted area could be any region of the body where we want to focus our attention: the hips, the spine, the legs, the shoulder, the arms, etc. The concept can be broadened to include nonphysical intentions as well, such as moving energy, paying attention closely to sensations, or refining your meditation. By thinking of your yoga practice this way, you will naturally evolve a functional approach to yoga over a purely aesthetic or performance-related view.

Often in a yoga class, a focus on the posture creeps into the cues given by the teacher. This is understandable because the postures are the tools we use, but the intention behind any posture should be to generate an effect in the body, not simply to perform the posture or look good doing so. This is the main difference between a functional approach to yoga and an aesthetic approach. When a teacher, or the student herself, starts to judge the pose by what it looks like, rather than what it feels like, then the intention of optimizing health is lost. How you look in a pose is irrelevant: what is important is what you feel in the pose.

We don't use the body to get into a pose—
we use the pose to get into the body.[65]

Realizing this simple fact frees us from dogma and images of perfection and allows us to deal with the body we have. We can focus on what we are really trying to accomplish in our yoga practice. Not everyone can do every pose, and that is fine: focusing on a functional approach to your yoga practice allows you to not even try to achieve a particular shape if it does not generate a health benefit for you or is dangerous for you, given your unique anatomical structure.

We have seen that stress can come in two forms: compression or tension. Fortunately if one pose doesn't generate the stress you desire, there are other poses you can try. Moving away from an aesthetically pleasing alignment is allowed! Feel free to wiggle. Move around to see whether some slight or more dramatic adjustment creates the sensations you are after. Remember, it doesn't matter what you look like—as long as there is no pain present, who cares what you look like? Another way of saying this is:

If you are feeling it, you are doing it!

Go to where there is an edge. Sometimes the adjustment you need may be very minor. Maybe using a block or a bolster will give you the support needed to find the edge. Sometimes all you need to do is back off a little bit. Surprisingly, for many people, backing out of a pose a little generates more sensation than going to the ultimate limit of their range of motion.

By adopting a functional approach to your yoga practice you are much more likely to achieve your intention of optimizing health while minimizing the risk of injuries. The functional approach to yoga also leads directly to another realization: your body needs your yoga. Focus on aesthetics has led the yoga world into a focus on alignment cues instead of functional cues. Since every body is different, how can one set of aesthetic cues work for every body? Unfortunately, it can't.

GENES: No two people have the same genetic structure. While we are similar to each other, we are also similar to chimpanzees. We share with chimps about 97% of the same DNA, but the other 3% is quite significant. Any two human beings share around 99.5% of their DNA, but that 0.5% is also quite significant. Our DNA is made up of millions of pairs of four kinds of bases, so a 0.5% variation translates into 16 million different pairs. The range of variation then is four to the $16,000,000^{th}$ power, which is about seven with a million zeroes after it![28]

VARIATIONS BEYOND THE GENES: Even if our genes were identical, which genes are activated varies greatly between individuals. Histones, which are spool-shaped proteins around which the long strands of DNA are wrapped so that they can easily fit inside the cell's nucleus, can affect which cells are activated.[30] Our genes can also be superseded by what our mothers and even grandmothers did while they were pregnant: if your grandmother exercised a lot and did not overeat, you have a very low chance of becoming obese. But if she took advantage of all the modern labor-saving devices available and bulked up on low-quality/high-calorie fast food, there is a much higher chance of you becoming fatter and less active than the average person, despite what your genetic structure might otherwise dictate.[31]

CHAPTER 3
The Value of Stress

What stops us is either a tensile stress, called tension, or a compressive stress, called compression. Unfortunately, the word "stress" has a negative reputation in our culture: we seem to think that stress is bad, but this cannot be—without stress, we would all die. Problems occur when we *over-stress* the body and do not allow enough time to rest and recover from the stress. For some reason, yoga teachers have decided that stretching is an okay form of stress, but compression is not. You will often hear even very experienced teachers warn students against compression. They will use very negative imagery to hammer home the point: "Don't *jam* into your lower back. Don't *collapse*. Don't *crunch*." We are cautioned against allowing our shoulders to rise up towards the ears because that would mean we were compressing the neck. The idea transmitted through this negative imagery is that compression is bad. This is not true.

If compression were bad, every massage therapist would be out of work, and walking would be one of the worst forms of exercise. We need to compress tissues in order to stimulate the body at a cellular level. Compression stimulates healing. Take bones, for example: we have known for over 100 years that bones can be coaxed into growing thicker and stronger if they are subjected to compressive stress. If we take the stress away, the bones atrophy. Space studies have shown that astronauts who experience no stress on their bones lose a significant amount of calcium, and their bones atrophy to the point that many astronauts cannot walk after coming back to Earth. (This is known as "disuse osteoporosis."[66]) When our muscles are denied stress, they atrophy. This also occurs to astronauts on orbit. All tissues atrophy without some stress.

Joints are comprised of bones, cartilage, ligaments and the joint capsule: all these tissues need stress to be healthy. Sometimes, a *distraction* occurs around the joint, which is a tensile pulling apart of the joint capsule, but often stress comes through compression.[67] Stressing the ligaments causes cells, called *fibroblasts*, to become active: they secrete hyaluronic acid, which forms a joint's synovial fluid and helps lubricate the joint's movement, and they secrete collagen to thicken and reinforce the joint capsule. Stressing the cartilage stimulates chondrocytes (which are cells that build cartilage) to secrete the collagen used to strengthen and repair the cartilage. Many other effects from stress help our tissues become strong and healthy—from the release of anti-inflammatory cytokines to the reduction of matrix-degrading enzymes.[68] We need to stress our joints! If we refrain from stressing our tissues, we risk creating fragility in the body (see It's Important: Antifragility, on pages 28–29). But we need to stress them appropriately: being yin-like tissues, bones, cartilage and ligaments do best when stressed in a yin-like fashion, which are long-held, static stresses. Repeated, rhythmic stress (which we can call yang-like stress) could damage these tissues in the same way a credit card is damaged by repeatedly bending it back and forth.

We can do too much of anything. Too little stress leads to atrophy. Too much stress can lead to tissue degeneration. We need to find the *Goldilocks Position*: not too much and not too little. This can be shown graphically: in figure 1.17 we see a classic n-shape curve that illustrates the danger of being outside the optimal bounds. Along the bottom axis we have the amount of stress being applied to tissues, and along the vertical axis we see the tissues' level of health.

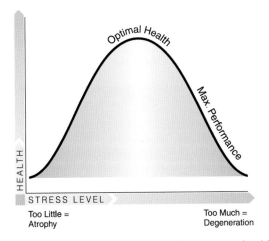

FIGURE 1.17 Stress versus health. To optimize health, we need an appropriate amount of stress—neither too much nor too little. This is the Goldilocks Curve.

IDENTICAL TWINS: As embryos, identical twins share exactly the same genetic structure, but from the moment of conception, they start to diverge. Through the process of epigenetic changes (changes due to environmental and other factors), small random mutations, and copy number variations (where segments of the DNA code are mistakenly duplicated or deleted), the genetic code may change with each reproduction of a cell. These changes accumulate over time, resulting in different genes being expressed or suppressed, perhaps causing one twin to be more susceptible to disease or to have a very different body shape than the other.[29]

If we apply too little stress to our tissues, they atrophy, become fragile and easily fail us. All living things require some stress to be healthy! If we apply too much stress, however, tissues degenerate. Numerous studies have verified the n-shaped curve shown in the graph.[69] We can call this the *Goldilocks Philosophy*. Some people do need to go to the far right, because their sport or occupation requires the maximum performance that their body can give: dancers, gymnasts, athletes and martial artists, for example, all have to maximize performance. But this comes at a cost: the focus on maximum performance can reduce overall health. Some of the most broken bodies that show up in a yoga class belong to retired dancers, gymnasts and professional athletes. They spent the first part of their lives over-stressing their tissues and suffer the consequences for the rest of their lives.

Stressing tissue initially reduces its tolerance level. This is what exercise is all about: we stress tissues to make them weaker, at least at first. Once we release the stress, the tissues recover and become stronger. If we apply too much stress, or hold the stress for too long, or do not allow enough rest between stresses, then we are in danger. Figure 1.18 shows how these three variables of stress, rest and time work together. The curve at the top of the graph shows the level of tolerance to stress that a tissue has before becoming

damaged. The lower peaks show the degree of stress being applied through either repetitive stresses or one prolonged, steady stress. The horizontal axis represents time.

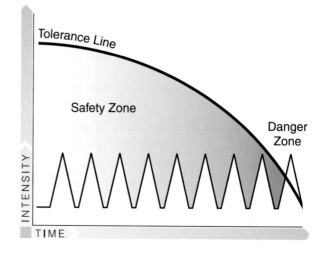

FIGURE 1.18 Our tolerance to stress decreases with continued stress.[70]

Notice how the amount of stress that our tissues can tolerate decreases with total stress and time. Eventually, if we continue to stress the tissues to the point where the two lines cross, damage will occur. This is known as the "last straw effect." It is a classic occurrence with low back injuries: you bend over at home to pick up your socks, and you throw your back out. Worker's compensation refuses to cover your injury because it occurred at home. What actually happened was that years of a repetitive or chronic stress at work reduced the tolerance of your tissues to the point that one last little stress created a serious injury. This "last straw effect" can also show up in yoga studios: this same person who has for years been reducing the tolerance of her tissues comes to a class and does, say, Pigeon Pose, and "snap!"—her hip or knee gives her searing pain. She then decides to sue the yoga studio for the injury; but in reality, it was all the other stresses she had been applying to the area over the years that set up the conditions for the injury to occur.

However, notice the graph in figure 1.19. Here we see the recuperative effect of a refractory period (called "rest"). If we stress and then rest the tissue, the tissue's tolerance level increases above what it was before. The key, then, is not simply to avoid over-stressing the tissue, but also to allow the tissue enough time to recover and grow stronger.

EYESIGHT, PART 1: Not everyone can see the same range of colors, and many people are blind to certain colors. An inability to see red or green shows up mostly in males and is caused by a variation in the X chromosome. Women have two X chromosome, so the odds of both having the same problem are small. Men, however, have only one X chromosome and hence no backup. The rate of color blindness in young boys depends upon ethnicity: one study found 5.6% of Caucasian, 3.1% of Asian, 2.6% of Hispanic and 1.4% of African-American boys had red/green color blindness.[33] Women and men are equally likely to have blue color blindness, but this is even rarer than red/green blindness, affecting only about 0.5% of the population.[34]

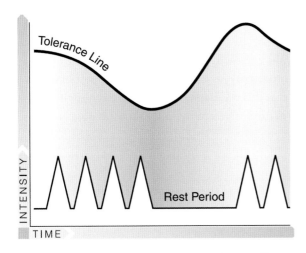

FIGURE 1.19 Rest restores and increases tolerance.[71]

All tissues need stress. Let's reemphasize that! *All tissues.* This includes our joints, our bones, our fascia, our muscles, our nerves, our organs, etc. All tissues. This means that we cannot afford to ignore some areas of the body out of fear of injury. To say, as many teachers do, that we should never stress our sacroiliac joint is not helpful—no stress there will cause the joint to atrophy, tighten and lose range of motion. Yes, too much stress could lead to arthritis and hypermobility, but this does not mean that we should entirely avoid stressing the area.

Chronic stress creates fragility; acute stress followed by rest builds *antifragility.* To quote Nassim Taleb, "Our antifragilities have conditions. The frequency of stressors matters a bit. Humans tend to do better with acute than with chronic stressors, particularly when the former are followed by ample time for recovery, which allows the stressors to do their job as messengers."[72] Stuart McGill observed that "loading is necessary for optimal tissue health. When loading and the subsequent degradation of tolerance are followed by a period of rest, an adaptive tissue response increases tolerance.... Avoidance of loading altogether is undesirable."[73] Thus, exposure to load is necessary, but as microtraumas accumulate, the applied loads must be removed (with rest) to allow the healing and adaptation process to gradually increase the failure tolerance to a higher level.

While some stress is good, either a lot of stress or chronic stress can be bad. How can we know the difference? Pain! The body will generally warn you when you are going too deep or holding the stress for too long. Some teachers, out of concern for their students' safety, will caution,

"Always bend your knees and never flex your spine when you do a forward fold, otherwise you will stress the vertebral joints," or, "Never do Pigeon Pose, because you will stress the SI joint." While these instructions or similar warnings are intended to help and protect students, they represent a misunderstanding of the nature and necessity of stress, and an ignorance of the causes of fragility. The teacher would be more helpful if she warned her students to avoid stressing any area of the body if they are feeling pain: even little tweaks are to be noticed and avoided, because little tweaks lead to big tweaks, and big tweaks lead to expensive operations, time off work and no yoga practice, which leads to yoga studios going out of business and yoga teachers being out of work, and our economy collapses—all because you weren't paying attention to pain. So, don't ignore little tweaks! This is a warning against any stress—including stretching, twisting and compression—that causes pain. But do not be afraid of compression per se! Tissues need to be compressed to stay healthy.

EYESIGHT, PART 2: Myopia (nearsightedness) affects people all over the world, but the variation in ability to see things far away varies by culture and education. The more reading a person does, the more liable he is to myopia. People with myopia have a greater risk of suffering macular degeneration, early cataracts, retinal detachment as well as glaucoma. One study found that over 24% of people with no high school education or other training were nearsighted, whereas 35% of high school graduates and vocational school graduates were nearsighted, and 53% of university graduates were nearsighted. Myopia affects 42% of people in the United States but up to 80% in Asian countries.[35]

IT'S IMPORTANT: Antifragility (or no strain—no gain!)

Aunt Trudy was always different: she loved frogs and she loved to collect frogs—the artistic, porcelain kind. She had her prized porcelain frogs proudly displayed in an open cabinet. Alongside them was a cast iron frog given to her by her niece one Christmas, and, occasionally, a live frog that her nephew would find for her. One day, a slight earthquake shook the cabinet, and they all fell to the floor. The exquisite porcelain frogs shattered upon impact, the iron frog merely bounced, while the real frog leapt to safety. The porcelain frogs were fragile—any chaos was bound to harm them. The iron frog was robust—no matter what happened, it would be unharmed but also not better than before. The real frog was antifragile and actually benefited from the exercise of jumping. Sedentary life with no challenge or change is harmful to the real frog, whereas the stress of life makes it stronger.

Human beings seem quite fragile: we break easily. But there are many respects in which we can be said to be *antifragile*. Antifragile is a word coined by the philosopher, writer and quant Nassim Nicholas Taleb and refers to a condition whereby an entity gains from randomness, stress and disorder.[82] We can use the example of our bones: compared to a beam of wood, which breaks down over time (the wood is fragile), our bones get stronger with repeated stress. They are antifragile: they gain strength, to a limit, with increasing stress. Something fragile suffers from chaos and change, as we saw in the story of Aunt Trudy's frogs. (See figures 1.20 to 1.23 for graphic representations of the fragility–antifragility spectrum.) Machines, such as computers or cars, are fragile—they wear out over time and with accumulating stresses. Living organisms, on the other hand, get stronger with time and stress. You are not a machine; stress (to a limit) makes you stronger, not weaker. You are antifragile in so many ways, as long as you continue to seek out an appropriate amount of stress in your life. Comfort is the opposite of stress. Modern living tends to seek stress-free conditions, where we are comfortable, but this comes at a terrible cost: fragility.[83] Said another way, comfort is fragilizing!

It may seem quite counterintuitive to suggest that someone who is injured (perhaps they have a fragile or damaged spine) should deliberately stress the injured area. The obvious course of action is to give it rest, leave it alone and take all stress off the damaged or weakened tissue. However, this debate has run its course in terms of women's recovery after childbirth. At the turn of the 20th century, the prevailing wisdom prescribed lots of bed rest to allow the new mother to recover her strength. In time, physicians realized that this was the worst thing for most mothers: instead, they needed to become mobile as soon as possible. Indeed, a study published in *The Lancet* suggests that bed rest is never a good idea for any condition.[84] This is not a license to overdo movement during recovery, but by subjecting ourselves to small amounts of stress, we become antifragile. Figure 1.23 shows this graphically: if we extend Nassim Taleb's logic to people who are injured, we find that they still need some stress or they will risk becoming increasingly fragile.

Something that is harmful in excess can build antifragility when given in small measure. To apply no stress will create fragility. Let's look at a few ways that we have, with the best of intentions, actually made our bodies weaker and more fragile by reducing stress.

Jaws: Human faces have become 5–10% smaller since the agricultural revolution. Many people by the time they are young adults will need to have their wisdom teeth removed. Their jaws are too small to accommodate all their teeth. This was not the case for our ancestors before the agricultural revolution. Today our food is easily chewed. It is comfortable to have well-prepared foods that require little work to masticate. But this has a cost: with less stress in our jaws as children, the jaw bones do not grow to their full extent. These smaller jaws no longer have space for all our teeth. Children who chew hard food have larger jaws and are less likely to require their wisdom teeth to be extracted as adults.[85]

Feet: The arches of our feet need stress to stay strong. If we do not walk and run, if we do not stress the arches of our feet, the ligaments become lax and the foot loses its arch, creating fallen arches and plantar fasciitis. Shoes with arch supports and sneakers that cushion each step reduce the stress needed to keep feet strong. Orthotics may be necessary for those whose feet have completely collapsed, but they can also lead to that very same problem for people whose feet are normal and can tolerate—indeed require—stress.[86]

Immune System: Our immune system develops through stress. As children, we need to ingest a certain amount of dirt and germs in order to develop a normally functioning immune system. David Strachan has called this understanding the "hygiene hypothesis." We need the occasional cold and flu to develop strength in our immune system. If we don't get enough exposure to bad stuff when we are young, we may start to overreact to benign substances when we are older, causing allergies and other immune system dysfunctions.[87]

Eyes: Children who spend more time indoors are more likely to develop myopia as adults. This condition is rare in hunter-gatherer communities, but as people spend more time inside, the rate increases.[88] A 19th-century Danish study found that outdoor laborers, like hunter-gatherers, only suffered myopia 3% of the time, compared with 12% for artisans and craftsmen and 32% for university students. Today, with the ubiquity of computers, these rates are undoubtedly worse. The eyes need the stress of focusing far away as well as close at hand to develop normally.[89]

Eating: Too much food or eating too regularly can be unhealthy. Hunger is a necessary stressor that our ancestors used, unwillingly and unknowingly, to keep the body lean and fit. When we occasionally starve ourselves, say for one to three days, the body starts to cannibalize its own tissues to get the protein it needs for daily living. It starts by re-consuming the weakest, most damaged cells and redeploys those nutrients. The process is called *autophagy*, and the body begins with the cells that are most likely to lead to problems later on, pre-cancerous cells, preventing them from harming us later in life. If we are never hungry, these cells are left to do their nasty thing.[90] Skipping a meal once in a while is not comfortable, but it may be quite healthy for you.

Marcus Aurelius once said, "Fire feeds on obstacles." The Roman poet Ovid wrote, "Difficulty is what wakes up the genius." Cut off the head of a hydra, and two more grow back! We could go on and on, describing many ways that *acute* stress is necessary to keep the body, heart and mind healthy and whole. (Remember: *chronic* stress is rarely so benign or helpful, nor is an acute stress that exceeds the body's tolerance.) This is known in the realm of exercise: we recognize that by stressing our muscles with ever-increasing weights, they will become stronger and healthier. We often fail, however, to make the link between the stress that is good for our muscles and the fact that we also need to stress our bones, our joints, our ligaments—in fact, all aspects of our being. Yes, you can do too much (remember the Goldilocks Philosophy), but no stress at all is also dangerous and unhealthy. Here is a useful mantra to memorize: "*No strain—no gain.*"[91] Stress is healthy and necessary, not an enemy to be avoided at all costs.

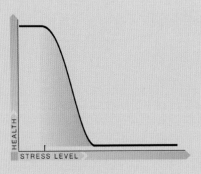

FIGURE 1.20 Fragile. Here we see how stress beyond a certain tolerance level can cause a fragile object to be shattered or broken. The transition is sudden once the tolerance level is reached.

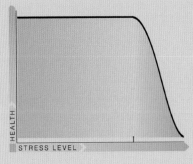

FIGURE 1.21 Robust. Here we see that regardless of the stress levels, a robust object is unaffected by any amount of stress. Up to a limit, it neither benefits from nor is harmed by the stress.

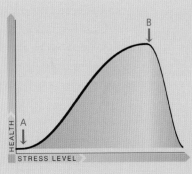

FIGURE 1.22 Antifragile. An antifragile object benefits from stress, up to a certain point. As stress increases, so too does the health and strength of an antifragile object. However, once a certain stress level is reached, the object is no longer antifragile and will suffer from greater stress. At this point (B), the object is again fragile. Note, too, that if the stress stays at the point A level, the object will be unhealthy.

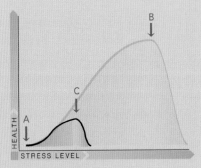

FIGURE 1.23 Fragility and antifragility of injured tissues. When tissues are damaged, the point at which they pass the threshold from antifragile to fragile moves to the left, to C. Clearly, if stress is applied at the B level, the tissues will be damaged, but if the stress level remains at point A, the tissues will remain fragile. Ideally the stress should be close to but not beyond the edge represented by point C.

IT'S IMPORTANT: The value of compression

Muscles, being more yang-like in nature, do better with yang-like forms of exercise: rhythmic and repetitive stresses. Connective tissues, like our bones, ligaments and joints, being more yin-like, do better with yin-like forms of exercises: static, long-held, tensile and compressive stresses.

In 1892, Julius Wolff released a paper called "The Law of Transformation of the Bone." Today we call his findings Wolff's Law. Wolff discovered that bones are transformed by the stresses placed upon them. When the stress placed upon bone increases, so too does the structural resistance of the bone: it becomes thicker and stronger. Especially effective is cyclical loading and unloading, which inhibits bone absorption and increases bone formation.[74] The process by which this happens includes both *mechanotransduction* and *piezoelectricity*. Mechanotransduction occurs when cells convert mechanical stress into biochemical and electrical signals. When the cells' membranes sense physical pressure, a cascade of events occurs within the cell: particular proteins are expressed, and the cell secretes certain chemical messengers.[75] Piezoelectricity is a small electrical current created when a material is deformed. (This is how the LEDs in some children's sneakers light up when they walk.) When we stress our bones, small piezoelectric currents flow through our tissues and signal specific cells to become activated or inactivated. This effect also happens when we stress our cartilage, teeth, tendons, blood vessel walls, muscles and even our skin. Stress is essential to health, and compressive stress sends signals throughout our matrix, including deep into the cytoplasm of individual cells.[76]

We need to compress our tissues in order for them to stay healthy and strong—*antifragile*—but for some reason this form of stress has come to be considered unhealthy or dangerous in the yoga world. We hear teachers use derogatory terms for compression: "crunching" or "collapsing." All compressive stress is lumped in with dangerous movements that may indeed cause problems, but not all stress is bad.

For example, a student will be told to move her shoulders away from her ears when she is doing a Down Dog pose (Adhomukhashvanasana) because she is "compressing the neck." So? Why is it bad to compress the neck? Our body is designed to allow us to bring our shoulders up to our ears. This is a natural movement. If someone asks you a question and you don't know the answer, you want to be able to shrug your shoulders up to your ears.[77] Similarly, many students are warned against "collapsing" into their lower spine when doing a back bend because they will be "crunching" their vertebrae together. Again, so? Why is it bad to compress the vertebrae? If we *never* compress the spinal bones, they will atrophy rather than remaining strong and healthy. Remember the Goldilocks Philosophy.

As always, it is possible to do too much of anything, so if compression leads to pain, then it is wise to modify what you are doing. Some people do have to take great care when doing backbends, to avoid overly compressing already damaged spines. If you are constantly moving the body and relying upon your ligaments to restrain your range of movement, rather than using your muscles to control how far you go, then you do risk the "credit card" effect. We all know what happens to a credit card that is bent back and forth repeatedly, 108 times every morning—eventually, it will weaken and break. That may be great for your finances, but it is not ideal for your lower back or wrists. Doing 108 drop-backs to Wheel Pose (Urdvadhanurasana) from standing every morning without learning to engage the muscles that stabilize your back, or if you have an inherent instability in your lower back, may injure the lumbar ligaments or the joints of the lumbar spine. This does not mean that a longer-held, static stress to these same ligaments is not healthy for most backs. *How* you exercise your tissues makes a big difference to them, but all tissues must be stressed to be healthy, and that stress includes compression.

NOTE TO TEACHERS: Stress when injured

When the intention of a yoga practice is to achieve optimal health, we must ask how deeply to stress the body. The answer is found in the fragility curves we saw earlier. If too little stress is applied, the tissues atrophy. If too much stress is applied, the tissues degenerate. If your intention is to gain and remain healthy, the curve in figure 1.22 shows that you need to apply a stress below the level of point B. However, for some students the intention is not optimal health but rather optimal performance: they will want to push the poses to the maximum of their physical and emotional limits.

All tissues need stress! This fact confuses the discussion of using yoga as therapy. A student who suffers osteoporosis in her lumbar spine may have been told not to stress her lower back at all in order to protect her spine. This advice was offered with the best of intentions, but it may not be wise, because if there is absolutely no stress on the spine (point A on our curve), the tissues will continue to atrophy. But clearly, too much stress (point B) will cause the bones to degenerate, leading to worse problems. So what to do? In these cases, it is best to think of the fragility curve as becoming narrower and shifted to the left.

Let's revisit figure 1.23: the fragility–antifragility curve for injured tissue. Notice in this graph that the area of safe stress is much smaller and there is a narrow margin of error between too little and too much (between A and C). The point is, all tissues need stress, but with injury or illness, the safe range of stress is very narrow. It is easy to go too far and hurt the student, but it is equally too easy to say, "Don't do anything," which also hurts the student. The student coming to a yoga class may be totally justified in wanting to take your class. A gentler restorative yoga class may not work for them: it may be too easy, or they may have only one area that needs care whereas the rest of their body wants a regular workout, or they do want to work into the damaged connective tissues to an appropriate degree and can only get that in a regular class.

The key word is appropriate. How does a teacher know when the stress is appropriate? Short of wearing X-ray glasses and having a portable MRI handy, you cannot be absolutely sure, but what you can do is teach the student how to pay attention to her edge. This is the answer you need to give the student who shows up unexpectedly at the beginning of your class, claiming that it will be good for her severe spinal stenosis: "Pay attention! Practice mindfully!"

Teach the student how to feel what is going on. This is not easy and takes time and practice. Advise her to go very slowly and very gently into each pose, feeling in detail all the sensations occurring. Tell her that pain is an inappropriate sensation. Unfortunately, she may answer that she always feels pain, in which case tell her to look for any increase in pain or changes in its quality. Make your caveats clear: this is not restorative yoga, and it may not be appropriate for her; you are not a doctor—but if she promises to take it really easy, do all the modifications that you will suggest and come out of the poses whenever it becomes too challenging, then you will let her try the class. Unfortunately, and there is no way around this, you will have to keep checking on her and offering appropriate options that fit her situation: that's part of the bargain you made when you accepted her into your class. (If you are not prepared or are unable to do this, don't let her in the class!) Also, don't let her slip away with the crowd after shavasana. Talk to her again after class; check in with her, see how she feels, and spend a bit more time explaining the ideal Goldilocks Position for her.

Finally, ask her to pay attention to how she feels over the next 48 hours. Sometimes the changes for good or ill do not show up right away. She needs to keep paying attention to what is happening within, then try to correlate any changes to what she has been doing. That is also part of practicing yoga mindfully.

IT'S COMPLICATED: Stress at the cellular level

Every move we make stresses our body, and our body is made up of trillions of cells. Thanks to the presence of our extra-cellular matrix, most of these cells are connected together. What we do to the body, we do to our cells, and that is a very good thing, because our cells require mechanical stresses to become activated. This process is called mechanotransduction. To understand how it works and why it is so important for our health and healing, we need to understand a little bit about the extracellular matrix (ECM).

The ECM is what is left in our body when we take away all the living tissues: the muscle cells, blood, organs and skin. What remains is a scaffold of collagen and other fascial fibers that give shape and support to the body. It was long thought that this inert matrix of dead proteins played no role in our healing process. However, it turns out that not only is the ECM an incredibly important part of our body, but it is absolutely essential for good health. The ECM does much more than give structure or stability; it has several functional roles.

Just as our body as a whole has a skeletal structure, every cell has its skeleton, too. Within the cells is a cytoskeleton, made up of the same types of collagen proteins that compose the ECM. As shown in figure 1.24, the cell's internal scaffold extends from the DNA within the nucleus out beyond the cellular membrane, and through these "integrins" the cell is connected with the ECM scaffold. Most of our cells are hardwired into the whole mechanical continuum of the body. Thus, when we stress our body, we are sending mechanical stress signals to the cells—and via each cell's own scaffold structure, to deep inside the cell as well, even to the DNA. The stress of mechanotransduction is one of the major communication pathways that cells use to sense the outside world (along with electrical, chemical and other signaling pathways).

Figure 1.24 depicts the internal skeleton of a cell, formed of collagen protein. Notice how the cytoskeleton is continuous with the outer cell integrins, which in turn connect to the ECM. While the ECM is more than simply wires, we have also discovered that cells respond to the stress along those wires. If we want to regrow tissues—say, cartilage to replace a meniscus that was torn, or a trachea

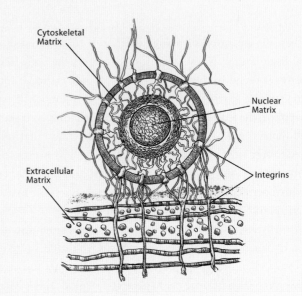

FIGURE 1.24 The cell's cytoskeleton is connected via integrins to the extracellular matrix.[78]

that became so damaged that a patient could not breathe—an artificial scaffold is necessary. This scaffold (sometimes taken from animals or human donors) guides stem cells to reproduce new cartilage in the right location. In laboratory experiments, however, the resulting structure was always much weaker than the body's own, original structure. Something was missing.

There is a mystery in medical science: Why do some injuries heal, but not fully? Why do injuries get better for a while, but the job is unfinished and some weakness or infirmity remains? The answer to this mystery is starting to be discovered: stress! The body needs stress in order for our cells to receive communication. Our ECM is under constant tension. The artificial scaffolds used in the laboratory petri dish were under no tension, so the stems cells were not getting the proper communication. They didn't know what to do. When researchers started applying stress to the ECM, the stem cells began behaving in the most remarkable ways. They multiplied and migrated to the right places on the scaffold where they could be most effective. But there was another surprise in store for the researchers: different levels of stress on the matrix caused the stem cells to differentiate into different tissues! A single scaffold could initiate stem-cell differentiation into a wide variety of different tissue

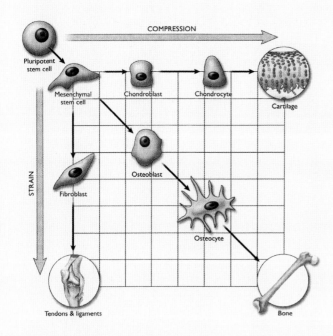

COMPRESSION

STRAIN

Pluripotent stem cell

Mesenchymal stem cell

Chondroblast

Chondrocyte

Cartilage

Osteoblast

Fibroblast

Osteocyte

Tendons & ligaments

Bone

FIGURE 1.25 How the cell's exposure to strain and compression determines its future.[80]

types, because at different locations within the scaffold's matrix, there were different levels of stress (see figure 1.25). It is now possible to regenerate a complete organ, with all its complexities of structure, blood vessels and nerves cells, through seeding a scaffold with only a few types of stem cells. Researchers have recently grown a complete kidney, which is a very complicated organ, and successfully implanted it into an animal.[79]

Stress is needed to stimulate our stem cells to be active, and depending upon the degree of stress, the cells can become the kind of tissue needed for the occasion. When a stem cell senses flowing movement, it will become a blood vessel. If the amount of stress is very slight, it becomes a nerve cell. If the stress is a bit stronger, it becomes a fat cell.

Stronger still and the stem cell will become a muscle cell. With even more stress, it becomes bone. Too much, too little or no stress and the stem cell doesn't respond at all.

Our extracellular matrix has Velcro-like hooks (called fibronectins) that latch onto the cell's integrins, selecting only the type it wants, holding them in place and transferring stresses deep inside the cell, where the nucleus can decode the signal and prepare whatever is needed. But the ECM has another trick up its sleeve: it also contains growth hormones that stimulate the growth of the new cells.

To quote science writer Bob Holmes, "This may explain why exercise and physical therapy are so important to health and healing—if cells don't get the right physical cues when you are recovering from an injury, for instance, they won't know what to do."[81] And this brings us back to yoga's magic ingredient: stress. All tissues need stress to remain healthy; remember our fragility curves. Sometimes the stress is blocked from reaching the cells: this can be the case when scar tissue has replaced the normal ECM structure. The tissues are too stiff. Cells may also not get the message when the stresses are too slight; instead of muscles, bones or fascia being regenerated, only fat is created, which does not help restore strength or range of motion to the injured area. We need to stress our tissues, but we need to do it in the right way and to the right degree.

We need to move, to walk, to breathe, to stretch, to work on strengthening the muscles and stressing our joints. When we move, when we breathe, walk, stretch or compress our body, we are sending mechanical signals throughout the matrix. Our trillions of cells are listening, waiting to hear what instructions we are sending. Think of this next time you are marinating in a long-held yoga pose. You are literally turning yourself on.

CHAPTER 4
The Physiology of Our Tissues

Earlier, we asked, "What stops me?" and discovered that our limitations arise due to either tension in the tissues or compression where the body contacts the body. These are very simple concepts to understand, but the experiences of them are not quite so simple to recognize. It takes practice; it takes intention; it takes attention. To differentiate tension from compression and when each is occurring, it is useful to understand the differences between the types of tissues we all possess. That is the purpose of this section: to introduce you to the kinds of tissues and other materials that make up our physical bodies.

Scientists love to break things down into categories, and subcategories, and sub-subcategories and so on. They have done this for our tissues, identifying four main kinds:
- Muscle Tissue
- Connective Tissue
- Nervous Tissue
- Epithelia Tissue

The body is made up of approximately 400 trillion cells—that's a 4 with 14 zeroes! However, about 90% of these cells are not human cells at all but symbiotic bacteria. Of the roughly 37 trillion *human* cells, there are only about 210 different kinds.[92] Some are migratory cells, such as red blood cells, which move around the body, and others are cells that form aggregates, which we call tissues. Depending upon the functions of these aggregates, we can divide the various types into the above four tissue categories.

Muscle tissues consist of an aggregate of contracting cells and their support structure. Their job is to produce movement, maintain posture (balance) and generate heat to maintain the body's temperature. Connective tissues—which include bones, ligaments, cartilage, tendons and fascia—are aggregates of cells that are found in an extracellular matrix, and they act like a scaffold to keep tension in the tissues and alignment between the cells. Nervous tissues are aggregates of cells specializing in transmitting electrical and chemical signals throughout the body. The epithelia tissues are the linings of the body, such as the outermost lining, our skin, and the inner ones, such as our blood vessels and digestive tract.

Muscle and connective tissues are the ones most often talked about in yoga teacher training because yoga asana practice deeply and directly affects these kinds of tissues. But yoga affects the other types as well. More importantly, our epithelia and nervous tissues can also affect our yoga practice and how flexible we are! (A study showed that even our skin contributes some resistance to the movement of a joint, albeit only 2%: that's the epithelia.[93]) All tissues contribute to our strength, mobility and overall health. Conversely, damage to or malfunction of these tissues creates issues that affect our health and mobility.

As we address more deeply the question of "What stops me?" we will discover many factors. Yoga is not only about our muscles; the emphasis in yoga teacher training on the names and functions of each muscle that we use in specific poses is but one part of the story. It is time to use what we have learned so far and see how tension and compression arise in other tissues. As we are about to discover, restrictions on our flexibility and range of motion can come from tension and compression in many different kinds of tissues but also from neurological factors, and from the ways our immune and endocrine systems behave.

MICROBIOME: While we are made up of 37 trillion human cells (some estimates are as high as 50 trillion), most of the cells inside and on us are foreign bacteria. We are a community of cells, of which only 10% are human, the rest being symbiotic guests.[42] There are more than 1,000 different kinds of non-human microbes found on or in our bodies, but most of these inhabit our intestines, where they perform vital functions that keep us healthy.[43] We are also a community of viruses, which outnumber our bacteria by a factor of 9 to 1. We are host to 1,000 trillion viruses, most of which are doing good work for us.[44] Obviously, no one has the exact same makeup of human cells, bacteria, fungi and viruses as anyone else.

Sources of Tension

So much of the focus of modern yoga classes revolves around stretching our muscles. We find the same emphasis in yoga teacher training and yoga anatomy books that focus on which muscles are targeted and affected in which postures. Unfortunately, this confuses the means with the ends. If the goal of your physical yoga practice is to increase your flexibility, to gain an optimal range of motion and regain your natural mobility (and by optimal and natural we mean *healthy*, not maximum), then it is important to understand that most of what is stopping you is not tension in your muscles. Focusing solely on lengthening muscles is not optimal: there are many more important reasons for your lack of mobility than short, tight muscles. We will investigate these sources of tension, but we will begin as most books do, by looking at the muscles. We will not stop there, however! We will also look at our fascia, our nervous system, our immune and endocrine

MUSCLES: There are seven major variations and many minor ones observable in muscles. These variations are in comparison to what is typically presented in anatomical textbooks, but this does not mean these variations are abnormal; they do happen, and we should be aware that their occurrence is not a pathology. In the seven major variants:

1. a muscle may be absent;
2. a muscle may be doubled;
3. a muscle may be divided into two or more parts;
4. a muscle may have an increase or decrease in its attachment number and locations;
5. a muscle may join neighboring organs;
6. a muscle or its tendon may have a deviant distribution; or
7. a completely new muscle may appear.[45]

IT'S IMPORTANT:
Millimeters versus inches

Scientists prefer to use metric standards when measuring things. That means they use millimeters and centimeters whereas many people still refer to inches. The translation between these two languages is pretty simple, however.

- 1 inch = ~2.5 centimeters or 25 millimeters
- 1 centimeter = 10 millimeters or ~0.4 inches
- 1 millimeter = ~0.04 inches

systems, other connective tissues such as tendons, ligaments and joint capsules, and at water. All these can be sources of tension, of restriction in our movements.

MUSCLES

Muscles make up 40–50% of our body mass[94]—pumping blood, expanding our lungs, causing our various tubes to open and close, heating the body from the inside, maintaining our posture and allowing us to run and jump. They come in a variety of shapes, which correspond to particular needs or functions (see Appendix B: Muscle Shapes and Functions for a more complete investigation). But to really understand our muscles—how they move us and restrict our movements—we will start really small, with the tiniest part of our muscles, and work our way outwards, towards a view of the whole body. We will begin with the muscle cell itself, which is also often called a *muscle fiber* or *myocyte*. These cells can range from one to 120 mm in length.[95] Muscles are very unusual cells, containing hundreds to thousands of nuclei in each cell.[98] They do not replicate in the normal way; they don't divide, so when the body needs more muscle cells, it recruits nearby cells, known as *myosatellite* cells, to reproduce and become muscle cells. The myosatellites first become *myoblasts*,[99] and these can either merge with existing muscle cells—repairing them or making them bigger—or, when we are very young, the myoblasts can become separate muscle cells. Muscle cell growth can be stimulated by injury or by exercise.

The contracting portion of a muscle cell is called a *sarcomere* (see figure 1.26). Contraction of the muscle resulting in a shortening of the sarcomere is called *concentric contraction*. Sometimes, however, the muscles *try* to contract, but they are lengthened while doing so: this is called *eccentric contraction*. That sounds strange because the muscle is not "contracting" at all, so a better term here would be *eccentric activation*. The muscle is activated, it is trying to contract, but it is becoming longer. This happens in our yoga practice quite often. For example, as we descend from a Plank Pose down into Chaturanga, where we hover above the floor, our triceps lengthen eccentrically: they resist the lowering while they are getting longer. The final activation option is where the muscle tries to contract, but it is held at a constant length: this is called *isometric contraction*, but again it is not really contracting, so let's use the term *isometric activation*.

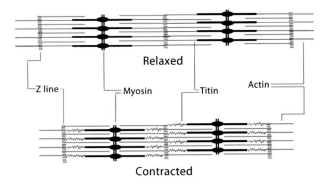

FIGURE 1.26 Sarcomeres in concentric contraction. The actin fibers are shown in red, the titin fibers in blue and the thick myosin in black.

A muscle can relax, and its titin does have a bit of elastic recoil, but the muscle cannot lengthen by itself; it requires an outside force to stretch it—either gravity or an opposing muscle. When the sarcomere is stretched, the ends of the sarcomere are drawn apart. This causes the actin proteins to pull away from each other, increasing the gap between them until the tips of the myosin align with the tips of the actin. Various studies have shown that the maximum amount a sarcomere can stretch without being damaged is about 67%.[100] At this point, what has elongated is the titin, which anchors the myosin. The myosin does not stretch. The titin in its contracted state is folded up like an accordion, but it unfolds when the sarcomere stretches. The titin's elasticity and ability to elongate are affected by several factors, including genetics. There are natural human variations in our DNA that can affect how easily the titin unfolds: not everyone's titin lengthens to the same degree and in the same way. (You are unique, remember, and how much your titin can expand is also unique.) However, once the titin is completely extended, going any further will cause it to rupture, injuring the sarcomere. Interestingly, titin can sense the stresses upon it, and it sends signals to the cell, leading to gene expression and muscle growth. We are discovering that this function of titin is important for the health of the sarcomeres in heart muscles.[101]

Another study has shown that if we take the sarcomere out of its fascial tubing, it can actually lengthen 240% before tearing.[102] Above I indicated that a sarcomere can stretch only 67% of its resting length, so why can it stretch further when it is not in the body? The study suggested that it is not the sarcomere itself, or its titin, that stops the muscles from stretching further; it is the fascial wrapper in which the sarcomere lives. The conclusion: when it comes to what stops us stretching further, the limiting factor is not the muscle's sarcomere but the fascia within and around the muscle cell.

We will look at the fascia in a moment, but clearly the *number* of sarcomeres in the muscle can be a limiting factor. If we string more sarcomeres together, end to end in a long series, the muscle will have more length and, indeed, more power. When a muscle can't stretch any further, the limiting factors are both the number of sarcomeres and the resistance of its fascia. With strength-building exercises, we can coax the body to add sarcomeres, which will result in longer muscles and thus a greater range of motion.

IT'S COMPLICATED:
Sarcomere contraction

Each muscle cell contains smaller fibers called myofibrils, which are made up of thousands of smaller units called sarcomeres (Greek: sarco = flesh; mere = unit) that are laid end to end along the whole length of the muscle cell. Sarcomeres are tiny, only about 2.2 micrometers (μm) long in their relaxed state. They are a collection of proteins arranged in a hexagonal lattice to allow filaments to slide. Figure 1.27 shows a simpler, two-dimensional view of how they work. Each sarcomere contains "walls," which are called Z-lines (sometimes called Z-discs when looked at three-dimensionally). In between the walls are three kinds of proteins: titin, myosin and actin. The titin anchors the myosin to the Z-lines, while the actin proteins are directly connected to Z-lines on either side. About 60% of the cell's protein is found in the myosin, the thickest of the three proteins. Actin is next: it contains 20% of the muscle's protein. There is a space between the two sides of actin, a gap that the myosin lies beneath.

According to the sliding theory[96] of muscular contraction, the myosin proteins "walk" across the actin filaments and draw the two Z-line walls closer together, thus contracting the muscle. When this happens, the titin proteins fold up like an accordion. Normally, muscles can contract in this manner to about 1.1 μm, or 50% of their resting length,[97] which corresponds to the length of the myosin filament; once the Z-lines hit either end of the myosin, further contraction is restricted.

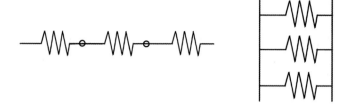

FIGURE 1.27 Sarcomeres added in series increase length; sarcomeres added in parallel increase force.

If a limb is immobilized and the muscle is fixed or held in a shortened position, then the cell reabsorbs sarcomeres and the muscle cell becomes shorter and weaker. This happens when a limb is placed in a cast: the muscles of the limb and its joints are not stressed or stretched, so the muscle loses length and strength. This is called *atrophy*. Muscular atrophy arises quite quickly when a joint or limb is immobilized, with changes occurring within the first 48 hours. Around 30% of muscle mass can be lost after only three days of immobilization, and this can rise to almost 50% within 15 days.[106] This is a key reason why you don't see as many

IT'S COMPLICATED: Adding sarcomeres

There are two ways to add sarcomeres. We can add them in *series* with the existing ones, which increases the length of contraction we can produce, but this does not increase the *force* of the contraction; or we can add them in *parallel* to the existing ones, which increases the force of the contraction but does not add length to the muscle (see figure 1.27).[103] Body builders generally do the latter, while yogis do the former.

In either case, adding sarcomeres through exercise increases the muscle's power, which is defined as force (F) times the change in length (L) over a certain time period (T). (So, power = FxL/T.[104]) In one case we increase the force (F) of contraction by adding sarcomeres in parallel, and in the other case we increase length (L) by adding the sarcomeres in series. In general, body builders have big, bulky muscles while yogis have long, lean muscles—but both may generate equal power when they engage their muscles![105]

casts around these days compared to 25 years ago; the risks of immobilization and its costs to the other tissues of the body are more fully appreciated now.

The amount of tension the contracting muscle can generate is due, purely from a muscle cell perspective, to the number of sarcomeres in each cell and the number of cells in the muscle. If the muscle is short, then it does not have enough sarcomeres to accommodate our desired range of motion. To reduce the tension that restricts our movement, we need to lengthen the muscles by adding sarcomeres, but we need to add them in series, not parallel. However, this is not the whole story—we have discovered that the fascia in the muscle also contributes greatly to tension and restrictions in range of motion.

MYOFASCIA

Around 30% of what we find in a muscle is fascia. Indeed, therapists more accurately refer to muscles as *myofascia*. When we zoom out from the sarcomeres, we can see why. Figure 1.28 shows the arrangement of the tubes within tubes that form our muscles. At the smallest level, we see the muscle cell (muscle fiber), which contains the sarcomeres we have been discussing. These fibers are encased in a tube of fascia called the *endomysium*. Notice how each fiber is part of a larger tube called a *fascicle* or a *fasciculus* (both words mean "a bundle"). The fascicles are also surrounded by fascia, called the *perimysium*. The perimysium is made up of the individual endomysia coming together to form a *septum*, which is Latin for "enclosure." Within the perimysium are arranged the blood vessels and nerves that support the muscle cells. The fascicles, in turn, are contained within the main tube of the muscle, which is surrounded by another tube of fascia called the *epimysium*; this consists of the perimysia flowing together. All these fascial coverings add up to almost 30% of the muscle.

It is the fascia that gives muscles their ability to transmit force to the tendons and thus to the bones, resulting in movement around the joints. The sarcomeres' contractions pull against the cytoskeleton within the muscle cell, which connects through the cell membrane to the endomysium surrounding the cell; in turn, the endomysium pulls on the perimysium, which pulls on the epimysium, which pulls on the tendon. There are also loose connective tissues between the individual muscle cells, which allow blood vessels and nerves to reach the cells.

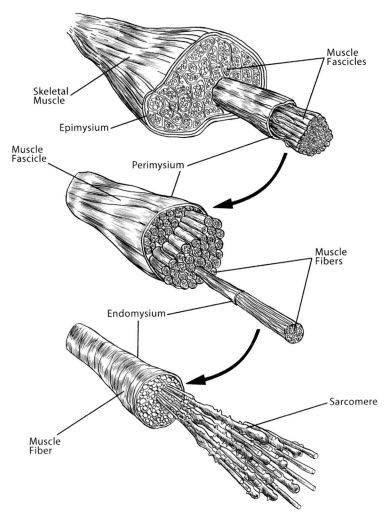

Skeletal Muscle
Epimysium
Muscle Fascicle
Perimysium
Muscle Fibers
Endomysium
Muscle Fiber
Muscle Fascicles
Sarcomere

FIGURE 1.28 Muscle cells are surrounded by tubes within tubes within tubes, all made up of fascia.

The fascia of the muscle limits how far it can be stretched. Fascia is made up of several types of proteins, but the most common one is called collagen, which is strong and inelastic. (Depending upon where the fascia is located and its function, it may also contain some fibers called elastin, which, as its name implies, is elastic. This kind of fascia is not as stiff as fascia made only of collagen.) Collagen resists stretching, but one fiber by itself is not very strong. When a large number of fibers join together, however, they become quite strong. Assisting in this stability are cross-links between the fibers, in the same way that the rungs of a ladder make the ladder stable. If a ladder had only one rung, the legs could easily be moved—it would be a very wobbly ladder. But if the ladder had a dozen rungs, it would be very difficult to move the legs—the ladder would be quite rigid. Exercise or other movement can decrease the number

of these rungs between collagen fibers and allow some sliding of the legs, thus allowing a greater range of movement.[107] After sliding has taken place, new cross-links form, restabilizing the fibers, but now the whole bundle of fibers is slightly longer. This remodeling of the fascia can result in longer tubes, space for more sarcomeres and thus greater muscle length and greater range of motion.

The muscle fibers also need to be able to slide along each other as they contract and stretch. If adhesions develop between the fibers, or between the fascicles, then movement will be restricted. This is a different form of tension that can develop in the muscle: restriction due to adhesions between the otherwise sliding surfaces. This source of tension has nothing to do with the number of sarcomeres, muscle cells or cross-links between the collagen fibers.

TENDONS

Often a nice, long tendon joins a muscle to a bone, but this is not always the case. Sometimes the muscle connects to the bones through a broad attachment, as we find, for example, with the tibialis anterior: it connects all along the tibia, not only at the ends. The vastus intermedius, in addition to joining the common tendon of the quadriceps, is also attached firmly to the femur through a layer of "bone paint": there is no tendon along the top of the femur where the muscle connects to it—rather, it is as if the muscle was painted onto the bone.[108] Sometimes the muscle joins to a wide sheath of fascia called an *aponeurosis*, which happens with the latissimus dorsi of our back: the muscle turns into the thoracolumbar fascia. Most of the time, however, the muscle's fascia becomes a tendon, which becomes the bone. There is no sharp beginning and end to these tissues in our body, but remember that scientists love to categorize things. It is like looking at a rainbow: we can definitely point to one region and say, "That is orange," and say of another region, "That is yellow," but we cannot precisely show where orange ends and yellow begins. A spectrum in nature has no sharp boundaries, but in science we like to make such assumptions. These are useful simplifications, but they are not reality. In reality, the fascia of the muscle *becomes* the tendon in the same way that orange becomes yellow in a rainbow. The place of becoming is called the *myotendinous* junction. It is here that muscle growth occurs when sarcomeres are added in series within the muscle cells, and it is here that most stress-related injuries to the muscle occur—because this area, which is neither fully tendon nor fully muscle, is weaker than either the muscle or the tendon.[109]

It is common in anatomy to speak of muscles having *origins* and *insertions*. These terms can change depending upon which bone is being moved or held still. The impression conveyed by these terms is that a muscle arises from one bone and then joins to another bone. If the first bone is fixed, the part of the muscle connecting there is called the origin, and the bone that moves (the second bone) hosts the insertion of the muscle. Confusingly, if the first bone is the one that moves, these terms might be reversed. Most often we use the term *origin* for the site of the muscle that attaches to the more stable bone, even if that bone can also move. This concept of origin and insertion is useful as long as we are not fooled into believing that it is reality; it is a conceptualization of the way the body works. In reality, as already discussed, the muscles can connect to the bone all along its length, such as with the tibialis anterior, which has a very broad connection to the tibia, as well as an origin at the top of the tibia and an insertion on the bones of the foot. Henceforth, we will avoid the confusing terms origins and insertions in favour of the more precise *proximal* and *distal attachments*. Proximal refers to the attachment closer to the core of the body, and distal refers to the attachment further away from the trunk or core of the body.

OUR WALK: Some people's gaits are very distinctive—think of John Wayne's swagger or Marilyn Monroe's seductive swaying. Indeed, everyone's walk is distinctive, thanks to the unique shape and width of our hips, the length of our legs, the size of our muscles, and the height and weight of our bodies. Everyone walks by moving one foot in front of the other, but our gait is so unique that we can be identified by it.

As the muscle evolves into being a tendon, similarly, the tendon becomes the bone: there is no sharp beginning or ending here either. Tendons are strongly anchored both to the surface of the bone—the *periosteum*—and deeper inside the bone's *cortex*. The site of the attachment, where the tendon becomes the bone, which is neither tendon nor bone, is another weaker area. Injuries may also arise here, usually preceded by some tweaky pain in the tendon near the bone. If these signals of mild pain are ignored and painful stress is allowed to continue to occur in this region, the tendon may tear. Such an injury takes much longer to heal than one

to the muscles, as there is less blood flow to these tissues. A muscle injury may resolve itself within days, but tendon injuries may take weeks, months or sometimes years to resolve if the student doesn't stop over-stressing the damaged area or doesn't receive appropriate advice or treatment in a timely manner.

As the muscle's fascia experiences the stress of activation, it transmits that stress through the tendon to the bone, which then moves—or resists movement, depending on the intention and situation. The tendon also experiences the stress that is flowing through it. Like fascia, it is made up predominantly of tubes within tubes within tubes of collagen,[110] and these tubes or fibers are lined up in the direction of the stress applied to the tendon. The tubes are quite inelastic, which is very important for providing fine control over our movements. We may want the muscles to be able to contract or expand, but not the tendon, and in this manner the stress generated by the muscles is precisely transmitted to our articulating skeleton. Indeed, if a tendon is stressed so much that it stretches beyond 4–10% of its normal length (beyond its elastic limit), it becomes injured.[111]

Don't take this range as gospel, because the statistic depends upon which tendons and which person. It is an average. Also, against this theory of "we must never stretch our tendons," a different view argues that the elasticity of our tendons gives us the ability to run and jump.[112] While tendons are relatively stiff compared to our muscles, they are not made of steel. They do store some elastic energy that, when released, can augment the power of the muscles. Kangaroos, gazelles and humans can all jump quite high thanks to the elastic nature of their Achilles tendons. (Curiously, other primates, such as chimpanzees and gorillas, cannot jump very well; homo sapiens is the jumping primate!) We can think of tendons like springs. When a spring is stretched, it converts the mechanical energy of stretching into potential energy; when the stress causing the stretch ceases, that potential energy is quickly released back into mechanical energy—the spring springs back, releasing its power. This ability of the tendon can be trained. This is good news because in sports (such as basketball and volleyball) and other activities that require spring-like action from our tendons, injuries of the tendons are much more frequent than in other activities that do not require such behaviour (such as swimming). Eccentric lengthening, stretching programs and ballistic exercise can increase the elasticity of the tendons, probably because the muscles are contracting while the tendons are being stressed, thus allowing more stress to get to the tendons.[113]

Normally, we are advised in our yoga practice not to target our tendons; we are warned that if the tension of a yoga pose is felt predominantly in the tendons, the pose is not doing any good. Modifications are offered to try to redirect the tension to the muscle. However, this may not be the best approach if we want to train the tendons and strengthen their elastic recoil ability. Some researchers are suggesting that deliberately stressing a tendon may be therapeutic when that tendon is injured, or to avoid injury in the first place.[114] The stress will stimulate a healing response. Like everything in life, you can do too much, but you can also do too little. Remember Goldilocks. What is important anytime you feel stress in a tendon is whether the stress is painful or not. If you experience any pain in a posture, the safest approach to avoid injury is to stop doing that pose and find some other way into the targeted area.

FASCIA

So far, we have seen the fascia show up throughout the muscle as the tubes that contain the sarcomeres and muscle bundles, but this is only one place that fascia is found. Fascia is a fascinating substance and has recently become recognized as an important contributor to our health and flexibility. Fascia used to be a term applied only to connective tissue that did not have any other specific term: any tissue that wasn't bone or ligament was fascia. Fascia was the miscellaneous, leftover connective tissue, and those interested in fascia were jokingly called *fascists*. However, our understanding of what fascia is

EARS: Just as we can be identified by our fingerprints or eyes, our ears are also unique. No two ears are alike, not even your left and right ears. Ears start out as six tiny bumps on the side of our head very early in the development of a fetus. These mounds gradually fuse, but their final shape is dictated both by our genes and by how the sides of our head are pressed against the walls of our mother's womb. Once formed, they do not change shape, but they do change in size.[37]

and what it does has grown considerably, and the term has been broadened to include almost anything made up of collagen: our tendons and ligaments now could be considered a kind of fascia.[115] Fascia may include collagen fibers as well as elastic fibers and the extracellular fluid that surrounds our cells. Today, people who study fascia are referred to as *fascinistas* or *fascinados*.[116]

Fascia is ubiquitous: it is found all over the body (see figure 1.29). We wear a full three-dimensional fascial body stocking under the skin (called the *superficial fascia*); fascia surrounds and invests our muscles; fascia surrounds and supports our organs (called the *deep* or *profound fascia*); fascia helps to guide the alignment of our blood vessels and nerves; fascia is the home for fat cells. It is connected to the immune system, and it is richly supplied with nerves and therefore connected to our nervous system as well. Fascia has several other functions, and we are discovering more as time goes on.

NOTE TO TEACHERS: Should we try to stress tendons?

Should we stress our tendons or not? It would be nice to have one prescription that would work for every body, but life is not so simple. The answer is "yes, no and maybe." Most yoga teachers will follow their training and advise against stressing the tendons. Unaware of any other options, they will tell their students to never feel the stress of the pose in the attachment zones of the muscles. That is what they were told, and that is what they will teach. For example, they may say, "During a forward fold, we want to feel a stretch in the belly of the hamstrings, not near the sitting bones where the hamstrings originate." But, as we have seen, for some people such stress is necessary to help strengthen the tendon. Stressing the

tendons builds their resilience and dynamic flexibility. Unfortunately, there are other students who should not do this, because their tendons are already weak and any stress could create a tear. Rather than dogmatically insist that no one should ever feel a stress in the tendons, it may be more skillful to teach your students to differentiate between healthy stress and what it feels like, and unhealthy stress and the pain that usually accompanies it. If the sensation in the tendon is a sharp, burning pain, stressing that tendon so much is not advisable. If the sensation is one of tugging or pulling, it may be quite healthy to allow it to continue.

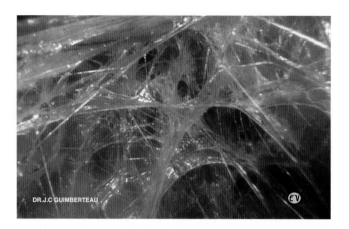

FIGURE 1.29.A Fascia is arachnoid (spider-web-like), wet and ubiquitous. Here we find the superficial fascia forming webs that contain fibers, fluids and aligning blood vessels. (Images from the DVD *Interior Architectures: Exploring the Architecture of the Human Body*, reproduced with kind permission of Jean-Claude Guimberteau.)

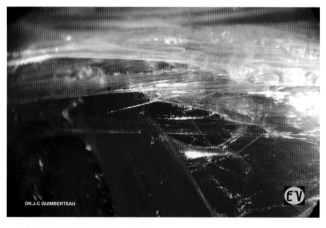

FIGURE 1.29.B Fascia surrounding muscle.

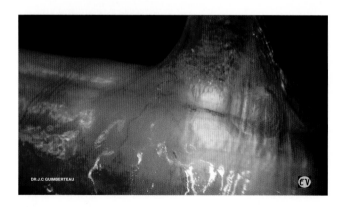

FIGURE 1.29.C Fascia being pulled away from a tendon.

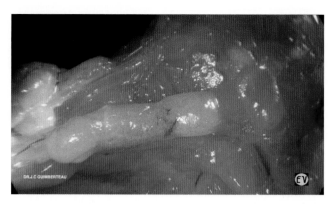

FIGURE 1.29.D Fascia surrounding fat.

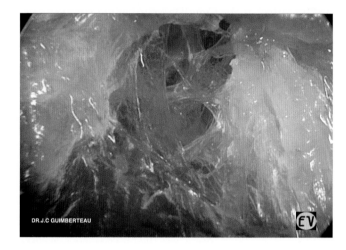

FIGURE 1.29.E Fascia investing the outside of bone tissue (the periosteum).

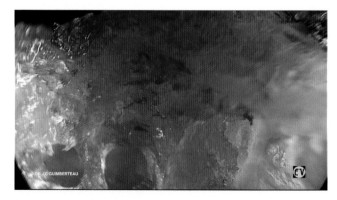

FIGURE 1.29.F Fascia within bone.

Adhesions

Understanding that fascia provides a sliding surface between muscles helps us realize how tension can arise in our tissues and is one answer to the question "What stops me?" For a muscle to contract or stretch, it has to be free to change its shape without interference or resistance from neighbouring tissues. Fascia is moist and slippery, which enables muscle groups to slide over each other's surfaces. However, if the fascia has sustained damage and scar tissue has built up between the otherwise sliding surfaces of the muscles, these *adhesions* can retard or even stop the muscles from moving.

Restrictions to movement due to adhesions will be felt as tension in the area of the adhesion, but they may also be felt as tension far away from that site! This may seem counterintuitive, but a simple example will show you why this can arise. Put on a shirt that has sleeves. With your left hand, grasp the bottom right corner of your shirt, by your right hip, pull it down as much as you can, then try to lift your right arm. Do you feel a restriction on the top of the right shoulder? You are pulling on the shirt down by the hip, so why would you feel tension in the shoulder? Because the shirt's fabric is not very elastic, the attempt to stretch the fabric when we lift the arm creates a stress that restricts the movement. Like our shirt, our body stocking of fascia can become chronically shortened, stuck or adhered in one area, but the effects of that stuckness may manifest in another area. You have felt similar constraints to movement when you donned tight blue jeans recently out of the dryer: you can't move because your body is encased in a tight sheath of material. If you feel tension reducing your range of movement, it may not be because of tight, short muscles but rather due to fascia that has become shortened or stuck together.

Thomas Myers wrote a pivotal book in the understanding of fascia as it affects movement, called *Anatomy Trains*. In it he explained how the web of fascia forms specific trains of stress, called *myofascial meridians*, that aid the body's movements. Myers also described how poor posture and pathological movement patterns can create unhelpful trains that restrict normal movement—analogous to our shirt example. By following this model, we can understand how constrictions in one area of the body can cause restrictions to movement around a distant joint.

An example can help to illustrate how important understanding the myofascial meridians is for yoga teachers and students. In figure 1.30, we see a student in Reclining Hero (Suptavirasana); highlighted are the areas where she is feeling tension: the top of the knees, the belly of the thigh, the front of the pelvis, and the stomach close to the lowest ribs, perhaps even the top of the feet and ankles. If your only tool for understanding where resistance to movement in yoga arises were an anatomical knowledge of the muscles, you would be unable to explain all the sensations created in this posture. You could not explain the tension in the ribs or at the front of the pelvis (the ASIS), because the thigh muscles do not reach these areas. However, understanding the fascial continuity of the front superficial line (FSL) myofascial meridian from the knee to the ribs does explain the tension felt, even across the bones of the pelvis and ribs. We are stressing not only the muscles here but all the fascia around them, which contribute to the FSL. (To learn more about these trains, read Appendix C: Myofascial Meridians.)

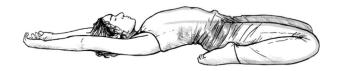

FIGURE 1.30 The myofascial meridians may create sensations far from the site of a primary restriction.

Myofibroblasts

Like a muscle, fascia can contract! Fibroblasts are cells that produce and secrete collagen—the protein that makes up our fascia, ligaments and tendons, among other structures. There are several types of fibroblast cells found within the fascia, one of which is the *myofibroblast*. This fibroblast can contract, like a muscle cell, but unlike a muscle cell, its reactions are very slow and persist for long periods of time. A fibroblast usually stays embedded in the collagen that it has secreted, becoming attached to these fibers like a spider in the center of its own web, sensing the strain that is placed upon the fibers. Again like the spider, a myofibroblast can remain connected to its fibers, but it can also contract, pulling on the fibers and thus shrinking the local region of tissues. This is very useful in wound healing: if we suffer a small cut, the myofibroblasts contract, reducing the area of damage, which makes it easier for skin stem cells to reseal the damaged area. However, this is not very useful if it is happening all the time.

Chronic pain in the neck or lower back often feels like tightness in the muscles, but individual muscle cells cannot stay contracted for very long. Myofibroblasts can and do. The chronic, painful tightness many people experience in their lower backs, shoulders, neck or other areas is often caused not by their muscles but by their fascia. This form of tension will also restrict range of movement, and it has nothing to do with tight, short or contracted muscles—it is fascial. Specifically, myofibroblasts have contracted, and if they stay contracted, the body will remodel the surrounding tissues to make that area permanently shortened and tight. One researcher discovered that people with chronic lower back pain have more myofibroblasts in their lower back than people who have no back pain. It is not clear whether this is a *cause* or a *result* of the pain, because pain creates psychological and physiological stress, and such stress can cause myofibroblasts to contract in an effort to protect an area.[117]

We Have But One Muscle

How many muscles do you have? Scientists, remember, love to break things down into simpler parts, but in a living system, the parts do not add back up to a whole. Estimates of the number of muscles we have range from 600 to 850, but consider: every hair follicle has a little muscle that can make it stand erect, and there are millions of those; every capillary has the ability to contract, so the capillary walls are muscles. The case can be made that we have tens of millions of muscles, but in terms of skeletal muscles, the case can also be made that we have only one! In this model, a single skeletal muscle is wrapped into many segments by the body stocking of fascia. Remember that muscle is also fascial—it is myofascia—so our one muscle is a ribbon of muscle and fascia strung together like so many sausages. When we engage one segment of the muscle, through the fascia the stress tightens nearby segments, which could be synergistic for other movements. As the muscle segment's fascia swells during contraction and presses against nearby muscle segments, a process called *hydraulic amplification*, these neighbouring muscle groups are pre-tensed, making them more effective and efficient.[118] In this model, tension is created and maintained not only by individual muscles doing their thing, but by the whole system of fascia.

LIGAMENTS

Ready for another generalization? In general, muscles and tendons move joints, while joint capsules and ligaments stabilize joints. However, sometimes muscles and tendons can stabilize a joint, when they act as an antagonist; and sometimes ligaments and joint capsules can increase a joint's mobility, when they release their contracture.

What stops me? If the joint moves too far in a particular direction, the ligaments on the other side of the direction of movement become taut. Remember we said that tendons generally connect a muscle to a bone, and it is the pulling of this muscle/tendon that moves the bone, articulating a joint. Ligaments, on the other hand, tend to limit the range of movement that a joint can undergo. They do this to protect a joint, to make sure that movement beyond the safe range of motion doesn't happen, because if the joint moves too much, that can damage the joint capsule. The simple diagram in figure 1.31 illustrates this concept. Here you see that in the direction of movement, the ligament becomes quite relaxed and slack, but in the other direction, the ligament becomes quite taut and restricts further movement. This tautness arises only at the extreme limit of movement. Where a tendon joins a muscle to a bone, ligaments join bone to bone. In this model, we see that ligaments and muscle-tendons operate in parallel, and the purpose of our ligaments is to protect the joint from too much mobility.

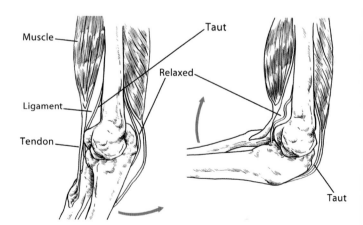

FIGURE 1.31 Ligaments can become slack or taut, depending upon the direction of movement. With extension of the joint, the ligament along the back of the joint becomes slack; when the joint is flexed, however, it becomes taut.

MYOFIBROBLASTS: People with chronic lower back pain have significantly more myofibroblasts in their lower backs than people without such pain. We don't know whether this difference is a cause of the pain or a consequence, but we do know that if you have more myofibroblasts, you may experience greater tightness in your lower back.[52]

However, this model is slowly being replaced by a more accurate model, one developed by Jaap van der Wal at the University Maastricht, in the Netherlands.[135] His work, based on a much more careful approach to dissecting the layers of tissues around a joint, has discovered that our ligaments work in *series* with the muscles, not in parallel! (See figure 1.32.)

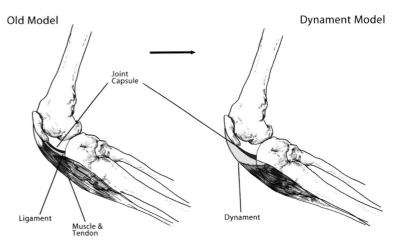

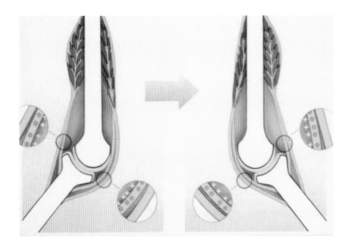

FIGURE 1.32 Ligaments are in series with the muscle-tendons, not in parallel, as was once thought.

This realization shows that ligaments are not passive structures that only come into play at the extremes of our ranges of motion, and only then to prevent too much movement. Instead, ligaments are part of a dynamic system, contiguous with muscles, tendons and bones. Van der Wal has called these units *dynaments* (from **dyn**amic liga**ments**).[136] (See figure 1.33.) While the old model still applies when ligaments directly connect bone to bone and no muscles are found (think of the cruciate ligaments in the knees), in most cases, ligaments are actively involved in determining the range of motion around a joint. Often, we are unable to differentiate where the tendon, ligament and joint capsules begin and end (again, think of the colors in the rainbow: we can't tell exactly where each color begins and ends).

FIGURE 1.33 The dynament model shows ligaments dynamically involved in determining the range of motion of a joint. Blue indicates the joint capsule, yellow the ligament and red the muscle and tendon.

Ligaments do not become tense only at the extreme range of the joint's movement; when the muscle tenses, the tendon and the ligaments both undergo stress. This stress may restrict our full range of movement long before the joint has reached its limits. We can no longer think of movement as being governed only by muscles. As we have already seen, the muscle is 30% fascia, which becomes the tendon. And now we see that there is no hard cutoff point between the muscle and our ligaments either. The newer model of an articulating limb is bone, fascia, muscle, fascia, bone—with the fascia consisting of the dynament of tendon and ligaments together. Tightness in the ligaments is simply one more form of tension that stops us.

Like tendons, ligaments are made up of fibers, but unlike tendons, the fibers in ligaments are not linear or lined up along one axis of stress. Instead, they are arranged in several directions, depending upon the variety of forces acting on the ligament. Joint capsules are similarly constructed. Also unlike tendons, ligaments come in a variety of shapes: cords, sheets and bands. While tendons are generally white, ligaments can be darker due to their mixture of elastic and finer fibers (elastin and collagen). Ligaments can be pliant

SCENT: We may not be able to use our scent as a password for online banking, but we certainly can recognize other people by their unique fragrance. One study found that our sweat contains over 5,000 chemicals, including acids, ketones and aldehydes. Forty-four chemicals were consistently found, but these varied so much in quantities that the researchers were able to create unique odor fingerprints for each participant.[39] A person's unique body odor also varies by location on the body and by the bacteria that have colonized the region.

and flexible in the directions where they are not binding the body, much like a credit card, which can be bent but not stretched. Ligaments are tough, strong and pliable yet mostly inelastic. The iliotibial band running down the outside of your thigh, for example, is strong enough to support the weight of a car without snapping! Not all ligaments are rigid along their lengths; some have a higher proportion of elastin than collagen. Elastin distributes stress instead of maintaining it in one place. Some ligaments along the vertebral column of our lumbar spine and in our necks are especially elastic in this way. The ligamentum flavum (an important spinal ligament) is one of the most flexible ligaments in our body.[137] When elastin fibers age, they become mineralized, cross-linked with other fibers and therefore stiffer. Thus, when our back ligaments age, they become much stiffer due to the increasing number of cross-links, restraining our range of movement.

THE NERVOUS SYSTEM

Our nervous system, like all systems, can be broken down into subcomponents. One of these is called the *autonomic nervous system* (ANS), which refers to all the things we do that are outside of our normal conscious awareness. The ANS in turn has two branches: the *sympathetic nervous system* (SNS), which controls our responses to stressful situations; and our *parasympathetic nervous system* (PNS), which activates the complementary responses to the SNS—our recovery and rest responses. The SNS is often called our *fight-or-flight* response, but it is broader than that: it can also trigger a *freeze* reaction[119] (whereby in the face of imminent danger, we freeze or faint), or, especially in women, a *tend-and-befriend* response (whereby in the face of danger, we seek out the company of others[120]). Such responses are adaptive; they help us to survive, and they helped our ancestors avoid the life-threatening dangers found all around them—predators on four feet and on two. The stress response, however, stops being adaptive and healthy for us if it becomes chronic. We will examine how the ANS contributes to "What stops me?" when we look at the immune system. For now, it is worth investigating another factor that reduces our mobility: the nervous system's interactions with our fascia and muscles.

There are 10 times more nerve endings in our fascia than in our muscle! This is a remarkable fact given how much fine control we have over our muscles. We make precise movements thanks to our nervous system's innervation of the muscles, and yet our fascia has far more nerve endings. What are they all doing? Providing feedback. This is called *proprioception*—we know what is going on within the body because of our nervous system's interaction with our fascia. Within the fascia there are several kinds of nerve endings: mechanoreceptors; nociceptors; Pacini, Ruffini, Golgi and interstitial receptors; and nerves connecting directly to our ANS. Embedded within the muscle fibers are *muscle spindles*, which measure stress within the muscle. Embedded in the muscular interface with our tendons (where the muscles become tendons) are *Golgi tendon organs*, which measure stress in this relatively weak area (these are different from the Golgi receptors found within the muscles and fascia). A brief review of these nerves can show how awake and aware our fascia is to what is happening within our body and during our yoga practice.

Mechanoreceptors sense stress. When we apply a stress to our body, whether through movement, posture or gravity, through tension or compression, through yoga or other exercise, through massage or through daily living, the stress reaches and affects our cells. Each cell's membrane (the outer wall of the cell) is studded with tens of thousands of proteins, called *integrins*, that reach up into the extracellular spaces and connect to the fascial fibers there (see Chapter 3). These integrins sense mechanical stresses in the environment, and based upon the strength of the stress, the cell makes different decisions about what to do—for example, which proteins to produce. Not only are the integrins connected to the external environment, but some of them reach down deep into the interior of the cell, even through the nucleus, right to our DNA. Signals from outside our body actually can communicate directly with our DNA! (See figures 1.24 and 1.25.)

Our cells also use mechanoreceptors to sense the flow of fluids around them. The cilia of the cells (those little hair-like projections that help a cell move) can feel the flow of extracellular fluids: if the flow is of a certain strength, stem cells will become blood cells. If fibroblasts feel a very slight flow of fluid, they will secrete an enzyme that can dissolve collagen and thus break down scar tissue.[121] This finding is quite exciting, as it promises new ways to perhaps get rid of scar tissue and other adhesions in the body through gentle massage and gentle movements.

The types of nerves innervating our fascia and muscles, called Pacini, Ruffini, Golgi and interstitial receptors, have different locations, functions and triggers, but they all sense pressure changes in the body's tissues. Based on which receptor is activated and the strength and location of the pressure applied, the body will react by: increasing or decreasing muscle tonus (the rigidity of the muscle); turning our autonomic nervous system up or down; changing the amount of fluid released into the extracellular matrix; and signaling to the brain where the body is and what it is doing (this is again proprioception).[122]

Nociceptors are the nerve endings that create the sensation of pain. Most low back pain, for example, is now known to be caused not by discogenic problems but by fascial problems.[123] The nociceptors in the lower back fascia are activated by chronic stress in the fascia and send pain signals to the brain. However, research has shown that these same nerves can also be activated even when there is no abnormal mechanical stress. This is because these cells also function as thermoreceptors (nerves that react to temperature changes) and chemoreceptors (nerves that react to changes in the body's pH level); hence, changes in the body beyond purely mechanical stress can trigger these cells, which then send signals that the brain interprets as pain.[124] Fortunately, there is a way to confuse nociceptors: because they are also mechanoreceptors, if we massage an area that is painful, the body reinterprets the signal from the nociceptors as a pressure signal. We have all experienced this. You bang your shin or stub your little toe. Ouch! What do you do? You rub the injured area, and it immediately feels better. By rubbing the area, you are changing the signal sent by the nociceptors from one of pain to one of pressure; the brain no longer registers the pain.

Muscle Spindles and Golgi Tendon Organs

Our nervous system is also constantly watching the state of stress in our muscles and tendons. If the muscle becomes stretched too much, or too quickly, receptors within the belly of the muscle, called muscle spindles, will send a signal to the spinal cord (technically called the horns of the spinal cord) or the brain stem (technically called alpha motor neurons). From there, a responding signal is sent to the muscle, causing it to contract so as to protect the muscle from being torn. Signals may also be sent to the antagonist muscles, ordering them to relax. This is a reflex action. (A reflex is an autonomic reaction of the body that is often not mediated by the brain. Sending a signal all the way up to the brain and waiting for the response may take too long and risks damage occurring while the body awaits the brain's signal; it is quicker to send the signal only to the spinal cord or brain stem and have the reaction come from there.)

Muscles normally have some degree of *tonus*: this is a state of slight activation of some of the muscle fibers. The whole muscle is never totally relaxed, except in special circumstances, such as under general anesthesia. The muscle tone is reported on by the muscle spindles. One of the sources of the tension that stops us, and which we experience in yoga, is the tone of the muscle: if the muscle is slightly activated, it will resist being stretched. If we can reduce that tone, we can get more stretch. If the tone is increased, by too much muscle spindle activation, we will have trouble stretching. Pathologies can arise in individuals whose muscle tonus is too high (hypertonia) or too low (hypotonia). Some people experience chronic rigidity or spasticity, which can limit their range of motion, because their muscle tone is too high or is unevenly turned on and off.

One way to reduce muscle tonus is to employ the Golgi tendon organs (GTO), located at the muscular junction to the tendons.[125] Just as muscle spindles watch to ensure that the muscles do not get stretched so strongly that damage occurs, the GTO monitor the level of stress in the area where muscle becomes tendon. If the stress becomes so high that the myofascial–tendon interface is at risk of rupturing, the GTO send a signal to the spinal cord, which sends a "cease and desist" order to the muscle to stop it contracting. This is the opposite signal to what the muscle spindles create: instead of contracting in self-protection, the muscle relaxes to protect itself.

Many physical therapists and yoga teachers employ these two ways to reduce muscle tonus to help increase the length of muscles and thus the range of motion. One approach develop in the 1950s by Herman Kabat, a neurophysiologist, is

GLANDS: The variations in the size of our glands have a bearing on our response to stress. The pituitary gland, for example, has a huge range of individual variation: one study found a 13-fold range, from 130 to 1800 milligrams.[49] Clearly not everyone's pituitary is going to release the same amount of stress hormones or growth hormones when it is activated. Since your pituitary is not the same size as everyone else's, how you react to stress, and the tension you experience in your tissues as a result, will be unique. The thyroid gland also can vary in weight from eight to 50 grams and can have a wide variety of shapes.[50] In some cases, the location of the thyroid is unusual: normally they are at the front of our throats, but some people have them at the base of the tongue. A healthy pancreas can be from 65 to 160 grams.[51] We could go on and list other glands, but the point is that all of our glands show ranges of variation in size and shape, which can affect their particular performance.

HEARTBEAT: Every heart has its own signature beat, and each beat is different. Waves of cascading electrical impulses flow through the heart muscles. These waves can be measured on an electrocardiogram (ECG) and vary depending upon the size, shape and electrical conductivity of each heart. No two ECG readings are exactly the same, and the electrical flow is not under conscious control. This uniqueness is being explored for security identification systems.[40]

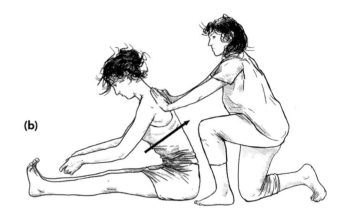

called *proprioceptive neuromuscular facilitation* (PNF). In PNF, a student pushes against a resistance applied by a teacher. For example, in seated forward-fold postures like Paschimottanasana, the student is often stopped from going deeper due to tension in the muscles along the back side of the body: the hamstrings or the large muscles in the back. As shown in figure 1.34, by pressing up against the teacher's hands, the hamstrings and back muscles are activated while in a lengthened position, creating a stress in their myofascial–tendon interface, activating their GTO, which in turn send a signal through the spinal cord back to these muscles, reducing the muscle tone. After pressing upwards for a few seconds, the student then relaxes and can fold deeper. This process is repeated several times, enabling the tonus in the hamstrings to become very low, which allows for a much deeper stretch. There are many variations of PNF, but one that shows arguably the best success is called *reversal of antagonists* (or, more popularly, *3S—scientific stretching for sports*). The 3S protocol uses the process of pushing against a resistance (either a machine or a partner) to engage the agonist muscle while it is in a lengthened position; then, while the agonist relaxes, the antagonist muscles are engaged for a few seconds to further lengthen the agonist, following which all muscles are relaxed. This whole cycle takes about 15 seconds and is repeated four times. Increased flexibility from 3S can be as good as or better than flexibility achieved from the static stretching employed in yoga; however, 3S does require special equipment or a trained partner.[128]

FIGURE 1.34 We can reduce muscle tonus and increase length through proprioceptive neuromuscular facilitation. In (a), the hamstrings have reached their edge and are tight. In (b), the student presses in the opposite direction against a resistance, triggering the Golgi tendon organs (GTO) to become activated. In (c), the GTO have told the hamstrings to reduce their tonus, allowing a deeper forward fold.

The nervous system plays an important role in how tension can stop us from increasing our flexibility and range of motion. The nervous system senses the state of our muscles, tendons and fascia and can either relax or increase muscle tone and/or turn on or off the activity of contracting myofibroblasts. Depending upon stress signals from our fascia, the autonomic nervous system can activate our endocrine system and our immune system. These two systems also affect our flexibility and mobility and produce tension in our tissues, so we will look at them next.

VOICE: The human voice is possible due to the complex shapes of the trachea and mouth, the position of the tongue, the shape of the larynx and the size of the vocal cords (more precisely called the vocal folds). Even the teeth will affect the sound of an individual's voice. With all the possible variations in these structures, it is understandable that each person's voice is unique (unless we decide to imitate someone else's voice). Our ability to change our voice and imitate others makes voice recognition for security applications a coarse tool that is usually backed up by other techniques (such as an iris scan).[38]

THE IMMUNE SYSTEM

Like our nervous system, our immune system has two key components: the *innate* system, which responds quickly to problems, and the *adaptive* system, which takes time to kick in but is more targeted in response to particular problems. The innate system is our *frontline* immune response: during times of stress, when the sympathetic nervous system is activated, the frontline immune system increases clotting factors in our blood (in case we get cut), increases cortisol levels (to boost glucose flow into the blood stream and decrease inflammation, which helps to improve blood flow), and releases cytokines, which attract specialized blood cells (such as macrophages and phagocytes) that target anything that is not "you," to combat infections. To assist with the initial response during acute stress, our heart rate, blood pressure and blood volume increase, helping to get the immune system's fighters to the front line. The frontline immune response is very fast but also very generic and often misses things. What gets missed is dealt with by the back line: the *adaptive* immune system.

Once a crisis has passed, our parasympathetic nervous system kicks in to counterbalance the work of the sympathetic nervous system. Our heart rate and blood flow decrease, our digestive processes resume, and the backline immune system adapts to any infections that evaded the frontline system. Specialized white blood cells—called killer T cells and beta cells—are created to hunt for these specific invaders; viruses and bacteria are rooted out from their hiding places, their disguises no longer working. If we suffered an injury, the damaged area is cordoned off through

ITS COMPLICATED: Our ground substance

The average man's body is 62% water. The average woman's body is 52% water.[126] In either case, we are mostly walking bags of water. Our *ground substance* is the nonfibrous portion of our extracellular matrix (the stuff outside the cells of our bodies) in which the living cells are held in place. The ground substance is made up of various proteins, water, and *glycosaminoglycans*. Water can make up 60% to 70% of the ground substance, and it is attracted there because of the glycosaminoglycans. One of the most important glycosaminoglycans is *hyaluronic acid* (also known as *hyaluronan*). The fluid in our joints (called *synovial* fluid) is a lubricant that is also made up substantially of glycosaminoglycans—predominantly hyaluronic acid, lubricin and two kinds of chondroitin sulphates. Various researchers have estimated that hyaluronic acid can attract and bind 1,000 times its volume of water.[127] When glycosaminoglycans combine with proteins, they are called *proteoglycans*, and it is in this form that they attach to water molecules and hydrate our tissues. The proteoglycans are very mobile and move about freely. However, being made of water, they also tremendously resist compression. The proteoglycans are shaped like brushes connected in tree-like arrangements, as shown in figure 1.35, and they wind their way through the collagen fibers of our fascia and cartilage. Our tissues can swell if too much water is absorbed by the glycosaminoglycans, but the tissue fibers resist and limit the amount of swelling that can occur. It is this interplay between the swelling of our tissues and the resistance of the fibers that creates tension and structure. This arrangement also is responsible for the ability of our articular cartilage to withstand repetitive forces.

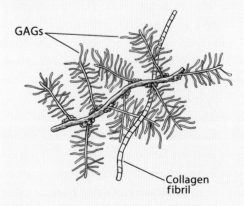

FIGURE 1.35 Proteoglycans consist of several glycosaminoglycans in multiple branches to help attract and structure water molecules.

inflammation, triggered by cytokines, which are small protein messenger molecules that function like hormones but are much smaller and more numerous. (Cytokines generally are released by a broad range of cells, whereas hormones are released by endocrine glands.) Inflammation restricts the infection to one small region and allows the adaptive system to be more efficient in resolving the problem. Inflammation is part of the backline immune system and is turned off by the frontline system.

This two-part response of the autonomic nervous system, which in turn triggers the two-part response of our immune system, is wonderful when it is triggered once in a while; however, if we suffer chronic stress activation, then the system starts to malfunction. Chronic exposure makes us intolerant to cortisol, which not only fails to control how glucose is released into the blood stream but also no longer can control the degree of inflammation we produce in the body. We become chronically inflamed, which creates a host of medical issues. Dr. Timothy McCall, in his book *Yoga as Medicine*, states: "It can be argued that stress is the number one killer in the Western world today." He goes on to say that "stress fuels some of the biggest health problems of our time, including type 2 diabetes, depression, osteoporosis, heart attacks and strokes as well as autoimmune diseases like multiple sclerosis and rheumatoid arthritis."[129]

When we are stressed, when we are sick, we lose physical mobility. We have all noticed this—when you have a cold or the flu, you feel stiff. You ache and cannot move as easily as you usually can. You have stiffened up and your body has become tight; there is tension all over. We can now start to understand why. One of the above mentioned cytokines released by our immune system is called TGF-β (transforming growth factor beta). TGF-β influences the growth of killer-T and beta cells, causes other cells to undergo apoptosis (cellular death), and increases the release of other cytokines. TGF-β is an important part of our immune function, but it has another effect unrelated to our immune response: it increases the production of myofibroblasts and causes them to contract.[130] Remember, myofibroblasts are found in our fascia, and when they tighten up, we feel the effects all over our fascial body stocking. When we are stressed or sick, when our immune system is ramped up, some of the chemical messengers being released cause our fascia to tighten. This may be beneficial in the short term—the body often contracts during times of injury to protect itself—but if we are chronically stressed or sick, then the contraction becomes chronic as well.

Again, let's ask What stops me? Well, we may have reduced mobility and range of motion due to our chronic state of stress or poor health! The connection between our immune system and our fascia is bi-directional. The mechanoreceptors we discussed earlier, the various interstitial receptors, send signals to the autonomic nervous system and can trigger a stress response.[131]

Another way that our autonomic nervous system and our immune system can lead to decreased mobility is through the release of water into the extracellular spaces between our tissues, through inflammation. This is yet another answer to WSM?. Inflammation causes the tissues to swell up, and we have all experienced the reduced mobility of a swollen area of the body. If we suffer chronic inflammation, we are going to experience less range of motion, not only in the inflamed area but, thanks to our fascial body stocking, all over the body. How water affects our mobility is our next area of investigation.

THE WONDER OF WATER

Water is sticky and loves to cling to surfaces. This is not so obvious in our macroscopic everyday world, but as we start to investigate the role of water within and between our cells, this fact becomes very obvious and very important. We call this stickiness *surface tension*. No doubt you have seen bugs that walk on water; this is due to surface tension. As small as these Jesus-bugs are, our cells are vastly smaller and much more susceptible to water's stickiness. As a layer of water becomes thinner, the surface tension increases, and therefore so does its stickiness. Water is also highly incompressible. When stress is applied to a bag of water, the water doesn't compress; instead, the tension is distributed throughout the bag. This phenomenon is known as *hydraulics* (which literally means "water in a pipe") and is used in everyday machines to amplify and distribute pressure—for example, in your car's hydraulic brakes. The final main point to know about water is that, within the body, it is structured: it forms layers upon layers that cling to each other, much like a bowl of gelatin. This *gel* state of water can also add tensile resistance to movements within and between cells. The other state of water found within the body and within cells is the *solution* state, when the water is in a more unstructured, bulk form and is free to flow and move around.

If you have ever had two pieces of flat glass laid on top of each other—perhaps you were preparing slides for a microscope—you may have noticed that with just a little bit of water between the two glass plates, they slid quite easily but were almost impossible to pull apart. You'll notice the same effect when you walk upon sand at the beach. Walk on dry sand, and your feet sink in, but walk on wet sand, and you don't sink—you are walking on water! The surface tension of the water glues the sand particles together, and these small particles of sand can now support your full body weight. Thus, water can lubricate our tissues, allowing gliding movements as with the glass slides, and water can bond our tissues together, creating rigidity and support, like the wet sand at the beach. How this happens is fascinating but beyond our scope of our investigation.[132] What we can investigate are the consequences of these facts about water, because it is the major component of the body's *ground substance*. (See It's Complicated: Our ground substance, on page 49.)

With water as its principal component, the ground substance is an excellent lubricant between fibers and fibrils, allowing them to slide freely past each other. Water gives our tissues a spring-like quality, permitting them to return to their original shapes once pressure has ceased. This is crucial to our tissues' ability to withstand stresses; however, a cyclical loading and unloading of the tissue, which we do in our yoga practice, is important for maintaining cellular health.[133]

When the extracellular matrix is well hydrated, cells, nutrients and other components of the matrix can move about freely. Toxins and waste products can be escorted out of the matrix into the lymphatic system and removed from the body. The ground substance, produced by the fibroblasts, is also helpful in resisting the spread of infection and is part of our immune system barrier.

Unfortunately, as we age, the body's ability to create water-loving proteins that keep our tissues wet (called *glycosaminoglycans*) diminishes. We have fewer fibroblasts available to us, and those we do have produce fewer glycosaminoglycans. Consequently, the extracellular matrix is increasingly filled with more and more fibers. As these fibers come closer together, they generate cross-links that bind them to each other. Our tissues thereby become stiffer, less elastic and less open to the flow of the other components in our matrix. Toxins and waste products are trapped in the matrix and cannot get out, and harmful bacteria can multiply freely. Immobility is one big cause of steep losses in hydration; immobilization can cause an up to 40% loss of hyaluronic acid—our most common glycosaminoglycan—in our joints, reducing the amount of water we have there and the ability of our tissues to slide across each other.[134]

What stops me? Well, one thing that makes us stiffer is a lack of water in the extracellular matrix. Without this lubricant between our tissues, we get stuck. However, if we have too much water, we can also become stiffer, just as a tube that is full of water is less flexible than an empty tube. Many women notice how their flexibility varies considerably throughout their menstrual cycle; this corresponds to the amount of water they retain at various times of the month. If they are retaining too much water, stiffness and restricted mobility result. When we suffer too much inflammation, we similarly have too much water in our tissues, which reduces our mobility.

Fortunately, exercise like yoga and massage, which stresses the extracellular matrix, can help us maintain the number of fibroblasts we have and keep them functioning properly, which assists in hydrating our extracellular matrix and our joints. These forms of exercise also allow the state of water to periodically change, from gel to sol and from sol to gel, which is important for the healthy functioning of our cells.

Sources of Compression

We have looked at a variety of sources of tension that can help us answer WSM? but there is another half to the WSM? spectrum of answers: compression. We have defined three kinds of compression:

- Soft—flesh hitting flesh
- Medium—flesh hitting bone
- Hard—bone hitting bone

GUTS: The term "guts" is rather imprecise and can refer to the whole alimentary canal, from ingest at the mouth to egress at the anus, but let's restrict the term to the intestines and colon, where most of digestion takes place. Human colons are smaller than chimpanzees' or gorillas', and smaller means less efficient. A 1925 study found that human colons varied in length by up to five feet.[46] The shorter the colon, the fewer calories extracted and the more gas released. The amount and quality of such gas is highly variable. In other words, your farts are quite unique to you. This expulsion of methane represents a loss of valuable, organic carbon, which longer intestines might have allowed you to capture.

Now that we have looked at the physiology of the softer tissues—muscles and fascia—it is time to look at the harder tissues, our bones and cartilage, to discover how they contribute compressive resistance to movement.

BONES

Our bones are struts of resistance and levers for movements: they resist compressive loads and provide attachment sites for our muscles. However, by themselves, the bones could neither support our body nor give it shape. They need the guy-wires of the muscles, ligaments and fascia to keep them connected and in alignment. Imagine a medical skeleton hanging in a corner; without its wires, the bones would simply collapse in a heap on the floor. This would happen in our bodies were it not for the tension provided by the "wires" of muscles and fascia. Together they form a *tensegrity* structure. Buckminster Fuller coined the word tensegrity to describe a tensional and compressional system.[138] Within our bodies, this is termed *biotensegrity*.[139] The muscles and connective tissues provide the continuous stress, while the bones contribute discrete compression sites.

There are two main components of bone: the *cortex* (from the Latin for "bark," as in the bark of a tree), which is the outer layer, and the *cancellous* (from the Latin for "lattice") inner structure (see figure 1.36). The cortical bone is quite different from the cancellous bone. Cortical bone is strong, hard and filled with collagen fibers, which provide the scaffold in which mineralized salts become embedded. These salts are made up predominately of calcium, but also present are phosphorus and traces of other elements, such as carbon, magnesium, zinc, copper, strontium, silicon, manganese and boron. As with everything else we have been looking at, we again find a wide range of human variation in these bone constituents. For example, the levels of boron in our bones can range from 16 to 138 parts per million.

SEXUAL ORGANS: It is no surprise that everyone's external sexual organs have different sizes and shapes. But did you know that there are important evolutionary reasons for this variability? One study found that men with smaller testicles made better dads. Testes can vary in weight in healthy men from 10 to 45 grams.[47] Parenting scores and MRI images both showed that men with smaller testicles scored higher as caring parents. The researchers could not, however, determine whether these better dads had smaller testicles to begin with or whether being more involved as a caregiver caused their testicles to shrink.[48]

This can have a dramatic effect on the strength of individual bones.[140] It is the strength of these mineralized areas along the length of the bone that provides the great resistance bones have to compression. However, bones can bend a little bit, which is useful when other stresses build up: it is better to bend a little than to break. Cortical bone is often called *compact bone*, and this living bone is white, like ivory. It is the cortical bone that gives bones their shape and structure, which are quite variable depending upon the function and placement of the bone in the body.

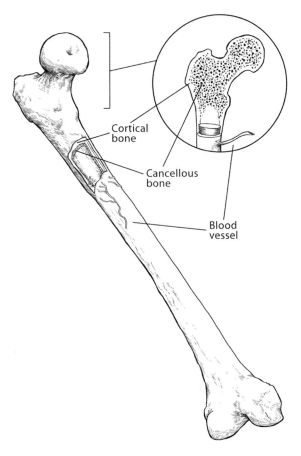

FIGURE 1.36 Bone has two main structures: the cortical (bark-like) outer portion and the cancellous (lattice-like) inner scaffold.

Inside the cortical bone, we find the open, porous, lattice structure of the cancellous bone, sometimes referred to as *trabecular* bone (which means, in Latin, "small beams"). These tiny struts give the bone rigidity but also make it lighter, since the inner bone is honeycombed rather than solid. As much as 60% of the compressive resistance our bones provide is due to the materials that make up our bones, but 40% is due to the architecture of the latticework, the arrangement of the materials inside the bone.[141] The ratio of cortical bone to trabecular bone can vary throughout the body. Our wrists may contain 80% cortical bone, while our vertebrae have only 33%. The necks of our femurs, which are subjected to great stress, are 75% cortical bone, but the shafts of the femur are 50% cortical bone.

Living bone contains significant portions of collagen and calcium salts. The mineral salts help us tolerate bone compression, while the collagen helps us resist tension that would bend or break the bone. If the bone was made only of mineral salt and was subjected to extreme pressure, it would snap the way a dead tree branch breaks: cleanly. However, healthy (especially young) bone, with a high degree of collagen meshing, breaks more like a living branch of a tree. If you have ever tried to snap off a living branch, you know that it doesn't break, it bends. To break it, you have to bend it back and forth, over and over again, until finally one side crumples while the other side frays apart.

Inside the spaces of the cancellous bone, also called the *marrow*, is room for blood stem cells (called *hematopoietic* cells) to create new blood—red blood cells and all the various white blood cells of our immune system. This requires that our bones be highly vascularized. Blood vessels flow into and out of the bones, providing nutrients to the bone cells and a pathway out of the bone for the new blood created within. As we age, or with injury or disease, the marrow may become filled with adipose tissue; fat replaces the blood-building cells, which affects our overall health. In some areas, such as in our sinuses, these honeycombed spaces are filled with air.

Growth and Aging of Bone

When we are newborns, our bones are not yet solid. How they solidify, a process called *ossification*, depends upon the type of bone and where it is. The flat bones, such as those found in our skull, jaw and clavicles, are formed by stem cells growing in a lattice of collagen. Virtually all of our other bones, including the long bones of the arms and legs, go through a cartilaginous stage, which provides a template for how the fully mature bone will look. Within neonatal bones are formed ossification centers. Cartilage is slowly, continuously deposited in these areas, making the young bone longer. Between these early ossification centers, a primitive trabecular bone is laid down. Eventually, the cartilage at the ends of the bone changes into mineralized bone, and the primitive trabeculae are replaced with mature trabeculae and marrow, which include the vascular and neuronal structures.

BRAIN WAVES: We start life with over 200 billion neurons, and as we age, this number is pruned to around 100 billion. But each neuron in the adult brain is connected, on average, to 7,000 other brain cells, equating to around 500 trillion synapses.[41] The resulting network is uniquely yours, and the ever-changing electrical fields created by your brain are unique to you as well. Your brain waves are unlike anyone else's, even though there are common frequencies that we all present at different times. These frequencies are grouped into clusters named alpha, beta, delta, theta and gamma waves, but even within these groupings, your brain waves are distinct.

The growing ends of the bone contain *epiphyseal plates*, where cartilage is deposited and then changed to bone. Once these epiphyseal plates become calcified, no more lengthening of the bone is possible. This happens between the ages of 18 and 25, depending upon the person and the bone. If the end of the bone becomes part of a synovial joint, some cartilage remains unossified, providing the cartilaginous surface that articulating bones need.

When our bones have finished growing, they are slightly hydrated: only about 10–20% of the bone is water. If we take out the water, 60–70% of what is left is mineralized salts, mostly crystallized calcium and phosphorous. Of the rest, 30–40% is collagen, which provides the scaffolding for the salts, and the remainder (about 5%) is glycoproteins and non-collagenous proteins and carbohydrates. Not surprisingly, these ranges of values vary considerably between individuals and by age.

With age, our trabeculae can become weaker. This loss of bone density is known as *osteopenia* (from the Greek, *penia*, which means "poverty"), but if severe it is termed *osteoporosis* ("porous bone"). This can happen in two ways: thinning of the trabecular struts making up the honeycomb of the inner bone, or loss of some of the struts altogether. The latter is more likely for women, whereas men are more likely to suffer only from thinning of the trabeculae.[142] In either case, the bone loses density and become weaker. (See Appendix D: Facts About Osteoporosis.)

Remodeling

Cells called *osteoblasts* (*osteon* is from the Greek for "bone," while *blastos* means "germ") secrete the collagen fibers and gylcoproteins that bind calcium into a cement. In time, osteoblasts turn into *osteocytes*—star-shaped cells with long tentacles that form channels through the bone, which can connect to other osteocytes. They can sense stresses in the bone and send out biochemical signals to initiate new bone creation or absorption. Bone absorption is done by cells called *osteoclasts* (*klasis* is from the Greek for "breaking"), which consume bone, recycling the calcium. These are huge cells: like our muscle cells, they are multinucleate, which means they have more than one nucleus. Some osteoclasts have over 50 nuclei. Osteoclasts are attracted to worn out, old or injured areas of bone and to areas where the osteocytes have died.[143] Our bones are a bank for calcium, and 99% of all the calcium we have is stored in this bank.[144] This process of deposition and reabsorption is called *remodeling*. It is under the control of our hormonal and immune systems, but it can also be affected by nutrition, genetics and external environmental factors, such as the amount of sunlight we get and the toxins we are exposed to.

Just as our bones can be remodeled from within, the cortical outer bone may also change on the outside. This happens when local stresses on the cortical bone persist, causing the bone to thicken in that region. This will often occur at a muscle attachment site. For example, the lesser trochanter is a bony prominence on the inner side of the femur's shaft, a little bit lower than the more famous greater trochanter of the femur. The lesser trochanter is the site of the attachments for the iliopsoas muscle. As figure 1.37 shows, everyone is different![145] Some people, perhaps because they were runners—constantly subjecting the lesser trochanter to a stress from flexing their legs as they ran—have much larger bumps here than their pedestrian friends who were not so active in that way. The larger the bumps, the more muscle tendon can attach to the bone, and this means the muscles can become bigger and thus stronger. This rule applies generally throughout our body. The greater the stress from the muscle's tendon to the bone, the larger the attachment site on the bone. And there is a gender difference: men, on average, have bigger bones than women due to larger muscular attachments, and men have larger muscular attachments because they have bigger bones. There is a circularity here of cause and effect beyond the basic nature of one's genetic predisposition. (Being stronger is not necessarily better or healthier; there is a trade-off between

greater strength, which creates stability, and lesser size, which allows more mobility.)

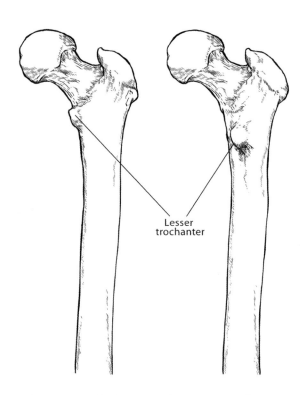

Lesser
trochanter

FIGURE 1.37 The lesser trochanter. Notice how its size and location can vary. The size can be affected by constant stress, such as that provided by running, but the location does not change after the bones have stopped growing.

Sometimes, unwanted bone depositions occur, creating *osteophytes*, more commonly called *bone spurs*. Why these deposits occur is not well understood, and they may be due to a number of conditions: aging, mechanical instabilities, diabetes, degeneration of the surrounding bone, or chronic inflammation such as is often found in osteoarthritis. If osteophytes occur along the spine, they may begin to impinge upon the spinal cord and can cause pain or numbness. In some instances, bone spurs may obstruct the free movement of a tendon, and as the tendon slides over the now rougher surface of the bone, clicking may result: the tendon gets temporarily stuck and then releases suddenly. (Many yoga students become aware of clicking noises as they move—this is often a benign sign of a tendon slipping over a roughened area of bone.)

While changes may occur within and on the surface of the bone as we age, its overall shape and structure will not change with either age or exercise once we are past puberty, in the absence of pathology or accidents. Yoga will

FEET: Women have a much wider range of foot movements than men, which may be a result of how much time our ancestors spent in trees. Girls, not boys, are the better tree climbers and spend more time playing on monkey bars at the playground. It is speculated that our early ancestors had a difference in gender preference for spending more or less time in trees: women, being lighter and more agile, climbed trees for their fruit and to escape predators, and preferred to sleep in the trees, while men preferred to sleep on the ground.[53]

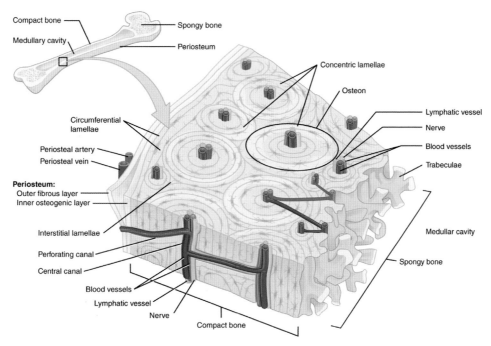

Labels in figure:
Compact bone
Spongy bone
Medullary cavity
Periosteum
Concentric lamellae
Osteon
Lymphatic vessel
Nerve
Blood vessels
Trabeculae
Circumferential lamellae
Periosteal artery
Periosteal vein
Periosteum:
Outer fibrous layer
Inner osteogenic layer
Interstitial lamellae
Perforating canal
Central canal
Medullar cavity
Spongy bone
Blood vessels
Lymphatic vessel
Nerve
Compact bone

FIGURE 1.38 The periosteum is continuous with the fascia of the ligaments and joint capsules and also dives deep inside the bone, becoming the endosteum.

not permanently bend our bones and create more room for movement. Yoga affects the softer tissues, building length and strength, and will affect the strength of our bones but not their length.

An illustrative example is the femur. When we are babies, our femurs are relatively straight with very little neck. As we begin to crawl and then walk, stress at the hip socket starts to guide the developing bone into a bent shape.[146] If we continue to lead a vigorous childhood with lots of walking, running, jumping and other physical work, the angle of the neck of the femur becomes more and more pronounced (see figure 1.9). Once the bone has finished growing, however, it will not change.[147] The growth plates have ossified, and only local remodeling of the bone surface is now possible.

Fascia and Bone

The fascia of our ligaments, which become the fascia of our joint capsules, do not simply "attach" to the bone, they *become* the bone. The outer lining of the bone, called the *periosteum*, is made up of fascia. The periosteum has a fibrous outer layer containing fibroblasts, and an inner cellular layer where we find the progenitor bone cells that develop into osteoblasts. Pain receptors (nociceptors) are found in the periosteum (which you have noticed anytime you banged your shin against a table), and the periosteum provides the pathway for the bones' blood vessels to and from the marrow, as shown in figure 1.38. The periosteum continues to the deep side of the cortical bone, where it is called the *endosteum*.

Within our bones, deep septa of fascia flow down, into and through the bones, in the same way that septa of fascia envelop and separate our muscles. Just as we can visualize our whole body as having but one muscle, like one long string of sausages drawn into connected compartments by our fascia, so too can we create a model of our body having but one bone, connected by fascia that becomes the joint capsule and then becomes the next bone.[148] And these ligaments are also continuous with the tendons of the muscles, the muscle's fascia and its septa. The same fascial network contains our viscera as well. Truly, we are completely integrated within and without, and it is only because we wish to aid our understanding by conceptualizing our total body as made of systematic components that we perceive separate features. The reality is much more complete and complex: we are a whole.

DIGESTING CARBOHYDRATES: Just as our ability to taste varies considerably, so too does our ability to digest carbohydrates. One particular gene, called *AMY1*, is involved in creating an enzyme in our mouths called amylase, which helps to break down starch before it goes into the stomach. A 2012 study found that people with multiple copies of *AMY1* created more amylase in their saliva and suffered a significantly lower spike in blood sugar after consuming a starch-laden drink than did participants with fewer copies of the gene. The lead author of the study noted, "Two individuals may have very different glycemic responses to the same starchy food, depending on their amylase levels." Based on this study, we can speculate that people with more copies of *AMY1* are less likely to develop diabetes or obesity than those with fewer copies.[56]

NOTE TO TEACHERS: Sources of compression

The final point to note about our bones, beyond the fact that yoga will not change their shapes, is that our ultimate range of movement is dictated by when our bones hit each other or squeeze other tissues in between them. Future volumes will look at this reality in detail for the major joints/segments of the body; but clearly, if the bones of two people have very dissimilar shapes, how far each person can move will also be quite different. For example, consider the two sets of lumbar vertebrae shown in figure 1.39. Notice the lengths and widths of the spinous processes (the bone projections coming up vertically from the body of the vertebrae) and the spaces between them. Obviously, the person on the left (let's call him Stiff Steve) will not be able to extend his spine (e.g., do a backbend) nearly as much as the person on the right (let's call her Flexy Flora), all other things being equal. By "all other things" we mean if these two people have the same tensile resistance on the front side of their body—for example, if their stomach muscles are equally flexible.

If Steve and Flora started doing yoga asanas together at the same time, they may well have had equally limited ranges of motion due to similar tensile resistances in the front portions of their bodies. However, as they worked through these areas of resistance, Flexy Flora kept going deeper and deeper into extension, while Stiff Steve quickly reached the point of compression (see figure 1.40). In frustration at not being able to go as deep as Flexy Flora, Stiff Steve may have quit yoga, thinking that there was something wrong with him. His teacher may also have reinforced the belief, secretly believing that if Steve had kept at it, he would have opened up more and more over time. She may have believed that he was a quitter! Unfortunately, this ignorance of human variation would have caused Steve injury had he continued to try to push his spine into the level of deep extension that Flora could easily manage.

It is dangerous for a yoga student to think that she can do any pose to any depth if she tries harder, and the risk of injury is made worse when the teacher believes the same thing. Our bones are as unique as anything else in our body. Depending upon their shape, structure and orientation, we will be more or less able to move as others do.

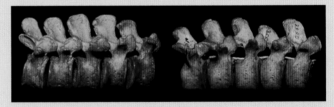

FIGURE 1.39 Stiff Steve's lumbar vertebrae on the left, Flexy Fora's on the right.

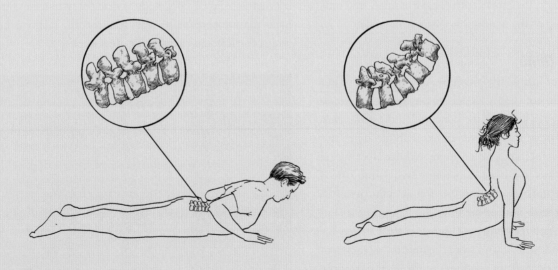

FIGURE 1.40 Flexy Fora's lumbar vertebrae allow a larger range of ultimate movement than Stiff Steve's do.

JOINTS AND CARTILAGE

The word joint is a noun, but it is helpful to consider the verb forms: to join, joining. Leslie Kaminoff considers a joint to be like a marriage—there exists a relationship, hopefully one that is strong and balanced.[149] To fully appreciate the beauty and function of a joint, we have to consider all the parties to the relationship and understand their contribution to the joining, how they assist mobility and how they assist in creating stability. All healthy relationships need both mobility and stability, and our joints are no exception. A joining consists not only of the bones and the connective tissues; it is a dynamic relationship that includes the muscles, superficial fascia, nervous system, circulatory system and the mental intention and attention provided by the owner of the joint.

A joint is restrained not only by ligaments, joint capsules and bony compression, but also by our muscles, which engage to limit movement, and our fascia, which creates hydrostatic tension that also bolsters stiffness. While we study the function and alignment of the connective tissue surrounding a joint, we must keep in mind the other contributors to the joint's stability, such as the cartilaginous articular surfaces of the bones. These articulating surfaces keep the bones apart, and the soft tissues around the joint keep the bones together. This is the case for all synovial joints, but these joints do vary in the degree to which the hard and soft tissues contribute to a particular joint's stability. Failure of the bones' articulating surfaces can lead to instability in the joint at least as often as failure of the ligaments or joint capsule.[150]

Stuart McGill says, "Stiffness is always stabilizing,"[151] and when a joint is bearing a load, it needs to become stiff. Our muscles co-contract around the joint to initiate the stiffness required. The other soft tissue of the ligaments, joint capsule and investing fascia also contribute to stiffness. Of course, we can overdo anything: the stiffness we seek is not rigidity. Stuart McGill found that healthy spines need stiffness all around the core of the body, but only at about 5–10% muscular engagement.[152] While in unhealthy spines this may need to increase slightly,[153] it is counterproductive to increase the muscular tension much higher than these levels. Too much stiffness from overly activating the muscles will increase the load on the joint and inhibit movement. Like yoga's bandhas, muscular engagement is necessary, but it needs to be more subtle than hard.

When stiffness is deliberately created, a joint cannot move through its full range of motion. To exercise a joint (so as to strengthen and thicken its joint capsule and associated ligaments and fascia), and to improve a range of motion, it is best to stress the joint when it is not bearing a load—when it is relaxed. It can be quite dangerous to combine load bearing and extreme mobility.

Joints Defined

A joining is not simple, but in science we like to simplify systems to help us understand the components. This is useful as long as we do not lose sight of the reality, which is much more intricate, complex and wondrous. We will follow the mechanistic approach and look at the traditional components of a joint, but please keep in mind that this is a simplification.

A joint (technically called an *arthrosis*, from the Greek word for joining) is the joining of two or more bones. There are many different kinds and functions of joints, as discussed in Appendix E: The Types of Joints. Normally, joints allow movement of the body to occur and also provide support and stability, but not always. Some joints are designed to prevent movement, such as the fibrous joints in your skull. For joints that are supposed to move, muscles, through their attachment to the bones, provide the force or leverage for the joint's articulation. Wrapping around this type of joint, called a *synovial* joint, is a fibrous capsule formed by fascia, tendons and ligaments that support and protect the joint. A cuff of the joint capsule connects to the bones quite close to their articulating surfaces, but in longer bones this attachment site may be quite far from the actual joint; thus, the joint capsule can be quite extensive.

IT'S IMPORTANT: Safely stressing joints

In general, we can propose the following philosophy on exercising joints:

1. When a joint is bearing a load, restrict its range of movement: stiffen the joint—engage the muscles.

2. To increase a joint's range of movement, move it to its natural limits when it is not bearing a load: relax the muscles.

Articulating Cartilage

The articulating surfaces of the bones in a joint are covered by a specialized form of cartilage called *hyaline* cartilage. (There are a few exceptions, such as the joining of the sternum and clavicle, and the acromion and clavicle, both of which have a dense fibrous connection.) Cartilage is softer and more pliable than bone because it has a higher ratio of proteoglycans (water-loving molecules) to collagen. Articulating, or hyaline, cartilage has a very low coefficient of friction (it is five to 20 times more slippery than ice![154]), resists wear and tear, is somewhat elastic and can be compressed slightly, which helps it withstand repeated stress, making it ideal for easy movement over similar surfaces. The thickness of the cartilage varies by individual and age: when we are young, the cartilage lining the ends of our bones may be as much as 7 mm thick in the large joints like the hips, but when we are older, that thickness may be reduced to only 1–2 mm.[155] In some people, the cartilage may have been worn away completely, a condition called *osteoarthritis*.[156] Once the protective covering of cartilage is gone, the ends of the bones start to grind upon each other, which is very painful and debilitating. The thickness of the cartilage also varies depending upon the shape of the bone being covered. If the bone is convex (bulging outward, like the head of the femur), the cartilage is thickest in the middle and thinnest at the edges. If the bone is concave (bulging inward, like our hip sockets), it is thickest at the edges and thinnest in the middle. This thickening at the periphery of the concave bone helps to form a lip of cartilage called a *labrum* (which is Latin for the rim of a bowl), found only at the hip and shoulder sockets. The function of the labra (plural for labrum) is not fully understood, but they may simply deepen the socket, making the joint more stable, or they may enable a greater spreading of the synovial fluid.[157]

Damage to cartilage may take a long time to heal due to the restricted availability of nutrients. Articulating cartilage has neither a direct blood supply nor nerve endings. It is not clear how cartilage is nourished, but one speculation is that the circulating synovial fluid brings nutrients to the cartilage-building cells (the *chondrocytes*), but some nutrition may seep in from neighbouring blood vessels in the bone. While we do not fully understand these mechanisms, it is clear that given this lower level of nutrients, damaged cartilage is slow to heal. It is also speculated that gently moving a joint that has damaged cartilage is important in order to enhance the flow of synovial fluid around the cartilage surface. Cyclical stressing of the cartilage, which occurs through simple activities like walking or riding a bicycle, improves its strength.[158]

Meniscus

In the knee, between the femur and the tibia, is a particular form of fibrocartilage called a *meniscus* (from the Greek "crescent"). This C-shaped half disc of cartilage is not covered by a synovial membrane. Menisci are also found in the acromioclavicular joint near the shoulder and in a few other places.[159] The exact function of the menisci is not known, but they probably act as shock absorbers and help to make the two irregular endings of the bones fit better.[160] As a shock absorber, the meniscus flattens out when a load bears down upon it, distributing the stress radially. The composition and orientation of its collagen fibers help to distribute the multidirectional forces it experiences. The menisci of the knee may also help to reduce the amount of sliding that the femur can do across the top of the tibia. In addition, menisci help spread lubrication within the joint, distribute weight over a broader surface and protect the edges of the bones' cartilage. Usually the menisci are connected at their edges to the fibrous joint capsule, such as with the medial meniscus of the knee, which is anchored to the medial collateral ligament, but not always: the lateral meniscus of the knee is not anchored to the joint capsule. Because there is no vascularization within the knee joint, damage to a meniscus is very hard to heal. Close to the outer edge of the meniscus, some nutrition is available from the joint capsule, but further inside the joint there is little and there are very few chondrocytes to replace damaged fibers. If the inner cartilage is torn or ruptured, usually the only recourse is surgery to snip out the damaged portion. However, for some people symptomatic relief has been achieved by stressing the knees passively through periods of sitting on the heels (called Thunderbolt or Diamond Pose—Vajrasana—in yoga), or placing dowelling or rolled up washcloths behind the knees while sitting on the heels.[161] Please remember, however, this won't work for every body!

IDEAL DIET: Nutrigenomics is the science that prescribes an ideal diet based upon your genes. Each body processes food differently, and how fast or slow our metabolism runs may be connected both to our genes and to the kinds of foods we favor. For example, a gene called APOE can affect how we break down fat, but one version of this gene is correlated with higher rates of cardiovascular disease and dementia. A different gene dictates how much vitamin B9 we need to be optimally healthy. Genes can also determine whether we like the taste of certain foods, like broccoli and Brussels sprouts.[55]

Intervertebral Discs

The cartilage found in the discs between the vertebral bodies of the spine is different from articulating cartilage. As with menisci, these discs distribute stress and help to join the two articulating bones together more solidly, but they also create, in effect, two joints lined up in series. These two joints allow a greater range of movement than one joint alone would. The intervertebral discs are more complex than menisci. As shown in figure 1.41, they have two major components: a ring of fibers called the *anulus fibrosus*, and an inner core of jelly called the *nucleus pulposus*. A good analogy is a jelly donut: the pastry of the donut is the fibrous cartilage of the disc, while the jelly is a gel-filled sac that helps to absorb stresses. The thickness of the discs varies throughout the spinal column: they are thinnest in the cervical spine and thickest in the lumbar region. The thickness of each disc varies within itself as well: the front of the discs in the cervical and lumbar spine is thicker than the posterior side. This contributes to the backwards curve of the spine, called *lordosis*. In the thoracic spine, the discs are equally thick on all sides. The forward curve of the thoracic spine, called *kyphosis*, is due solely to the shape of the vertebrae, not the discs. Similar to menisci, the intervertebral discs are connected to ligaments. Along the front and back of the spine run two long ligaments to which each disc is connected: the anterior longitudinal ligament and the posterior longitudinal ligament. The thoracic discs are also connected laterally to intra-articular ligaments.

Overall, the discs contribute about 25% of the total length of the spine. This can vary with the time of day: in the morning, the discs are the most hydrated and thickest, but by bedtime at night, they are the least hydrated and thinnest.[162] For this reason, stresses on the spine first thing in the morning are not recommended because the tension along the spine is already very high due to the hydration that occurs as we sleep. (It is not a good idea to begin your yoga practice in the first 30 minutes after rising in the morning!) As our day progresses, gravity provides natural compression to the discs, causing them to lose some hydration and shrink, which reduces the stress along the spine. Most people feel much more flexible at night than first thing in the morning. As we age, the discs' contribution to the length of the spine also changes. Perhaps surprisingly, our discs actually become thicker as we grow older, but they're also less resilient.[163] The shrinking of the spine and the loss of body height that occur with age are due to the vertebrae getting thinner, not the discs. Here again we should note the wide

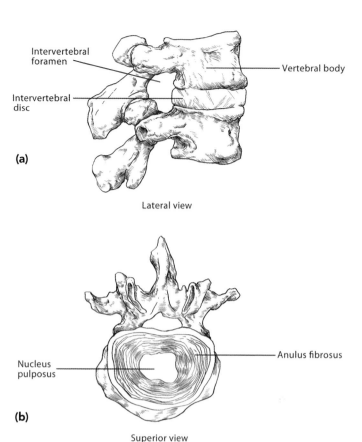

(a)

Lateral view

Intervertebral foramen

Intervertebral disc

Vertebral body

(b)

Superior view

Nucleus pulposus

Anulus fibrosus

FIGURE 1.41 The intervertebral discs. (a) shows the two components of the disc—the inner gel-like nucleus pulposus and the outer anulus fibrosus.

range of human variation; not everyone's discs are the same size or have the same ability to withstand stress.

The nucleus pulposus is quite developed in the cervical and lumbar spine but much less so in the thoracic region. At birth, the pulposus is very large and soft, but as we age, it loses its ability to retain water, and thus its gel-like properties. It becomes more fibrous, which makes it less able to withstand stress. The increasing fibrosis also causes the nucleus pulposus to grow thicker, even though it is weaker.[164] For some people (even as young as 26 years old) the pulposus disappears completely. This is yet another example of how we are all different.

FINGERPRINTS: This is a well-known variation between people, but your unique fingerprint is not totally dependent upon your genes. During your time as an embryo, your fingerprints were being shaped by your mother's movements, which in turn changed the pressure and flow of the amniotic fluid surrounding you. A tiny percentage of people do have the same fingertip patterns as other members of their families, because they actually have no fingerprints at all! This is due to a very rare genetic mutation.[36]

IT'S COMPLICATED: Other parts of our joints

Sometimes *bursa*, formed from *synovium* extrusions (also called the *synovial membrane*), are located under the ligaments or tendons. These small sacs contain synovial fluid and help to reduce the friction of ligaments and tendons sliding over the joint capsule. Inside a synovial joint may be found synovial fluids or cartilage, or both, depending upon the type of joint and its function.

Figure 1.42 illustrates the synovial joint of our knee, showing the bones, the cartilage covering the ends of the bone, the space between the cartilage, and a thin layer of lubricating fluid called the *synovia*, as well as the covering fascia forming the joint capsule, which in turn merges into the tendons and ligaments. The synovial fluid is made up of special glycosaminoglycans such as hyaluronic acid, chondroitin sulphate and lubricin. In reality, the space between the two bones and their cartilage is much smaller than shown here and the layer of synovial fluid is very thin.

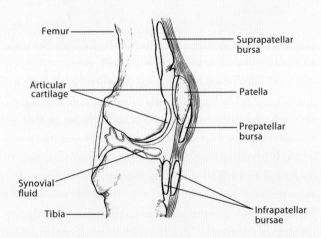

FIGURE 1.42 The knee is a synovial joint containing the articulating bones, covering articular cartilage and a synovial space filled with synovial fluid, all wrapped by the joint capsule, which may be contiguous with the ligaments.

Some joints, like our knees, have folds of fibers inside the joint capsule, such as discs, menisci, intra-articular ligaments (for example, the cruciate ligaments in the knees) and fat pads; these all help to fit the two ends of the bones more snugly or securely together. Fat pads vary in size and are located between the joint capsule and the synovium, not within the synovia. They are prominent in the elbow and knee joints. Fat pads serve to make the joint capsule fuller, helping to fill in any recessed spaces caused by incomplete conjunction of the bones forming the joint. This in turn reduces the amount of synovial fluid required in the joint. The intrajoint pads and folds are also quite elastic, flexible and deformable, which helps to distribute some of the stress in the joint. Another name for folds within the synovial joint is *plicae* (Latin for "folds"). In the knee, these plicae are remnants of embryological development and usually are greatly diminished when we are adults, becoming unobtrusive synovial folds. However, in some cases, plicae can adhere the patella to the femur, preventing full movement of the knee. Sometimes, the plicae can also become inflamed, which may cause them to thicken and thus be more likely to get snagged on the femur, restricting movement.[165] On the other hand, plicae can increase the surface area of the synovia, allowing greater range of movement.

At times, these fibrous incursions into the joint can get caught up with other fibers or become fixated to the cartilage of the bones and momentarily stuck. When they get unstuck, they make clicking, cracking or popping sounds. Debris, from pieces of fibers or fragments of cells broken off by wear and tear over time, can accumulate inside the joint, floating in the synovial fluid; this may cause grinding sensations or sounds. The joint capsule is not always one solid covering encasing the joint; it may have nerves, blood vessels, ligaments and tendons passing through it, such as are found in the knee and shoulder joints.[166] Synovial fluid can also be found outside the joint capsule, covering tendons and ligaments, making their sliding movements easier. However, the function of synovial fluid is not limited to reducing friction between moving surfaces; it is also involved in nourishing the cells found in the cartilage.[167]

Close-Packed and Loose-Packed Positions

When the joint is maximally congruent, usually at the end range of its movement, it is in a *close-packed* position. In this position, the ligaments supporting the joint are taut, as is the joint capsule. This means that the joint is maximally supported by the associated connective tissues, so the least amount of accessory muscular action is required to maintain this position. This is often found in the lower body when the limbs are in the typical standing position: the knees are locked straight, and the femur heads are tightly bound into the hip sockets. In this symmetrical standing position, we expend a minimum amount of energy to maintain our posture. Due to a spiral twisting action of the hip capsular ligaments, in this fully congruent position the femur and the pelvis are literally screwed down together. This maximum stability makes the two bones act almost as one, as if there were no joint, in terms of the distribution of the stresses along the bones. If the joint were to undergo further movement now, injury would occur to the joint structure.

In the loose-packed position, the joint has the least amount of congruency and the associated ligaments and joint capsule are lax. This usually occurs around the middle of the joint's range of movement. At this point, the joint could be pulled slightly apart due to the laxity of the supporting structures. It is in the loose-packed position that movements such as roll, slide and spin can occur. (See Appendix F: The Biomechanics of Joint Motion for the details of these kinds of movement.) The contact area between the articulating surfaces is now minimal, which reduces the friction of any movement and thus erosion. In the knee joint's loose-packed position, where the knee is flexed 90°, the ligaments are lax enough to allow some spinning of the tibia. This twisting of the lower leg allows for some movements that would be prohibited or even dangerous in the close-packed position, such as turning the feet outward while the knee points straight ahead. We will look at this in detail in Volume 2 when we examine the knee joint, but it means that sometimes it is possible to move the body in certain ways, depending upon the laxity of the ligaments and joint capsule, when at other times such movements are not a good idea.

Contracture in the Joints

There are several possible sources of tension arising from the joint itself and the joint capsule that may restrict or reduce our range of motion. A lack of synovial fluid may make the joint stiff. The cartilage may no longer freely slide along the surface of the neighbouring cartilage. Eventually, as we noted earlier, the surface of the cartilage may erode away, causing *osteoarthritis*. If the erosion continues, the cartilage may be worn completely away so that now the ends of the bones start to erode as well.

Another source of tension in the joint capsule is a process called *contracture*, whereby the collagen of the joint capsule tightens and is remodeled into shorter strands. Professor Laurence Dahners, from the University of North Carolina, studied this phenomenon. He discovered a mechanism in which the body shrink-wraps our joints by removing materials from our ligaments.[168]

An example of shrink-wrapping contracture occurs when the shoulder becomes immobilized. For example, Grandma falls and breaks her arm, the bone is reset, and the arm rests in a sling for several weeks. When the sling is removed, the bone has healed, but the shoulder is stiff and can't move. What happened? In this case, the cause of the reduced range of motion is the lack of use of the shoulder joint: immobility. The body took away materials no longer used so that when the time came to use the shoulder again, it couldn't respond.

One treatment for shoulder restrictions caused by immobility is, not surprisingly, mobility. A study of contracture repair contrasted short, intense stresses, such as we find in active yoga practices, with long-held, mild stresses, such as we find in a yin yoga practice.[169] The researchers

THE PERCEPTION OF NORMAL: The average American woman is 5'4" tall and weights 140 pounds, and the average fashion model is 5'11" and weighs 117 pounds.[57] What is normal? Certainly not the fashion models, and yet in the minds of many American women, their own bodies are not normal: they want to be like the fashion models. Our concept of normal gets mixed up with our desire to look a certain way. Yet the definition of beauty is culturally variable and has changed dramatically over the centuries. In the same way, the range of flexibility we see in yoga teachers and yoga magazines can unconsciously make us believe that their bodies are normal, and ours are inadequate, inflexible mannequins, terribly stiff and lifeless. In reality, normal is not what we *want* to look like, normal is what is healthy for our individual bodies. What we should really be asking is: what is normal for me, given my biology and biography?

concluded: "The longest period of low force stretch produces the greatest amount of permanent elongation, with the least amount of trauma and structural weakening of the connective tissues. Consequently, permanent elongation of connective tissue results in range of motion increases for the patient." In other words, longer and gentler stresses were better for restoring the health of the joint than more forceful but shorter stresses.

What stops me? If our ligaments or joint capsules have become shortened, through contracture or any of the many other causes we have already looked at, we will experience tension in the joint itself. Again, this tension is not caused by short, tight muscles, and the experience of tension in the ligament or joint capsule will be quite different from the experience of tension caused by the muscles. It will be in a different location, more localized and subtle, and harder to detect than muscular tension. Should we try to lengthen these structures? Many physical therapists, yoga teachers and fitness professionals advise against stressing the joints and ligaments, fearing joint destabilization. Remember, one model posits that the purpose of our ligaments is to restrain a joint from moving too far and damaging itself. However, we have seen that often, our range of motion and mobility is too restricted; we are not in danger of going too far—we are suffering from not being able to access our natural and normal range of movement. The only way to regain our lost mobility is to target the structure that is stopping us, to exercise our ligaments and joints, but we must do so in a way that won't harm these areas.

The Goldilocks Philosophy applies here. Yes, it is possible to go too far and damage a joint, but this does not mean that the other extreme is healthier. To never stress a joint is to invite atrophy, pathology and fragility. We have to find the middle path of not too much and not too little.

VOLUME 1
Summary

There are many answers to the question "What stops me?" The causes can be arranged into a spectrum, with two major divisions. We are stopped either due to tension in our tissues, which prevents us from going any further, or due to compression arising from tissues hitting tissues. We have been investigating the sources of tension and have found that this can arise in a number of different ways: we may experience tension in our muscles, within the smallest muscle cell and up to the entire length of muscle; within the fascia inside the muscle and within the deep fascia outside the muscles, which forms a full body stocking of collagen, enveloping and investing all our organs and other tissues; within our tendons; within our ligaments; within our joint capsules; from responses of the nervous system due to stress or pain; from immune system responses; and from a lack or surplus of water in our joints, muscles and fascia.

Just as we know that no two people look exactly the same on the outside, no two people are exactly the same on the inside either. We have seen that the amount of water we retain affects our flexibility. Our water content varies from 46% to 70%.[170] Since water contributes to a significant degree of tension in the body, your individual water content will affect how flexible you are. Also remember that this is not a constant: some days we have more water in our body than other days, which means that some days we are going to be more flexible than other days.

We have also seen that our immune system, working with our nervous system and our endocrine system, can affect the degree to which myofibroblasts are produced and activated. The degree of psychological stress we each have in our life, and the way we react to this stress, are also quite unique; when we are stressed, our endocrine system is activated, and hormones, steroids and cytokines are released into our blood system. The famous hypothalamus, pituitary and adrenal axis is stimulated, but not everyone reacts the same way to stress. The variations in the sizes of our glands have a bearing on our response to stress. The pituitary gland, for example, has a huge range of variation between individuals: one study found a 13-fold range, from 130 to 1800 milligrams.[171] Clearly, not everyone's pituitary is going to release the same amount of hormones when it is activated. Your pituitary is not the same size as everyone

else's, you react to stress differently from the average person (who does not actually exist), and the tension you experience in your tissues as a result will also be quite unique.

The number of nerve endings we have also varies from person to person. There is a distinct difference in the number of myofibroblasts in the lower back of people with chronic lower back pain than in people without such pain. Whether the increase in myofibroblasts found in lower back pain sufferers is a cause of the pain or a consequence is unknown, but it is known that if you have more myofibroblasts, you will have greater tightness.[172]

Is the tension you experience when you reach your edge in a yoga pose due to the makeup of your fascia? Maybe. And, just as our fascia is uniquely constructed, so too are our ligaments and joint capsules. All these tissues have the capacity to contract, and that capacity is uniquely determined by nature and nurture, by our biology and our biography. The number of nerve endings in our muscles and tendons is unique, as is the make up of the sarcomeres and their sliding filaments that control and allow muscular contraction and elongation.

The range of human variations, when we look at all the factors that contribute to tension, is enormous. It is pointless to say what an average is, to define what normal is, to say "this is what everyone should do," when there are so many ways that we are each unique. All we can do is point out where your edges *may* arise, to make you aware of the sources of the tension and compression that may be stopping you, so that you can decide what is the best course of action for you, given your uniqueness.

There is a myth in the yoga community that everybody can do every posture, if they just work hard enough, long enough, with the right teachers and supplements, and a matching yoga outfit and mat. This is a dangerous myth. We have seen that the science of human variation and the reality of ultimately reaching compression mean that you cannot do every posture, and trying to go past where your body can take you will lead to injury, not progress.

Remember, our *ultimate* stopping point is reached when we hit compression, which we will be exploring further in Volume 2 when we look at the architecture and variations found in our lower body.

APPENDIX A
The Forms of Stress

What we have been calling stress engineers often call load; when a structure is bearing a load, it is under stress. Stresses are often categorized into five different kinds. In figure 1.43 we see a bone undergoing compression, tension, torsion, shearing and bending. These five kinds of stress usually occur in combinations. Tension is the stress that tries to pull a structure apart or elongate it. Compression works in the other direction—compressive stress pushes the structure into itself. Whereas tension and compression are stresses in opposite directions along an axis running through a structure, shear is stress applied in two parallel but opposite directions at once. In this way, shear is similar to compression, but in shear, the two compressing forces are not lined up—they are slightly offset. Torsion is the stress that causes a structure to twist. Torsion is similar to shear, but it is applied in a circular or radial manner, and generally the sources of the stress are further apart than in shearing, often at the ends of the structure. Finally, bending is the stress that causes a structure to curve; this results from a combination of tension and compression on opposite sides of the resulting curve. Compression occurs on the inner part of the curve, while tension occurs on the outside of the curve, which is the location of fracturing if the structure's materials become overly fatigued and start to fail. Fractures occur on the outside of bending curves. For our purpose—answering "What stops me?"—it is sufficient to consider the stresses arising in yoga poses to be either tension or compression. This is a simplification, but it works.

Consider the load acting upon a wooden beam supported by two walls, something you could imagine finding in an old log cabin where the roof has a supported beam (see figure 1.44). Here we find all five forms of stress: the weight of the beam, acting in the middle of its length, bends the beam slightly, which is basically the stress of compression on the top side of the beam and tension along the bottom. Closer to the supporting ends of the beam, torsion occurs; this twist in the wood arises because the ends of the beam are fixed but the load in the middle of the beam is trying to move the beam downwards. There is also a shearing stress right at the points above where the beam is supported, as part of the beam wants to come down, but the supports push up against that load, creating shear.

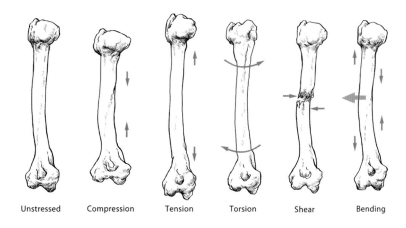

Unstressed Compression Tension Torsion Shear Bending

FIGURE 1.43 The five types of stress.

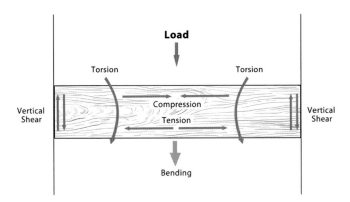

FIGURE 1.44 A supporting beam undergoes all five forms of stress.

The same stresses occur in our tissues when we do a physical yoga practice. Let's visualize what is happening to our front femur during Triangle Pose (Trikonasana). As figure 1.45 shows, there is a shearing in the joint at the knee as the femur tries to slide past the tibia. There is a torsion or twist all along the femur as we anchor the foot and knee and then try to externally rotate the hip. The weight of the body creates compression through the length of the femur. There is a bending along the length of the femur, just as there was in the wooden support beam in our above analogy. This bending includes both tension and compression. In Triangle Pose, we stay in the posture for several breaths. This creates a static loading on the tissues. The other possible kind of loading occurs while we are moving—for example, when we flow through vinyasas or through Sun Salutations (Suryanamaskar); this creates dynamic loading of the tissues, sometimes called cyclic loading. Either kind of loading affects our tissues and if done to excess may result in fatigue of the microscopic structures and eventually failure, resulting in injury and pain. However, there is a big difference between a beam of wood supporting a roof and our femur supporting us in Triangle Pose. The body is self-repairing. The stresses we apply to our tissues create a cascading series of changes at the cellular level, which result in the stressed tissues becoming stronger.

Stress, Strain, Sprain and Creep

Stresses can be generated in our tissues by our muscles, by gravity or by bearing weight beyond that of our own bodies—for example when we use a sandbag, or from a teacher or partner pushing on us.

Stress is not the same as stretch; often, we may be subjected to a stress, but no movement occurs—we neither lengthen nor shorten. The stress in these cases is being balanced by an internal resistance due to the resilience of our tissues, bones, fascia, ligaments, etc. When the stress exceeds this internal resilience, then some deformation occurs: we stretch or compress—we move. The amount of movement is technically called a strain. Consider an elastic band. With no stress, it is at a certain resting length. With a little stress, it may stay at that original length, but it will become taut. With a bit more stress, now it starts to stretch. The amount of stretch it undergoes is called the strain, usually measured as a percentage of its resting length. The ratio of the stress

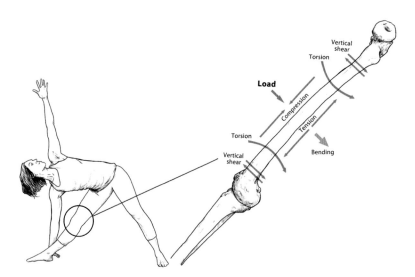

FIGURE 1.45 Our femurs also experience the five forms of stress in a variety of standing postures.

to the strain is called the material's *stiffness*, as shown in figure 1.46. Different materials have different stiffnesses. The strain occurring in an elastic band is more than the strain that would occur in a piece of metal, such as a spoon, undergoing the same stress. The spoon is stiffer than the elastic. The same thing happens in our tissues: passive muscles can easily stretch under a stress, but a bone, being much stiffer, will not stretch at all under the same stress. Ligaments and tendons will exhibit a bit of strain when under stress, but not nearly as much as a muscle. Fascia is somewhere in between the stiffness of muscles and of ligaments.

We can generalize and say that muscles are elastic, which means that after the stress ends, they return to their original length, while ligaments and tendons are plastic, which means they won't stretch very much at all; but if the stress exceeds the ability of the material to resist stretching, they will remain stretched. This is a generalization, and it doesn't work for all levels of stress. If a small amount of stress is applied to a ligament, creating a small amount of strain, ligaments (and tendons) can be considered elastic. As long as the strain does not exceed 4–10%, the ligament or tendon will elastically return to its original length. But once this critical threshold is surpassed, the ligament is plastically deformed and will not return to its original length. This permanent elongation is referred to as a *sprain*. Any ligament that has been subjected to a stress that exceeds its elastic limit (yield strength) and has become plastically deformed has been sprained. It will not return to its original length. For example, when someone rolls an ankle and stresses the lateral ligaments, they are said to have sprained their ankle; the ligaments were taken beyond their elastic limit and remained stretched. (To be confusing: muscles can also be subjected to too much stress and be pulled beyond their elastic limits. This may happen if the muscle is stretched beyond 50% of its resting length.[173])

When a static stress is applied to a plastic material like a ligament or tendon, over time the length of this tissue will increase slowly (see figure 1.46). This is known as *creep*. The material will remodel itself to accommodate the stress. If the stress continues for too long, fatigue will set in and the

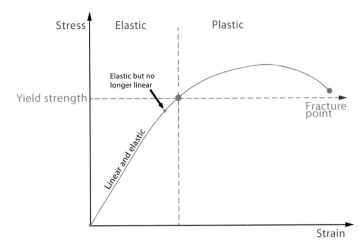

FIGURE 1.46 The relationship between stress and strain determines a tissue's stiffness, which can be either elastic or plastic. Up to a certain level of strain, the tissues can rebound back to their original length: that is elastic. Past the tissue's yield strength, the tissue behaves plastically and remains stretched.

structure may fail, but if the stress ceases before that critical time, the resulting elongation is maintained. This is valuable in living tissues, as long as it is not overdone.[174] The result is that the ligament or tendon may increase its length, and thus the range of motion of a joint may increase slightly, but the tissue is temporarily weaker. Over time, the body will restrengthen the tissues through the buildup of new collagen fibers. Obviously, this does not happen in nonliving systems like buildings or bridges; creep occurring in these structures makes them more liable to failure.

Creep is one example of a more general condition called *viscoelasticity*. It is beyond our scope to investigate the viscoelastic properties of our tissues, but this simply refers to the way the stiffness changes as the stress changes. All of our tissues are viscoelastic. This is a good thing! For example, the cartilage in our knees changes stiffness as the rate of stress changes; when we go for a run, the transient stress on the knee joint is quite high with each step, but fortunately, because our knee's cartilage is viscoelastic, the stiffness of the cartilage increases with each quick, jarring step, thus protecting the joint from damage.[175]

APPENDIX B
Muscle Shapes and Functions

Several factors determine the strength of our muscles. These include the number of muscle fibers we have, the size of the fibers, the age of these fibers (which atrophy over time and are replaced with fat and collagen), the nervous system interaction with the fibers, the blood supply (and thus the quality of nutrients and hormones flowing to the fibers), as well as the degree of tension in opposing muscles. Obviously, some of our muscles need to be stronger than others. The tiny muscles that move our eyes do not need to be as strong as the leg muscles that move our whole body. The leg muscles, being stronger, are also considerably bigger: the strength of these muscles is proportional to the cross-sectional area of all the fibers. In some places it is not possible to simply keep adding fibers. An architectural change to the orientation of the fibers occurs that increases the cross-sectional area of the muscle. This results in different shapes for our muscles.

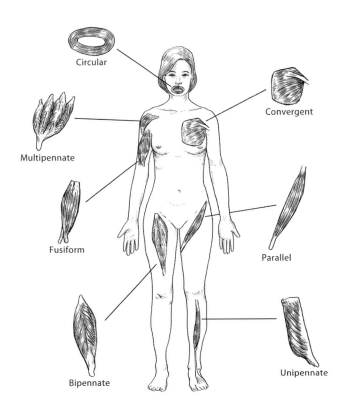

FIGURE 1.47 Muscles can form several shapes to increase their pulling power.

We can divide the shapes of our muscles into several categories, and different researchers pick different ways of doing this (see figure 1.47). We will use the following four categories:

1. **Parallel**. Also known as *strap* muscles or *fusiform* (from the Latin for "spindle"), these muscles have long fibers, all running in parallel, such as the sartorius muscle. Some texts will list the fusiform as a separate category; here the muscles are shaped like spindles and have bellies wider than their ends (called the *origin* or *proximal attachment*, where a muscle arises, and insertion or *distal attachment*, where it terminates), such as the bicep brachii. Most skeletal muscles tend to be fusiform muscles.[176]

2. **Circular**. Sometimes called *radial*, such as the muscles around the eye, mouth or our various sphincters.

3. **Convergent**. Also known as *triangular* or *fan-shaped* muscles, these have a large origin but a smaller insertion, such as the pectoralis major.

4. **Pennate**. From the Latin for "wing," and sometimes called *pinnate* (from the Latin for "feather"), these muscles have shorter fibers, running at an angle to the primary direction of the muscle. This orientation allows for a higher cross-sectional area of the muscle, making it stronger. However, the tradeoff for this added strength is that these muscles will operate more slowly due to their shorter length.[177] It is also possible for hypertrophy, in which the muscle grows by adding sarcomeres in parallel, to alter the angle of pinnation. There are three subcategories of pennate muscles:

   i. **Unipennate**: one row of muscle fibers runs diagonally from a long tendon towards the direction of force, such as the semimembranosus hamstring muscle.

   ii. **Bipennate**: two rows of muscles fibers run diagonally from a long, central tendon towards the direction of force, such as the rectus femoris of the thigh. This arrangement resembles a feather or leaf.

APPENDICES

iii. **Multipennate**: multiple parallel fibers fan out from a central tendon, such as the deltoid muscle of the shoulder, which has anterior, middle and posterior sections.

In addition to these arrangements of the fibers within the muscle, the muscles also may vary in their number of attachments and bellies, as shown in figure 1.48. (Note: ceps is from the Latin for "head," so bicep means two [bi] heads, and triceps means three [tri] heads.)

- Two-headed muscles, such as the bicep brachii, have two proximal attachments and only one distal.
- Three-headed muscles, such as the triceps brachii, have three proximal attachments and only one distal.
- Four-headed muscles, such as the quadriceps, have four proximal attachments and only one distal.
- Two-bellies, such as the diagrastic muscle, under the lower jaw, have two bellies but only one distal and one proximal attachment.
- Multiple-bellies, such as the rectus abdominis, in the abdomen, which has four bellies, three of which, on each side of the stomach, are easily visible in athletes with "six-packs."

A point worth reiterating is that the "heads" of the muscles, located at the so-called origins or proximal attachments, are not always so clear and separate as they are presented in anatomy books. The artist decides how to depict the muscle, depending upon what he wants to illustrate. For example, the proximal attachment of the semitendinosus muscle of the hamstring is usually shown separately from the attachment of the long head of the bicep femoris. However, in reality, these two "heads" are one and the same.[178] They are not different structures, but they can be carved up to show separate structures if the illustrator so chooses. Again, in science, we often simplify reality to make it easier to comprehend, but this does change the underlying reality.

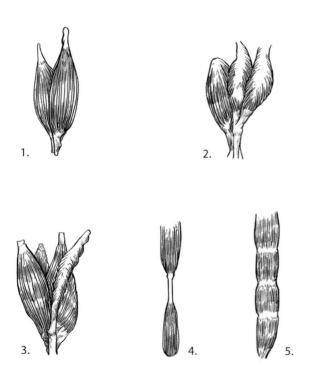

FIGURE 1.48 1. a two-headed muscle; 2. a three-headed muscle; 3. a four-headed muscle; 4. a two-bellied muscle; 5. a multi-bellied muscle.

APPENDIX C
The Myofascial Meridians

In *Anatomy Trains*, Thomas Myers describes trains of myofascial continuity that run through the body, from head to toe. He coined the term *myofascial meridians* to emphasize that these lines of connection run all over the body. Rather than us looking purely at the local effects of muscles in a narrow region of the body, considering these myofascial meridians offers us a longitudinal awareness. To remove any confusion, Myers is not using the term "meridian" as found in the Eastern energetic paradigm of traditional Chinese medicine, but rather to describe, as he says, "lines of pull, based on standard Western anatomy, lines which transmit strain and rebound, facilitating movement and providing stability."[179]

Myers identified 12 myofascial meridians, which are summarized in table 1.3 and illustrated in figure 1.49.[180] In answering "What stops me?" we direct attention to the "restrictions" column of the table; malfunctioning of the myofascial meridian, such as chronic contractions, or scar tissues and adhesions anywhere along the meridian, can restrict movements far away.

TABLE 1.3 The myofascial meridians and their role in answering "WSM?".[181]

MERIDIAN	ROUTING	FUNCTION	RESTRICTIONS
Superficial Front Line (SFL); figure 1.49a	The front side of the body from the toes, along the front of the legs and torso, along the side of the neck, to the back of the skull.	To flex the core and hips, extend the knees and dorsiflex the foot.	Restricts extension of the whole body above the knees or in localized areas.
Superficial Back Line (SBL); figure 1.49b	Starting on the soles of the feet, the SBL covers the back side of the body: the calves, hamstrings, along the spine, the back of the neck, to the front of the skull, to the eyebrows.	Creates extension and hyperextension of the body but flexion at the knees and below.	Limits flexion of the whole body above the knees or in localized areas.
Lateral Line (LL); figure 1.49c	From the outside of the foot, the LL runs along the side of the legs and torso, along the side of the neck, to the base of the skull.	Posturally balances front and back, and side to side. Can create lateral flexion of the torso and creates abduction of the legs.	If one LL is tight, it may restrict movements on the opposite side. May cause leg adduction restrictions and chronic lumbar side flexion. Postural compensation may occur, such as genus varum or valgus at the knees.

MERIDIAN	ROUTING	FUNCTION	RESTRICTIONS
THE HELICAL LINES			
Spiral Line (SPL); figure 1.49d	The SPL creates a loop. From the top of the foot, the SPL runs up the front of the leg, moves to the outside of the thighs, crisscrosses in the abdomen, and wraps the rib-cage and upper back. From there it descends down most of the SBL to join the feet again. Much of the my-ofascia found here also participates in the SBL, SFL and LL.	Maintains body balance in all three planes. Helps to create the spiral movements of the body.	Problems here can show up in restrictions along the SBL, SFL and LL. A chronic rotation to the body can occur.
Front Functional Line (FFL); figure 1.49e	The two FFL crisscross from one shoulder to the opposite leg, be-ginning at the top of the humerus, then going along the outer edge of the pectoralis major, to the lateral sheath of the rectus abdominis, to the pubis, and along the adductor longus to its attachment on the femur, the linea aspera.	Normally used in athletic movements when one side of the body requires support from its opposite side, such as throwing a ball. In yoga, these lines are used to stabilize the upper appendicular body on the axial core anytime the arms are above the head.	Can shorten to bring one shoulder closer to its op-posite hip across the front of the body. Repetitive one-sided movements can overtone this line (e.g., repeated throwing with one arm).
Back Functional Line (BFL); figure 1.49f	The two BFL crisscross from one shoulder to the opposite leg. They begin at the upper back of the hu-merus, then run down through the latissimus dorsi to the sacrolumbar fascia, through the gluteus max-imus, the vastus lateralis and the subpatellar tendon, ending on the tibial tuberosity.	Normally used in athletic movements when one side of the body requires support from its opposite side, such as throwing a ball. In yoga, these lines are used to stabilize the upper appendicular body on the axial core anytime the arms are above the head.	Can shorten to bring one shoulder closer to its op-posite hip across the back of the body. Repetitive one-sided movements can overtone this line (e.g., repeated throwing with one arm).
Ipsilateral Functional Line (IFL); figure 1.49g	The two IFL traverse each side of the body, beginning at the top of the humerus, following the outer edge of the latissimus dorsi, going along the back side of the external obliques to the anterior superior iliac crest, then along the sartorius to the inner knee.	Normally used in athletic movements when the upper body requires support from the core, such as the overhead stroke in swimming or a gym-nast working on the rings.	Chronic tension here can lead to flexion of the core or an anterior tilting of the pelvis.
THE ARM LINES			
Deep Back Arm Line (DBAL)	From the spinous processes of the lower cervical vertebrae, down the medial scapula, across the head of the humerus to the olecranon of the ulna, to the outside of the little finger.	Working with the DFAL, similar to the leg's LL, controls the an-gle of the elbow and side-to-side movement of the torso.	Problems in the arm lines can manifest as challeng-es in the neck and ribs and can affect breathing. Shoulder problems in all directions can be inhib-ited.

MERIDIAN	ROUTING	FUNCTION	RESTRICTIONS
Superficial Back Arm Line (SBAL)	From the nuchal ligament at the back of the head, along the spine of the scapula, along the posterior humerus to its lateral epicondyle, to the back of the fingers.	Controls backward movements of the arm, behind the body, and abduction of arm and shoulder. Also balances and limits the action of the SFAL.	Restrictions in the SBAL can affect extension and abduction range of motion.
Superficial Front Arm Line (SFAL)	Like a fan starting from the clavicle and the front costal origins of the thoracic ribs, the lines come together in the front of the armpit, along the medial humerus, to the medial condyle, to the palm and front of the fingers.	Exerts a wide control on movement of the arm to the front and side. Adduction and extension are important in swimming and overhead tennis strokes, as well as arm movements in yoga.	Shortening or tightening of the SFAL can restrict extension and adduction of the arms.
Deep Front Arm Line (DFAL)	From the third, fourth and fifth ribs to the coracoid to the radial tuberosity, along the radius, to the outside of the thumb.	Provides myofascial continuity between the pectoralis minor and the arm muscles of the biceps brachii and the coracobrachialis, when the arms are above the horizontal. Stabilizes the limb from thumb to chest, such as is found in yoga plank postures.	Shortness can pull the scapula into an anterior tilt, resulting in the rounded shoulders effect.

THE CORE

MERIDIAN	ROUTING	FUNCTION	RESTRICTIONS
Deep Front Line (DFL); figure 1.49h	This is the core layer of deep fascia, sandwiched between the SBL and SFL, and between the two LL. It runs from the sole of the foot, behind the knees and along the inner thigh, then splits into two paths; one runs along the front of the pelvis and lumbar, the other along the back of the thigh, through the pelvic floor to the lumbar. From here it stays internal, surrounding the organs up to the cranium.	The DFL ties the movements of our organs to our muscular activities (e.g., breathing with walking). Important functions include stabilizing the legs and pelvis, supporting the lumbar spine, balancing the head on the neck. The DFL is also important in hip adduction.	The effects of problems in the DFL are subtle. Failures of the DFL actions are covered up by compensation in the other myofascial meridians but over time take a toll on the joints. Defects in the DFL show up as a loss of gracefulness in motion.

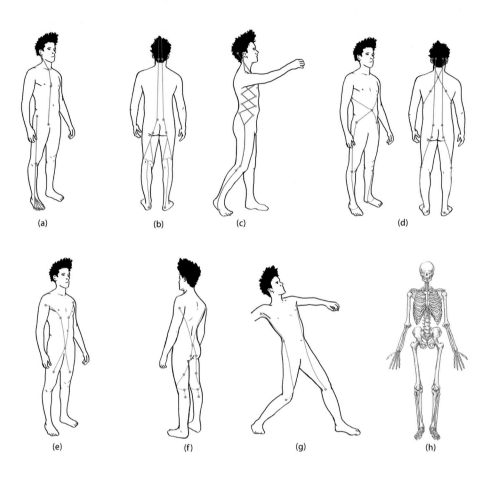

FIGURE 1.49 The cardinal and helical myofascial meridians: (a) superficial front line; (b) superficial back line; (c) lateral line; (d) spiral line; (e) front functional line; (f) back functional line; (g) ipsilateral functional line; (h) deep front line.

APPENDIX D
Facts About Osteoporosis

Osteoporosis means "porous bone." The milder form is called osteopenia, which means "lack of bone." Once the bone becomes thin enough to be considered osteoporotic, there is a high risk of fracture. Statistics for the USA show that one out every two women over 50 years of age will develop osteoporosis. The statistics are not much better for men: one out of four men over 50 will also develop osteoporosis.[182] More men will suffer hip fractures than prostate cancer, and more women will suffer hip fracture than the combined number of those who will have ovarian, breast or uterine cancer![183] A broken hip does not sound as deadly as breast cancer, but more women will die from a broken hip, due to the changes in lifestyle that occur after the fracture.[184] After 50, the odds of dying in the first year after fracturing your hip are 25%.[185] And the hips are not the only area where osteoporosis can occur; they are not even the most common site. Of the 1.5 million fractures occurring each year in the USA due to osteoporosis:

* 47% occur in the spine
* 20% occur in the hips
* 17% occur in the wrists
* 16% occur in other areas.[186]

All this points to the fact that osteoporosis is a challenging health problem. Our body's cells need calcium to function properly. They acquire calcium, when needed, from our bones. It is from the trabecular bone that most of our calcium is retrieved and stored for later use, so having less stored there means less is available for the cells when they need it. If too much calcium is lost, the bone becomes too porous. The bone density of our femurs can range from 5% porosity at age 20 to around 30% by the time we are 80 years old. This increase in porosity—which is another way of saying decreased bone density—means that the bone is not as strong as it once was. In the neck of the femur, which bears the weight of the upper body, porosity can range from 70% when we are 25 years of age to 95% when we are elderly. That makes this region of the femur very susceptible to

fracture.[187] A bone's risk of fracture is dependent upon both the number of trabecular struts we have and how thick they are. As we age, we lose struts and thickness—quality and density.

It is not only our trabecular bone that becomes weaker as we age. Our cortical bone also loses density; its ability to withstand stress declines at about 2% per decade after the age of 25.[188] The amount of energy needed to break our bones is far less when we are older than when we are young. Hence, the more we can put into our "bank account" when we are young, the longer our bones will stay strong as we age. This means the most important time to protect your bones is when you are young. If you stressed your bones a lot when you were a child and as a teenager through exercise and sports, that will pay you dividends later in life.

There are many potential causes of osteoporosis: diet, genes, hormones, lack of exercise and immobility. NASA discovered that due to a lack of stress on the bones while in orbit, astronauts can lose 1.5% of their bone density for every month they spend in space. However, NASA experiments with controlling nutrition, vitamin D levels and resistance exercises have shown that it is possible to maintain bone mineral density even in conditions of microgravity.[189] The same tools are available down here on Earth: proper diet with essential minerals, adequate vitamin D either through judicious and regular exposure to sunlight or through eating oily fish or supplements, and stress of the bones through a yoga practice or other forms of resistance (weight) training. The longer the bones are stressed, the greater the beneficial effect. However, even a stress as short as eight seconds can stimulate physiological changes in the bone and prevent degeneration.[190] A good resource to discover how to use yoga to combat osteoporosis is *Yoga for Osteoporosis* by Loren Fishman and Ellen Saltonstall. However, as these authors point out, prevention is far better and much easier than remediation. Whatever your age, start now to stress your bones.

APPENDIX E
The Types of Joints

Remember, it is easier to understand the body if we break the systems into subsystems (but also remember that despite this analytical trick, the body is not simply a collection of subsystems). There are several ways we could choose to classify our joints. We could classify them by how much movement they allow, or by the kind of movements available. Or we could choose to classify them by how they are joined together. Following this last approach, we can define three basic kinds of joints:

1. **Fibrous joints**, also called *synarthroses*, where the bones are held together by dense, irregularly arranged connective tissues. An example of this kind of joint is the joining of the plates of our skull. No movement is desired here, so the joints are fibrous, held tightly together. The rigidity of the joined bones allows forces to be transmitted widely throughout the combined structure.

2. **Cartilaginous joints**, also called *amphiarthroses*, where the bones are held together by cartilage, which allows some slight movement. Examples of these kinds of joints are the pubic symphysis (where the two ends of the pubic bones are connected by cartilage), the joining of our vertebrae (most commonly called the "disc" or the "intervertebral disc," but sometimes called the "intervertebral symphysis"), and, for a few people, where the ribs meet the sternum.[191] Slight movement is allowed in all these areas, but large ranges of movement are not desirable.

3. **Synovial joints**, sometimes called *diarthroses*, have a space (the synovial cavity) between the bones, unlike the first two categories, which are non-synovial joints. Synovial joints provide the greatest degree of movement and do so in a variety of ways.

We don't want any movement in fibrous joints, and the small range of motion available in our cartilaginous joints is usually sufficient. While yoga practice may generate stress on cartilaginous joints, which is a healthy thing to do, the intention is not to make those joints more mobile, unless some pathology is present there. If a cartilaginous joint has become immobilized and there is no movement at all, then with specialized care we may use our yoga practice to help resolve the problem.

TYPES OF SYNOVIAL JOINTS

We can further divide the synovial joints into seven subcategories (see figure 1.50):

1. **Ball-and-socket joints** (also called *spheroidal* joints), such as the hip and shoulder. Here one bone forms a deep concavity and is the stable part of the joint. The more mobile bone has a convex spherical shape. This arrangement allows a wide range of movement in all three dimensions—flexion/extension, abduction/adduction and rotation—as well as combinations of these movements (i.e., circumduction). In the shoulder and hip sockets, an extended lip of cartilage (the labrum) makes the socket even deeper, thus more stable. The shapes are actually slightly ovoid, and thus there is a perfect fit between the two bones in only one position, which is at the further end of common movement.[192]

2. **Condyloid joints**, such as the knee (also called *bicondylar* joints—*condyle* means knuckle). These are similar to ball-and-socket joints, but the depth of the curved surfaces is much shallower. Instead of the three-dimensional movements allowed in a ball-and-socket joint, condyloid joints allow movement in two directions. For example, in the knee, flexion and extension are allowed, as is some twisting when the knee is flexed. When the knee is extended, however, there should be no rotation. What is never desired in this joint is abduction or adduction. Collateral ligaments support the knee joint to prevent those movements. Condyloid joints are also found in the fingers as well as at the jaw and the first two cervical vertebrae.

3. **Ellipsoid joints** (many authorities include this type under the condyloid category) have one bone's end

shaped as an elongated, convex oval (an ellipsoid), while the matching bone's end is a concave ovoid. This allows movement primarily in two dimensions—flexion and extension as well as abduction and adduction—but little or no twisting. However, these four allowed movements can be combined into a cone-shaped circumduction. An example of this joint is found at the distal end of the radius bone where it joins the carpal (wrist) bones.

4. **Saddle joints** (also called sellar joints) resemble a saddle. The bones have convexity and concavity orientated in orthogonal directions (at 90° angles to each other). They are called saddle joints for this reason: a saddle is concave from front to back but convex from side to side. The articulating bone has corresponding smaller surfaces shaped the same way. This allows movements of flexion and extension as well as abduction and adduction. Rotation is not allowed. The thumb (between the metacarpal and carpal bones) is a prime example of a saddle joint, but this kind of joint is also found at the ankle joint and calcaneocuboid joint, which is the joint between the heel and the cuboid bone in your foot.

5. **Hinge joints** (also called *ginglymoid* joints) act like a door hinge, allowing flexion and extension in only one plane. To prevent movements in any other directions, these joints have strong collateral ligaments. Unlike an ordinary door hinge, though, hinge joints are not perfect cylinders but rather have slight spirals; thus, the movement around a hinge joint is not perfect rotation. The elbow and finger joints display this kind of movement.

6. **Pivot joints** (also called *trochoid* joints) allow rotation of one bone around one axis, like a doorknob turning. In the elbow joint, the pivoting radius has a ring around its head, called the anular ligament, within which it rotates. Alternatively, the ring may rotate around the bone, as happens with the atlas, the first cervical vertebra, as it rotates around the dens of the axis (the second cervical vertebra).

7. **Gliding joints** (also called *plane* joints) have two relatively flat surfaces, which allow some twisting or sliding (called *translation*), like a car skidding on ice. While the surfaces are almost flat, there is some small curvature, which may affect the ease of movement in the joint. Resistance to movement in these joints comes from the supporting and restricting ligaments. Examples include the sacroiliac joint, which may have articulating surfaces shaped like ridges or rails to guide the glide, as well as the wrist joints. While there is a wide variety of movement, not much distance is allowed, so the range of motion is restricted to a small area.

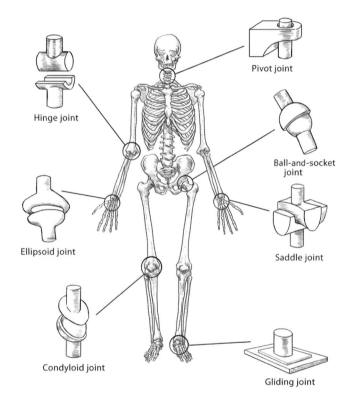

FIGURE 1.50 The seven kinds of synovial joints.

APPENDIX F
The Biomechanics of Joint Motion

Synovial joints bear loads, provide stability and allow for movement. Two main kinds of movements occur at a joint: translational (gliding or sliding) and rotational (turning). Simple movements are rare; usually, movements involve a combination of translation and rotation, and the axis of rotation changes as the joint moves. The resulting movements can be described as:

- **Translation**. A gliding of one surface over the other without any rotation—for example, the wrists and ankles.
- **Angulation**. A change in the angle of the bones creating the joint—for example, the elbow's flexion or extension.
- **Flexion**. Generally used to describe movements of the front sides of the body towards each other.
- **Extension**. Generally used to describe movements of the back sides of the body towards each other.
- **Abduction**. Generally (but not always) describes movement in the frontal plane where the two bones move away from each other.
- **Adduction**. Generally (but again not always) describes movement in the frontal plane where the two bones move towards each other.
- **Circumduction**. A sequential combination of flexion, abduction, extension and adduction, causing a circular movement whereby the moving bone draws a cone with the apex of the cone in the joint—for example, the shoulder or hip sockets.
- **Axial rotation**. A movement around the long axis of a bone. However, the joint often is not aligned so that the long axis of the bone lines up with the center of the joint. Axial rotation is therefore more complicated than the simple definition suggests. It depends upon both the movement of the bones and their orientations.

Arthrokinematics is the term used to describe movement between the articulating surfaces of a joint. Where slight movement is allowed, the articulating surfaces are generally equal in size. Where a large range of movement is allowed,

the more stable bone's articulating surface is generally larger. Many joints involve one convex surface (like the head of the femur) and one concave surface (like the hip socket). This relationship assists in building congruency between the surfaces of the articulating bones, which means the areas of the surfaces that are in contact are maximized. When the joint surfaces are not fully congruent—which means the surface area in contact is not maximal—we can depict the movements as spin, roll and slide, as shown in figure 1.51:

- **Roll**. Many points on one articulating surface come into contact with many points on the other surface, like a car's tire driving over pavement.
- **Slide**. One point on one articulating surface comes into contact with many points on the other surface, like a car's tire skidding over the road when braking quickly.
- **Spin**. One point on one articulating surface stays in contact with one point on the other surface, like a fast-spinning toy top that stays in one place.

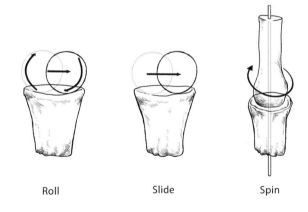

Roll   Slide   Spin

FIGURE 1.51 When the surfaces of the joints are not fully congruent, movements can occur, such as rolling, sliding or spinning, or some combination of these.

Rolling and sliding often occur together in a joint movement, again to maximize surface area contact. This happens, for example, at the knees and at the shoulders. As shown in the shoulder example in figure 1.52, when the humerus is abducted to the side, it rolls in the shoulder socket, but it also slides down a bit so that the surfaces stay in contact. If this sliding did not happen, the humerus would ride up in the socket and begin to pinch a bursa between it and the acromion of the scapula.

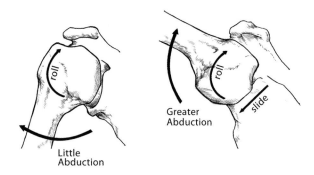

FIGURE 1.52 The shoulder joint uses only rolling when a little abduction occurs but includes sliding as well when the movement is larger.

The knee requires a similar motion, as shown in figure 1.53. When the femur flexes over a fixed tibia, it rolls downwards, but the condyles slide forward on the tibial plateau. When it extends, it has to roll up, but the condyles slide backwards over the tibia.

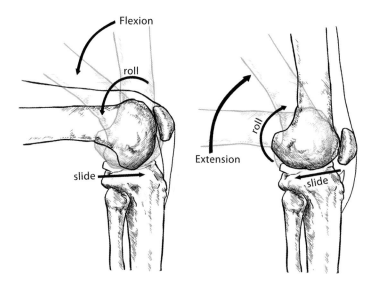

FIGURE 1.53 The knee joint utilizes both sliding and rolling in flexion and extension.

In the shoulder example when we move only the arm, and when we move the femur, we have a convex surface moving on a concave surface, and thus the roll and slide are in *opposite* directions. Interestingly, when we have a concave surface moving along a convex surface, the roll and slide are in the same direction, which occurs when we extend the tibia (the concave surface) under the femur (the convex surface) to straighten the knee (see figure 1.54).

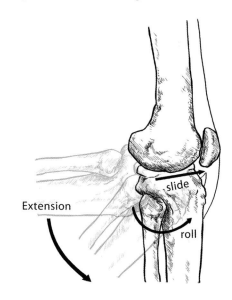

FIGURE 1.54 When a concave surface moves under a convex surface, the rolling and sliding occur in the same direction as when the tibia extends beneath the femur.

If the surface areas are small, then sliding and rolling must both happen together; only if a larger surface area is available is it possible to have independent sliding and rolling. We see this in the shoulder: a little abduction causes only rolling to occur, but greater abduction requires both rolling and sliding. To avoid too much sliding in the knee, we have several ligaments providing restraint, such as the cruciate ligaments.

Volume 1 Endnotes

1 See Roger Williams, *Biochemical Individuality* (New York: McGraw-Hill Professional, 1998).

2 Cited in Roger Williams, *Biochemical Individuality*, 1–2.

3 Stuart McGill, *Ultimate Back and Fitness Performance*, 5th ed. (Waterloo, Canada: Backfitpro, 2014). www.backfitpro.com

4 What time of year you were born indicates the seasons your mother experienced during her pregnancy, which determines how much sunlight she may have received, the freshness of the food she ate, how active she was and many other qualities that can affect a developing fetus.

5 Roger Williams, *Biochemical Individuality*, 3.

6 See C.D. Fryar, Q Gu, and C.L. Ogden, *Anthropometric Reference Data for Children and Adults: United States, 2007–2010*. Vital and Health Statistics, series 11, no. 252 (Atlanta: National Center for Health Statistics, 2012).

7 Due to epigenetic changes and mutations, our DNA structure changes over time.

8 See *The Collins English Dictionary*, online edition, www.collinsdictionary.com.

9 See Jonathan D. Schoenfeld and John P.A. Ioannidis, "Is Everything We Eat Associated with Cancer? A Systematic Cookbook Review," *American Journal of Clinical Nutrition* 97.1 (January 2013): 127–34. doi:10.3945/ajcn.112.047142.

10 See Schoenfeld and Ioannidis, "Is Everything We Eat."

11 "Although the configurations of human innards do not vary nearly as much as do those of our outards . . . they nevertheless reveal unmistakable variations among individuals—and only surgeons ever find out about them" (Sherwin Nuland, *The Mysteries Within* [New York: Simon & Schuster, 2001], 24).

12 This drawing is inspired by the drawing in Frank Netter's *Atlas of Human Anatomy*, 3rd ed. (Teterboro, NJ: Icon Learning Systems, 2003), plate 275.

13 Anne M. Gilroy, Brian R. MacPherson, and Lawrence M. Ross, *Atlas of Anatomy*, corrected reprint (Harrogate, UK: Thieme, 2010), 367.

14 This figure was derived by averaging the three North American sites surveyed in John Y. Anderson and Erik Trinkaus, "Patterns of Sexual, Bilateral and Interpopulational Variation in Human Femoral Neck-shaft Angles," *Journal of Anatomy* 192 (1998): 279-285. doi:10.1046/j.1469-7580.1998.19220279.x.

15 Anderson and Trinkaus, "Patterns," 282.

16 Ibid., 280.

17 Ibid., 281.

18 Drawing inspired by the drawing on page 58 in Loren Fishman and Ellen Saltonstall, *Yoga for Osteoporosis* (New York: W.W. Norton, 2010).

19 Barry J. Ansons, *An Atlas of Human Anatomy* (Philadelphia, PA: W.B. Saunders, 1963), v.

20 Roger Williams, *Biochemical Individuality*, 49.

21 Roger Williams, *Biochemical Individuality*, 29.

22 I. Gilligan, S. Chandraphak, and P. Mahakkanukrauh. "Femoral Neck-shaft Angle in Humans: Variation Relating to Climate, Clothing, Lifestyle, Sex, Age and Side," *Journal of Anatomy* 223.2 (2013): 133–51. doi:10.1111/joa.12073.

23 Anderson and Trinkaus, "Patterns."

24 Graphic reproduced with the kind permission of John Anderson, from Anderson and Trinkaus, "Patterns."

25 Quoted in Kate Douglas, "Reaping the Whirlwind of Nazi Eugenics," *New Scientist*, July 14, 2014. https://www.newscientist.com/article/mg22329770-800-reaping-the-whirlwind-of-nazi-eugenics/.

26 See Roger Williams, *Biochemical Individuality*, 53.

27 See Michael J. Sheehan and Michael W. Nachman, "Morphological and Population Genomic Evidence that Human Faces Have Evolved to Signal Individual Identity," *Nature Communications* 5 (2014): article 4800. doi:10.1038/ncomms5800.

28 See Caroline Williams, "One and Only You," *New Scientist* 215.2875 (2012): 32–26.

29 See Mario F. Fraga et al., "Epigenetic Differences Arise During the Lifetime of Monozygotic Twins," *Proceedings of the National Academy of Sciences* 102.30 (2005): 10604–9.

30 See Pauline N. C. B. Audergon et al., "Restricted Epigenetic Inheritance of H3K9 Methylation," *Science* 348.6230 (2015):132–5. doi:10.1126/science.1260638.

31 Edward Archer, "The Childhood Obesity Epidemic as a Result of Nongenetic Evolution," *Mayo Clinic Proceedings* 90.1 (2015), 77.

32 See Caroline Williams, "One and Only You."

33 See John Z. Xie et al., "Color Vision Deficiency in Preschool Children," *Ophthalmology* 121.7 (2014): 1469–74. doi:10.1016/j.ophtha.2014.01.018.

34 From "Color Blindness: Prevalence," http://www.colour-blindness.com/general/prevalence.

35 See Alireza Mirshahi et al., "Myopia and Level of Education," *Ophthalmology* 121.10 (2014): 2047–52. doi:10.1016/j.ophtha.2014.04.017.

36 See Janna Nousbeck et al., "A Mutation in a Skin-Specific Isoform of SMARCAD1 Causes Autosomal-Dominant Adermatoglyphia," *American Journal of Human Genetics* 89 (2011): 302–7.

37 See Caroline Williams, "One and Only You."

38 Ibid.

39 See Dustin J. Penn et al., "Individual and Gender Fingerprints in Human Body Odour," *Journal of the Royal Society Interface* 4 (2007): 331–40.

40 See Apple's application for a patent on a seamlessly embedded heart-rate monitor: http://patft.uspto.gov/netacgi/nph-Parser?Sect1=PTO2&Sect2=HITOFF&u=%2Fnetahtml%2FPTO%2Fsearch-adv.htm&r=2&p=1&f=G&l=50&d=PTXT&S1=%28600%2F509.CCLS.+AND+20131224.PD.%29&OS=ccl/600/509+and+isd/12/24/2013&RS=%28CCL/600/509+AND+ISD/20131224%29.

41 D. Drachman, "Do we have brain to spare?" (2005). *Neurology* 64.12 (2005): 2004–5. doi:10.1212/01.WNL.0000166914.38327.BB.

42 See "Human Microbiome Project: Diversity of Human Microbes Greater than Previously Predicted," *Science Daily*, May 21, 2010, http://www.sciencedaily.com/releases/2010/05/100520141214.htm.

43 See D.C. Savage, "Microbial Ecology of the Gastrointestinal Tract," *Annual Review of Microbiology* 31 (1977): 107–33. doi:10.1146/annurev.mi.31.100177.000543.

44 See Tina Hesman Saey, "The Vast Virome," in *Science News*, December 27, 2013, https://www.sciencenews.org/article/vast-virome.

45 This list is from F. Kopsch, *Rauber's Lerbuch der Anatomie des Menschen* (Leipzig: Georg Thieme, 1908). See http://www.anatomyatlases.org/AnatomicVariants/Introduction.shtml.

46 See Edward L. Miloslavich, "Contributions to Anthropological Splanchnology: Racial Studies on the Large Intestine," *American Journal of Physical Anthropology* 8.1 (1925): 11–22. doi:10.1002/ajpa.1330080102.

47 Roger Williams, *Biochemical Individuality*, 98.

48 See Jennifer S. Mascaro, Patrick D. Hackett, and James K. Rilling, "Testicular Volume is Inversely Correlated with Nurturing-related Brain Activity in Human Fathers," *Proceedings of the National Academy of Science* 110.39 (2013): 15746–51. doi:10.1073/pnas.1305579110.

49 Roger Williams, *Biochemical Individuality*, 102.

50 Ibid., 90.

51 Ibid., 94.

52 See Robert Schleip, "Lumbar Fasciae: A Frequent Generator of Back Pain. Latest Research Findings and Clinical Implication," paper presented at the Europäisches Symposium der traditionellen Osteopathie, February 7–10, 2013.

53 See Gordon H. Orians, *Snakes, Sunrises, and Shakespeare: How Evolution Shapes Our Loves and Fears* (Chicago: University of Chicago Press, 2014).

54 See Colin Barras, "Lifespan Boost for Mice that Feel Less Pain," *New Scientist*, May 31, 2014.

55 See Catherine de Lange, "Unravel Epicurean Genes to Let Us All Eat Healthily," *New Scientist*, June 7, 2014.

56 See Monell Chemical Senses Center, "Enzyme in Saliva Helps Regulate Blood Glucose," http://www.monell.org/images/uploads/amylase_final.pdf.

57 See Patrick Grimm, "Body Image," lecture 8 in *Philosophy of Mind: Brains, Consciousness, and Thinking Machines* (Chantilly, VA: The Great Courses, 2008).

58 The Serenity Prayer is attributed to the American theologian Karl Paul Reinhold Niebuhr.

59 See this Finnish study on the physiological effects of emotions: Lauri Nummenmaa, Enrico Glerean, Riitta Hari, and Jari K. Hietanen, "Bodily Maps of Emotions," *Proceedings of the National Academy of Sciences* 11.2 (2013): 646–51, http://www.pnas.org/content/early/2013/12/26/1321664111.abstract.

60 This sentiment was eloquently expressed by Joseph Campbell; see *Myths to Live By* (New York: Penguin, 1993), 207.

61 Kudos for this saying to Eoin Finn, a master yogi and blissologist.

62 Richard J. Johns and Verna Wright, "Relative Importance of Various Tissues in Joint Stiffness," *Journal of Applied Physiology* 17.5 (1962): 824–28.

63 In a yin yoga practice, dull and achy sensations can arise that are not an indication of trauma to the tissues; they are often to be expected when a long-held traction is applied. However, if these sensations arise in short-held Hatha postures, that may not be a good sign.

64 This may not work if the sensation is painful, due to the pain possibly being referred from some other area of the body.

65 The original source of this quotation is unknown, but it is a great piece of wisdom and advice. Thank you, whoever coined this saying!

66 See S. Takata and N. Yasui, "Disuse Osteoporosis," *Journal of Medical Investigation* 48.3–4 (2001): 147–56.

67 Distraction, or pulling apart the bones, stimulates the growth of the bones and their associated ligaments. See S.S. Natu, I. Ali, S. Alam, K.Y. Giri, A. Agarwal, and V.A. Kulkarni, "The Biology of Distraction Osteogenesis for Correction of Mandibular and Craniomaxillofacial Defects: A Review," *Dental Research Journal* 11.1 (2014): 16–26.

68 See Daniel J. Leong and Hui B. Sun, "Mechanical Loading: Potential Preventive and Therapeutic Strategy for Osteoarthritis," *Journal of the American Academy of Orthopaedic Surgeons* 22 (2014): 465–6. doi:10.5435/JAAOS-22-07-465.

69 Some researchers invert the graph and call it a "u-shaped relationship," but it represents the same understanding. See Stuart McGill, *Low Back Disorders: Evidence-Based Prevention and Rehabilitation*, 2nd ed. (Champaign, IL: Human Kinetics, 2007), 32.

70 Inspired by the graphic in McGill, *Low Back Disorders*, 13.

71 Inspired by the graphic in McGill, *Low Back Disorders*, 14.

72 See Nassim Nicholas Taleb, *Antifragile: Things that Gain from Disorder* (New York: Random House, 2012), 58.

73 See McGill, *Low Back Disorders*, 14.

74 See R.L. Duncan and C.H. Turner, "Mechanotransduction and the Functional Response of Bone to Mechanical Strain," *Calcified Tissue International* 57.5 (1995): 344–58.

75 Paracrine factors may signal osteoprogenitors to produce osteoblasts, the cells that secrete bone. Insulin-like growth factors and prostaglandins may also be released. See Duncan and Turner, "Mechanotransduction."

76 See James Oschman, *Energy Medicine in Therapeutics and Human Performance* (Edinburgh: Elsevier, 2003), 62 and 92.

77 There may indeed be valid reasons for suggesting a student not keep her shoulders up by her ears while in the Down Dog posture, but fear of compressing the neck is not one of them. If the reason is to prepare the shoulders and arms for flowing from Down Dog to Up Dog, this may be a valid instruction.

78 This drawing is inspired by a drawing in Oschman, *Energy Medicine*, 46.

79 See Andy Coghlan, "The Matrix: The Secret to Superhealing Regeneration," *New Scientist*, September 12, 2013.

80 Graphic reproduced with the kind permission of Loren Fishman and Ellen Saltonstall, from their book *Yoga for Osteoporosis* (New York: W.W. Norton, 2010), 76. Their graphic was based on T. Matsumoto, M. Kawakami, K. Kuribayashi, T. Takenaka, and T. Tamaki, "Cyclic Mechanical Stretch Stress Increases the Growth Rate and Collage Synthesis of Nucleus Pulposus Cells In Vitro," *Spine* 24.4 (1999): 315–9.

81 See Bob Holmes, "Healing Touch: The Key to Regenerating Bodies," *New Scientist*, February 16, 2010.

82 See Taleb, *Antifragile*.

83 For a more complete analysis of fragility and yoga, see Bernie Clark, "Are Yoga Teachers Making Us Fragile? An Essay about Iatrogenesis, Yoga and Fragility," at http://www.yinyoga.com/newsletter23_Fragile.php.

84 See C. Allen, P. Glasziou, and C. Del Mar. "Bed Rest: A Potentially Harmful Treatment Needing More Careful Evaluation," *Lancet* 354 (1999): 1229–33.

85 See E. Lieberman, *The Story of the Human Body: Evolution, Health and Disease* (New York: Pantheon, 2013), 305–9.

86 See Lieberman, *The Story of the Human Body*, 326–7.

87 Ibid., 309–14.

88 Ibid., 330.

89 See M. Tscherning, *Studier over Myopiers Aetiologi* (Copenhagen, 1882).

90 See Nassim Nicholas Taleb, *Antifragile: Things That Gain from Disorder* (New York: Random House, 2012), 277.

91 Please notice, this is *not* saying "no pain—no gain"! Pain is an indication that your stress has gone too far and you are now starting to damage your tissues.

92 The basis for this number can be found in Eva Bianconi et al., "An Estimation of the Number of Cells in a Human Body," *Annals of Human Biology* 40.6 (2013): 463–71, doi:10.3109/03014460.2013.807878.

93 Johns and Wright, "Relative Importance."

94 See Henry Gray, Susan Standring, and B.K.B. Berkovitz, eds., *Gray's Anatomy*, 39th ed. (London: Elsevier, 2005), 112.

95 See Michael Alter, *Science of Flexibility* (Champaign, IL: Human Kinetics, 1996), 17. Alter puts the upper limit to length at 4.0 cm, but Alan McComas extends this range to 12 cm (Brian MacIntosh, Phillip Gardiner, and Alan McComas, *Skeletal Muscle: Form and Function*, 2nd ed. [Champaign, IL: Human Kinetics, 2015], 5).

96 It is important to note that this is just one theory of how a muscle contracts. There are other theories, most notably the theory of phase transition. Muscle cells contain water locked into the sarcomeres, forming a gel. According to Gerald Pollack, this gel state can change, and the proteins within the sarcomere then undergo shortening. The titin shortens first, providing a low degree of contraction, but if greater force is required, the myosin contracts, which generates greater force. See Gerald H. Pollack, *Cells, Gels and the Engines of Life: A New, Unifying Approach to Cell Function* (Seattle, WA: Ebner and Sons, 2001), chapter 14.

97 See Alter, *Science of Flexibility*, 29.

98 See M.J. Cullen and D.N. Landon, "The Normal Ultrastructure of Skeletal Muscle," in J. Walton, G. Karpati, and D. Hilton-Jones (eds.), *Disorders of Voluntary Muscle* (New York: Churchill Livingstone, 1994), 87–137; B.S. Tseng, C.E. Kasper, and V.R. Edgerton, "Cytoplasm-to-Myonucleus Ratio and Succinate Dehydrogenase Activities in Adult Rat Slow and Fast Muscle Fibers," *Cell Tissue Research* 275 (1994): 39–49.

99 A blast cell is a precursor cell, which means this cell can become something different. However, it is a unipotent cell: it can become only one type of cell. A myoblast can become a muscle cell, an osteoblast can become a bone cell, and so forth.

100 See Alter, *Science of Flexibility*, 31.

101 See Wolfgang A. Linke, "Sense and Stretchability: The Role of Titin and Titin-associated Proteins in Myocardial

Stress-sensing and Mechanical Dysfunction," *Cardiovascular Research* 77.4 (2008): 637–48.

102 See L.E. Holt, T.E. Pelham, and J. Holt, *Flexibility: A Concise Guide* (Totowa, NJ: Hanawa Press, 2008), 118 and their reference to E. Fox, R. Bowers, and M. Foss, *The Physiological Basis for Exercise and Sport*, 5th ed. (Madison, WS: Brown and Benchmark, 1993).

103 The ends or terminal tips of skeletal muscle fibers have been shown to be the site of longitudinal growth. See H.J. Swatland, *Structure and Development of Meat Animals and Poultry* (Lancaster, PA: Technomic, 1994); M. Zhang and I.S. McLennan, "During Secondary Myotube Formation, Primary Myotubes Preferentially Absorb New Nuclei at Their Ends," *Developmental Dynamics* 204 (1995): 168–177.

104 There are other ways to look at this formula: force x length is also defined as energy—or another way to say this is that energy is expended when a force moves an object. Energy per unit of time is power. We could also look at the movement over time, L/T, which is also known as velocity. Power then would be force times the velocity of movement.

105 Muscle grows stronger not by adding more muscle cells but by adding more sarcomeres within the existing muscle cells. This is called hypertrophy. Prenatally, and in early life, we can add muscle cells (called hyperplasia), but most researchers believe that this ability ends as we grow up. Whether hyperplasia can occur in adults is still being debated. See P.J. Abernethy, J. Jürimäe, P.A. Logan, A.W. Taylor, and R.E. Thayer, "Acute and Chronic Response of Skeletal Muscle to Resistance Exercise," *Sports Medicine* 17.1 (1994): 22–38.

106 See M.A. Shaffer et al., "Effects of Immobilization on Plantar-Flexion Torque, Fatigue Resistance, and Functional Ability Following an Ankle Fracture," *Physical Therapy* 80.8 (2000): 769–80.

107 See Alter, *Science of Flexibility*, 41.

108 The term "bone paint" was coined by Gil Hedley; see Erik Dalton et al., *Dynamic Body: Exploring Form, Expanding Function* (Oklahoma City, OK: Freedom From Pain Institute, 2011), 67.

109 See Mark Lindsey, *Fascia: Clinical Applications for Health and Human Performance* (Farmington Hills, MI: Delmar, 2008), 96.

110 See Alter, *Science of Flexibility*, 40. These tubes are microfibrils, subfibrils, fibrils and fascicles.

111 See Alter, *Science of Flexibility*, 50.

112 See E. Witvrouw, N. Mahieu, P. Roosen, and P. McNair, "The Role of Stretching in Tendon Injuries," *British Journal of Sports Medicine* 41 (2007): 224–6, doi:10.1136/bjsm.2006.034165.

113 See Witvrouw et al., "The Role of Stretching in Tendon Injuries."

114 Ibid.

115 "[A]ll fibrous collagenous connective tissues, which are part of a body-wide interconnected tensional network, are recognized as fascial tissues. Joint capsules, intramuscular connective tissues, ligaments, and tendons are seen merely as local specifications of this tension-resistant fibrous network" (from Robert Schleip and Divo Gitta Müller, *Fascial Dysfunction: Manual Therapy Approaches—Use It or Lose It* (Pencaitland, Scotland: Handspring Publishing, 2014), 127.

116 Credit for popularizing these terms goes to Thomas Myers, who mentioned them at the Third International Fascia Research Congress, held in Vancouver, Canada in 2012.

117 See Schleip, "Lumbar Fasciae: A Frequent Generator of Back Pain."

118 See F.H. Willard, A. Vleeming, M.D. Schuenke, L. Danneels, and R. Schleip, "The Thoracolumbar Fascia: Anatomy, Function and Clinical Considerations," *Journal of Anatomy* 221.6 (2012): 507–36.

119 See Stephen W. Porges, "The Polyvagal Perspective," *Biological Psychology* 74.2 (2007): 116–43.

120 See Shelley E. Taylor, *Fight-or-Flight versus Tend-and-Befriend: The Significance of Gender Differences in Stress Responses* (November 2003), retrieved from http://obssr.od.nih.gov/pdf/taylor_slides.pdf.

121 According to Robert Schleip, the flow of water has to be less than 6 dyne/cm²; see Schleip, "Lumbar Fasciae."

122 See Robert Schleip, "Fascial Plasticity—A New Neurobiological Explanation: Part 1," *Journal of Bodywork and Movement Therapy* 7.1 (2003): 11–19, retrieved from http://www.sciencedirect.com/science/article/pii/S1360859202000670.

123 See Schleip, "Lumbar Fasciae."

124 See Schleip, "Fascial Plasticity."

125 This was reported by their discoverer, Camillo Golgi. See *Intorno alla distribuzione e terminazione dei nervi neitendini dell'uomo e di altri vertebrati*, reproduced in C. Golgi, *Opera Omnia* (Milan, Italy: Hoepli, 1903), vol. 1, 133–42, and *Sui nervi dei tendini dell'uomo et di altri vertebrati e di un nuovo organo nervoso terminale muscolo-tendineo*, 171–98.

126 See Williams, *Biochemical Individuality*, 53.

127 See E.F. Berstein, J. Lee, D.B. Brown, R. Yu, and E. Van Scott, "Glycolic Acid Treatment Increases Type I Collagen mRNA and Hyaluronic Acid Content of Human Skin," *Dermatology Surgery* 27.5 (2001): 429–33.

128 See Holt et al., *Flexibility: A Concise Guide*, 15 and 16.

129 See Timothy McCall, *Yoga as Medicine: The Yogic Prescription for Health and Healing* (New York: Bantam Books, 2007), 49.

130 See Schleip, "Lumbar Fasciae."

131 See Schleip, "Fascial Plasticity."

132 For those interested in learning more, a great starting place is Pollack, *Cells, Gels and the Engines of Life.*

133 See "Coming Soon to a Knee Near You: Cartilage Like Your Very Own," *Science*, 322.5907 (2008), 1460-1.

134 See Alter, *Science of Flexibility*, 54.

135 See J. van der Wal, "The Architecture of the Connective Tissue in the Musculoskeletal System—An Often Overlooked Functional Parameter as to Proprioception in the Locomotor Apparatus," in *Fascia Research II: Basic Science and Implications for Conventional and Complementary Health Care*, ed. Thomas W. Findley and Robert Schleip (Munich: Elsevier, 2009).

136 See Thomas Myers, "Dynamic Ligaments: The Revolutionary Re-Vision of Jaap van der Wal," *Freedom From Pain Institute*, retrieved from http://erikdalton.com/media/published-articles/dynamic-ligaments/#comment-998.

137 The ligamentum flavum is 80% elastin and 20% collagen; see McGill, *Low Back Disorders*, 63.

138 See R.L. Swanson, "Biotensegrity: A Unifying Theory of Biological Architecture with Applications to Osteopathic Practice, Education, and Research—A Review and Analysis," *Journal of the American Osteopathic Association* 113.1 (2013): 34–52.

139 See S. Levin, "Tensegrity: The New Biomechanics," in *Textbook of Musculoskeletal Medicine*, ed. M. Hutson and R. Ellis (Oxford: Oxford University Press, 2006).

140 See George V. Alexander, Ralph E. Nusbaum, and Norman S. MacDonald, "The Boron and Lithium Content of Human Bones," *Journal of Biological Chemistry* 192 (1951): 489–96.

141 See "Cortical and Trabecular Load Sharing in the Human Vertebral Body," by S. K. Eswaran and A. Gupta et al., Journal of Bone and Mineral Research 22 (January 2007): 149-157.

142 See Heather M. Macdonald, Kyle K. Nishiyama, Jian Kang, David A. Hanley, and Steven K Boyd, "Age-Related Patterns of Trabecular and Cortical Bone Loss Differ Between Sexes and Skeletal Sites: A Population-Based HR-pQCT Study," *Journal of Bone and Mineral Research* 26.1 (2011): 50–62.

143 See Loren Fishman and Ellen Salonstall, *Yoga for Osteoporosis* (New York: W.W. Norton, 2010), 29.

144 See Gray et al., *Gray's Anatomy*, 87.

145 See Leslie Aiello, ed., *An Introduction to Human Evolutionary Anatomy* (Waltham, MA: Academic Press, 2006), 463.

146 See Jean-Luc Jouve et al., "Anatomical Study of the Proximal Femur in the Fetus," *Journal of Pediatric Orthopaedics B* 14.2 (2005): 105–10.

147 Consider how difficult it is to change the shape of the jaw bones. Anyone who has worn braces knows that it takes many years of constant stress to make even a small change, and after years of wearing braces, a person must still wear retainers because of the bone's tendency to return to its original shape. A few hours of yoga every day is not going to change the shape of your vertebrae or femurs.

148 See Deane Juhan, *Job's Body: A Handbook for Bodyworks* (Barrytown, NY: Station Hill, 2003), 100.

149 See Leslie Kaminoff's video *What Do Your Marriage and Your Knee Have in Common?*, retrieved from http://yogaanatomy.net/joints.

150 See John Goodfellow and John O'Connor, "The Mechanics of the Knee and Prosthesis Design," *Journal of Bone and Joint Surgery* 60-B.3 (1978): 358–69.

151 See McGill, *Low Back Disorders*, 117–18.

152 Ibid., 174–5.

153 Ibid., 152.

154 See Donald A. Neumann and A. Joseph Threlkeld, "Basic Structure and Function of Human Joints," in *Kinesiology of the Musculoskeletal System: Foundations for Rehabilitation*, ed. Donald A. Neumann (St. Louis, MO: Mosby, 2010), 34.

155 See Gray et al., *Gray's Anatomy*, 108.

156 Another reason someone's cartilage may be diminished is due to old surgery techniques. Surgeons used to remove cartilage from the joints. Surgeons today try to avoid doing this or avoid surgery altogether because of the long-term effects, which include accelerated development of osteoarthritis.

157 See Gray et al., *Gray's Anatomy*, 110.

158 Cyclical loading and unloading of the cells is required to positively affect tissues. With each loading, a cell responds by releasing calcium and ATP (the molecule that provides energy for our bodies at the cellular level) into the extracellular space. However, the cell soon depletes itself and needs to rest to be able to generate more ATP and calcium. See B.P. O'Hara, J.P.G. Urban, and A. Maroudas, "Influence of Cyclic Loading on the Nutrition of Articular Cartilage," *Annals of the Rheumatic Diseases* 49 (1990): 536–9.

159 Such as the sternoclavicular and temporomandibular joints, as well as the radiocarpal joint.

160 See Gray et al., *Gray's Anatomy*, 110.

161 See Bernie Clark, "Yin Yoga for the Knees," *Yin Yoga Newsletter* 7 (July 2011), retrieved from http://www.yinyoga.com/newsletter7_yinyoga_knees.php.

162 We can lose 19 mm in height over the course of a day, and over 50% of that loss comes in the first 30 minutes after rising (T. Reilly, A. Tyrrell, and J.D. Troup, "Circadian Variation in Human Stature," *Chronobiology International* 1.2 [1984]: 121–6; cited in McGill, *Low Back Disorders*, 96).

163 The opposite occurs as we are growing in early life. From ages seven to 20, the vertebrae grow, whereas the discs change

minimally; see I.A. Stokes and L. Windisch, "Vertebral Height Growth Predominates over Intervertebral Disc Height Growth in Adolescents with Scoliosis," *Spine* 31.14 (2006): 1600–4.

164 When we are young adults, our nucleus pulposus is 65% proteoglycans, but by our 60s that has dropped to 30%; thus, we have dried up. See Jim Borowczyk, "Spondylosis, Facet Joint Arthropathy and Pain," presentation at the General Practice Conference and Medical Exhibition South, August 4–8, 2010, Christchurch, New Zealand, retrieved from http://www.gpcme.co.nz/pdf/GP%20CME/Friday/C5%201630%20Borowczyk.pdf.

165 See Donald A. Neumann, "Getting Started," in *Kinesiology of the Musculoskeletal System: Foundations for Rehabilitation*, ed. Donald A. Neumann (St. Louis, MO: Mosby, 2010), 27.

166 See Gray et al., *Gray's Anatomy*, 108.

167 Ibid., 108.

168 There are similar functions in many areas of our body; one part creates materials (like the osteoblasts in our bones, which create bone tissue), and another part consumes or removes materials (like the osteoclasts, which dissolve bone). Health is the balance of these two functions.

169 See George R. Hepburn, "Contracture and Stiff Joint Management with Dynasplint™," *Journal of Orthopaedic and Sports Physical Therapy* 8.10 (1987): 498–504. Shorter, more intense stresses were observed to result in "a higher proportion of elastic response, less remodeling, and greater trauma and weakening of the tissue." The elastic response occurs when the tissues return to their original lengths.

170 See Williams, *Biochemical Individuality*, 53.

171 Ibid., 102.

172 See Schleip, "Lumbar Fasciae."

173 In these cases, the muscle is said to be *strained* rather than sprained. This is a second, but different, use of the word strain. A strained muscle is one that has been deformed such that it does not return to its original length. Thus, we sprain ligaments, but we strain muscles. While technically muscles are not sprained, medical professionals will often say a muscle is sprained, so we don't have to be dogmatic in insisting upon the correct term being used.

174 See G.M. Thornton, N.G. Shrive, and C.B. Frank, "Ligament Creep Recruits Fibres at Low Stresses and Can Lead to Modulus-reducing Fibre Damage at Higher Creep Stresses: A Study in Rabbit Medial Collateral Ligament Model," *Journal of Orthopaedic Research* 20.5 (2002): 967–74, retrieved from http://www.ncbi.nlm.nih.gov/pubmed/12382961.

175 See Neumann, "Getting Started," 13.

176 See McComas, *Skeletal Muscle*.

177 Ibid., 5.

178 See Dalton et al., *Dynamic Body*, 64.

179 From Thomas Myers, *Anatomy Trains: Myofascial Meridians for Manual and Movement Therapists*, 3rd ed. (New York: Elsevier, 2014), 5.

180 See Myers, *Anatomy Trains*, chapters 3 to 9.

181 The table is the author's summary of Myers's work, and any factual errors here are due to mistakes by the author, not Thomas Myers.

182 See Fishman and Saltonstall, *Yoga for Osteoporosis*, 5.

183 See H.W. Minne, W. Pollähne, M. Pfeifer, B. Begerow, and C. Hinz, "Weeks of Pain, Vertebral Body Fractures During Sleep, Invalidism: Save Your Osteoporosis Patient from This Fate," *MMW Fortschritte der Medizin* 144.44 (2002): 41–4.

184 See S. Khosla and L.J. Melton III, "Osteopenia," *New England Journal of Medicine* 356.22 (2007): 2293–3000.

185 See D.M. Kado, T. Duong, K.L. Stone, K.E. Ensrud, M.C. Nevitt, G.A. Greendale, and S.R. Cummings, "Incident Vertebral Fractures and Mortality in Older Women: A Prospective Study," by *Osteoporosis International* 14.7 (2003): 589–94.

186 See M.M. Iqbal, "Osteoporosis: Epidemiology, Diagnosis and Treatment," *Southern Medical Journal* 93.1 (2000): 2–18.

187 See T.M. Keaveny, E.F. Morgan, and O.C. Yeh, "Bone Mechanics," in M. Kutz (ed.), *Standard Handbook of Biomedical Engineering and Design* (New York: McGraw-Hill, 2003), retrieved from http://server0.unhas.ac.id/tahir/BAHAN-KULIAH/BIO-MEDICAL/NEW/HANBOOK/Bone_Mechanics.pdf.

188 See A.H. Burstein, D.T. Reilly, and M. Martens (1976), "Aging of Bone Tissue: Mechanical Properties," *Journal of Bone and Joint Surgery* 58A.1 (1976): 82–6.

189 See S.M. Smith, M.A. Heer, L.C. Shackelford, J.D. Sibonga, L. Ploutz-Snyder, and S.R. Zwart, "Benefits for Bone from Resistance Exercise and Nutrition in Long-duration Spaceflight: Evidence from Biochemistry and Densitometry," *Journal of Bone and Mineral Research* 27.9 (2012): 1896–1906.

190 See Fishman and Saltonstall, *Yoga for Osteoporosis*, 62.

191 Sometimes, but not always. Again, due to the reality of human variation, most people have a synovial joint between the second to seventh ribs and the sternum, while many others have cartilage connecting their first to seventh ribs to the sternum. Imagine the difference if you have cartilaginous joints connecting your ribs to your sternum where most people have synovial joints there, which allow for deeper movements. For you, the movement of your ribcage, involved in breathing deeply, may be much harder than for these other people.

192 See Gray et al., *Gray's Anatomy*, 112.

VOLUME 2
The Lower Body

The Consequences of Human Variation and the Sources of Tension and Compression

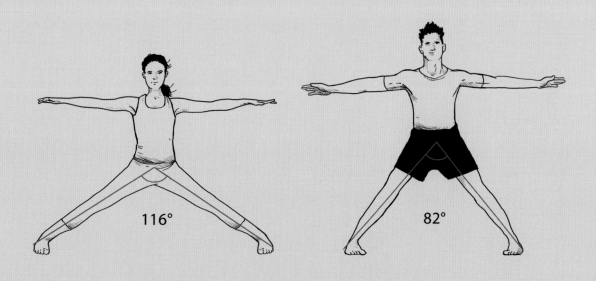

116°   82°

Intentions

How many yoga poses can one person do? Krishnamacharya, often thought to be the grandfather of modern Western yoga, knew 3,000 asanas, but he claimed that his teacher knew 7,000.[1] This was the state of the art back in the 1930s; since then, creative teachers, many with a dance, martial arts or gymnastic background, have continued to develop more and more postures, variations and movements. Perhaps no one knows exactly how many asanas the human body potentially can do, but it clearly is in the tens of thousands. How do we begin to get a grip on understanding what all these asanas are doing to our body—and how do we understand which ones are safe for us and which ones we are better off avoiding?

We can do what all good scientists do: break the problem down into components. Fortunately, while there may be thousands of postures, there are really only a few targeted areas that we need to focus on to understand what we are doing biomechanically during asana practice. We could look at the 850 or so muscles of the body. That would be easier than looking at 7,000 asanas one at a time, but still, 850 is an unreasonably large number. Besides, it is not possible to target each individual muscle on its own. We could group the muscles into major areas, reducing the number we need to analyze. Since all human movements occur at or around a joint, we could simplify the analysis even more by looking only at the major joints of the body. Ten major joints-segments in the body are used and affected by a yoga practice. This is a much more manageable number than 7,000, so our approach will be to look at the possible ranges of motion of each of these 10 joint segments and investigate what allows and what prevents movements at these locations. The 10 joint segments are:

- The Ankle–Foot Segment
- The Knee
- The Hip
- The Sacroiliac
- The Lumbar Spine
- The Thoracic Spine
- The Cervical Spine
- The Shoulder Segment
- The Elbow Segment
- The Wrist–Hand Segment

The first three comprise the lower body joints, which we will explore here in Volume 2. The next four joint areas, consisting of the sacrum to the cervical spine, will be looked at in *Volume 3: The Axial Body*. The final three areas will be investigated in *Volume 4: The Upper Body*. Finally, *Volume 5: Proportions and Asymmetries*, will be dedicated to looking at the relative lengths of the upper, axial and lower body and will examine the frequency and implications of our asymmetries.

Clearly, we have more joints than these 10—we have dozens of joints in our hands and feet alone—but it is not necessary to go into that level of analysis. These 10 joint segments will be sufficient to fully investigate the range of motion our body will move through in our yoga practice, and the restrictions to those movements.

For each joint segment, we will begin by examining the architecture: the shape and structure of its bones, the connective tissue binding the joints, the major ligaments, and the muscles and tendons that serve to articulate, restrain or support the joint. We will look at the average bones often depicted in yoga anatomy books, but we will also look at the range of human variations likely to be present within students in an average class. Based on the structure of the joint and the shape of the bones, we will examine the range of motion available at that joint, the tissues that restrain the possible movements (sources of tension), and where compression may arise that will prevent further movement (sources of compression). The sources of tension and compression will be illustrated for an "average" body but also for a number of people who do not fit the norm. Finally, we will look at what this means for our ability to increase range of motion in a number of yoga postures that require movement in this joint.

Through this process of investigation, you will be able to understand how your unique anatomical structure affects and dictates your yoga. Hopefully, you will be able to identify when no further progress is possible; you may thereby learn to accept and live with the reality and limitations of your own body.

Many readers may want to review only one particular joint segment, and for that reason, the sections are written to stand on their own. However, we will spend more time in the first joint-segment section (the hip joint), explaining the basic concepts of tension, compression and human variation as these manifest in and around a joint. Regardless of which joint segment most interests you, it will be valuable to read the hip-joint section first.

CHAPTER 1
The Bare Bones of Yoga

We examined in Volume 1 the answer to the question, "What stops me?" We have seen that restrictions to our range of motion can come from numerous and diverse sources, not only from short, tight muscles, which most yoga teachers seem to target. Resistance falls into two broad categories: *tension*, where certain tissues resist movement through their reluctance or inability to lengthen or to allow sliding movements; and *compression*, where body parts come into contact with each other and prohibit further movement in a particular direction. Tension can arise due to:

- short muscles
- short, tight fascia that envelops the muscle fibers
- tightness in the fascial bags that envelop the whole muscle group
- fascial restrictions distant from the local muscle group
- nervous system interactions with the muscle, tendon and fascia
- immune system responses that tighten the fascia
- shrink-wrapping of the joint capsule
- contracture of the ligaments and tendons
- water retention in the tissues
- several other factors, including our emotional state of mind

Compression is much simpler, as it is caused by the body coming into contact with the body, which stops movement regardless of any additional muscular efforts applied. Tension can be worked on, and over time reduced, but compression is an ultimate determinant of how far we can go in any particular direction. Sometimes we can go around the point of compression by changing the posture we are in, or by subtly or grossly changing the direction in which we are moving, but ultimately, compression will be reached in most directions. Once you have reached that final point, no further advancement is possible, and to try to go further may cause increasing frustration, not to mention injury.

As mentioned above, many yoga practices and texts identify a single cause of tension that limits progress in a yoga posture: short, tight muscles. Such texts are useful for understanding which muscles support limb articulation and which ones restrict movement around a joint. However, they provide an incomplete picture of what is happening and what is stopping us. They do not show the effects of the anatomical structure of the joint or its surrounding tissues, nor do they allow for the ever-present reality of human variation. This volume addresses the bare bones of yoga asanas, showing you where tension and compression can arise, and how it may manifest differently in different students. Knowing this will help yoga students and teachers understand when further progress is possible and when it is wiser to accept that an ultimate depth in a particular posture has been reached.

The Planes of Movement

A map is a handy device for navigating around unfamiliar landmarks. To use a map, we need to know the cardinal directions—where north is, for example. Normally, a map is a two-dimensional representation of space, but to navigate within our bodies, it is more useful to employ a three-dimensional representation. A 3D map will help us understand how yoga postures move our bodies, and how our unique skeletal variations affect those movements.

In figure 2.1, we see an image of a person depicted in 3D space. She is standing in the *anatomical position*, a term used by anatomists to depict a standard, reference posture. We will return to this term, so it is worth taking time to understand it. In the anatomical position, the body is erect and facing forward, the arms are at the side with the palms turned forward so the thumbs are pointing to the side, and the feet are together. It looks a bit like Mountain Pose (Tadasana) but with the palms facing forward and the feet slightly turned out. Theoretically, of the standing postures, this one requires the least amount of muscular engagement. As we will discover, though, for many people, this is not the most energy-efficient standing posture; due to their unique anatomical structure, they may find it preferable to stand with the feet turned more inward or more outward,

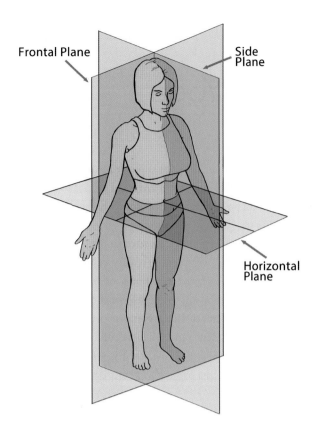

FIGURE 2.1 The anatomical position, with the three planes of the body.

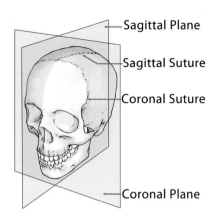

FIGURE 2.2 Two planes of the body are named after sutures in the skull.

the palms rotated more forward or more backward, and the knees more extended or less.

Anatomists have found it useful to describe the body in 3D planes, but they confusingly use several different names for the planes. We will use the simple terms *frontal plane*, *side plane* and *horizontal plane*. The side plane is technically called the *sagittal* plane because it follows a line on the cranium called the *sagittal suture*, which goes from about the middle of the skull to the back of the skull (see figure 2.2). The frontal plane is technically called the *coronal plane* because of a line that goes from one side of the skull to the other, called the *coronal suture*. The horizontal plane is also called the *transverse plane*, but sometimes it is called the *axial* or *transaxial plane*. In short:

- the frontal plane separates front and back
- the side plane separates left and right
- the horizontal plane separates top and bottom

As we will see, though, life is not as simple as pure movement in three planes, because each day, we move in multiple planes at once, often in combination.

THE DIRECTIONS WITHIN THE PLANES

A great number of the strange terms in anatomy have arisen because there are so many directions for movement within the body's three main planes. Sometimes we use different terms, depending upon what part of the body we are focusing on. As shown in figure 2.3, in general, the direction towards the head is called *superior*, while towards the feet is called *inferior*; inferior here does not mean lesser or unimportant, only that it is below. Towards the front of the body is called *anterior*, and towards the back of the body is called *posterior*. Towards the middle of the body is called *medial*, while towards the side of the body is called *lateral*.

You may also come across terms that are used in more localized areas, such as *distal* (which means away from the body's core or trunk) and *proximal* (which means closer to the body's core or trunk). If we move into studying the body's tissues, we may come across terms such as *superficial* (which means more towards the surface) and *deep* or *profound* (which mean more towards the body's center). While standing with our arms at our sides and the palms facing our thighs, we can *pronate* the hands—this means rotating the palms inward and backwards. Relative to the feet, pronation means to move the soles down and out while pointing the foot slightly upward (figure 2.4a). We can also *supinate* the hands or feet by rotating the palms forward (as shown in figure 2.1) or turning the soles inward and up while pointing the feet down (figure 2.4b). Paul Grilley offers a simple way to remember when to say pronate and when to say supinate for hand movements: if you want to become a

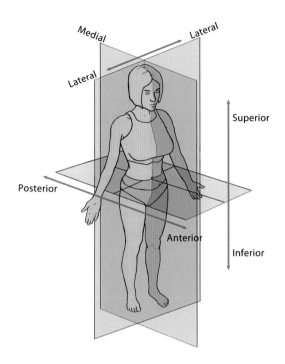

FIGURE 2.3 The main directions.

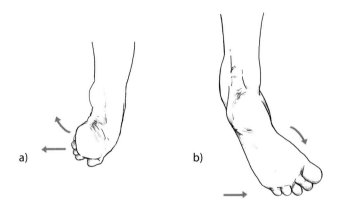

FIGURE 2.4 Pronation (a) and supination (b) of the left foot.

"pro" basketball player, you have to learn to dribble, which requires you to turn your palms towards the floor. That is how you become a pro—by pronating. However, if you are Oliver Twist and you want more "soup" for supper, you have to hold your bowl in your palms, which have been supinated: "Please, Sir, may I have some more soup?"

This is not an exhaustive exploration of the anatomical directions, but it will serve us well enough. (The interested reader can peruse Appendix A: List of Anatomical Directions for a more detailed account of possible movements and directions.) The most common directional terms we will come across in our yoga practice are flexion and extension, abduction and adduction, and internal and external rotation. These terms are applied to movements of the limbs with respect to each other or with respect to our axis, but we can also apply the terms (in a more limited degree) to movements of the body's core.

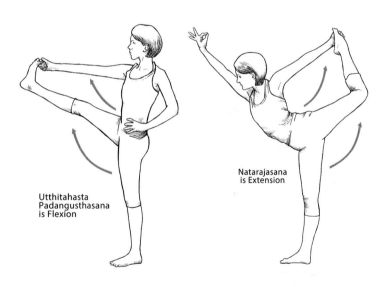

Utthitahasta Padangusthasana is Flexion

Natarajasana is Extension

FIGURE 2.5 Flexion and extension of the limbs.

FLEXION AND EXTENSION

It is simpler first to look at each plane of the body separately and then to define terms for the possible directions of motion. As shown in figure 2.5, in the side plane, if we move an arm or a leg anteriorly (forward), that is termed *flexion*. If we move the limb posteriorly (backwards), that is termed *extension*.

Often, a yoga teacher will tell her class, "Extend your arms up to the sky," which is poetical but not correct to an anatomist. It may seem strange to use the term flexion for raising arms forward and up, but anatomically speaking, it is accurate. Extending the arms means moving the arms backwards. There are typically few anatomists in yoga classes, so most teachers can get away with saying, "Extend your arms up," but better might be: *Raise your arms to the sky.*"

For these two movements as shown in figure 2.5, we keep the torso still, but we could choose to keep the limbs still (see figure 2.6). If we bend the upper body forward, for example as in Dangling Pose (Uttanasana), this is also called flexion at the hips, and to a lesser degree of the spine, even though we have not moved the legs. If we bend the upper body backwards, as we do in Cobra or Sphinx Pose (Bhujangasana), this is still extension, this time of the spine, and to a lesser degree of the hips, for some students.

INTERNAL AND EXTERNAL ROTATION

When we rotate our limbs inwardly in the horizontal plane, this is called *internal rotation* or *medial rotation*. When we rotate our limbs outwardly, that is called *external rotation* or *lateral rotation*. To feel this, stand in Mountain Pose with your heels apart and move your toes towards each other; that is internal rotation of the femur in the hip socket. Move the toes away from each other and the heels together; that is external rotation. Which term we choose is determined by what happens to the more distal segment of the limb—in this case, the foot.

This can also occur in the arms: the humerus can rotate in the shoulder socket. We use internal rotation in Cow Face (Gomukhasana) when we bring one arm down and behind our back. We do this also in binding twists. We use external rotation for the top arm in Cow Face, or when we draw our arms up and back for Wheel Pose (Urdvadhanurasana). In figure 2.7, we see internal and external rotation of the arm at the shoulder for Cow Face, as well as external rotation of both femurs in the hip socket.

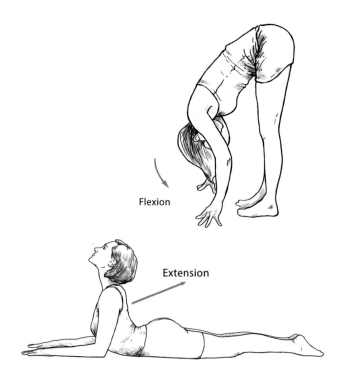

FIGURE 2.6 Flexion and extension of the core of the body.

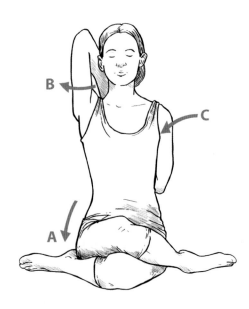

FIGURE 2.7 Cowface pose (Gomukhasana), with external rotation of the legs at the hip joint (a), external rotation of the top arm (b) and internal rotation of the bottom arm (c).

We frequently use external rotation of the arms in the shoulder joint when we come into postures like Down Dog (Adhomukhashvanasana). Athletes also do this when they throw an object, as shown in figure 2.8; a pitcher first externally rotates his arm at the shoulder as much as possible (usually adding some extension of the spine to develop more torque), then flows into internal rotation as he throws the ball.

In figure 2.9, we see a yogi in the pose called Goddess (Utkatakonasana) externally rotating her femurs in the hip socket and externally rotating her arms in the shoulders. In the Eagle Pose (Garudasana), we see her internally rotating her legs while maintaining an external rotation in the arms. It may be hard to understand that the arms are still externally rotated here, because they are wrapped around themselves; but she has kept the external rotation shown in Goddess and simply adducted the arms together. This brings us to the final two movements: abduction and adduction.

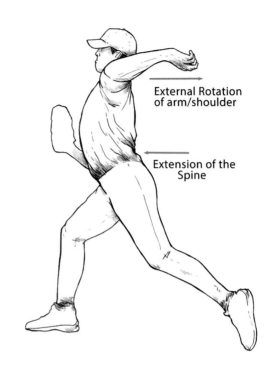

FIGURE 2.8 External rotation of the arm while throwing a ball.

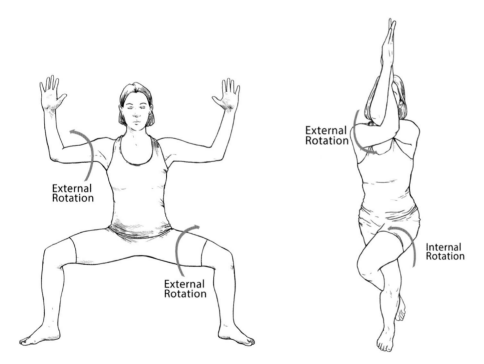

FIGURE 2.9 Both arms and legs are externally rotated in Goddess Pose (left), but the legs are internally rotated in Eagle Pose (right).

ABDUCTION AND ADDUCTION

In the frontal plane (which divides the front and back sides of the body), moving the most distal parts of our limbs laterally, away from the body, is called *abduction*, and moving the limbs medially, towards the body, is called *adduction*. Abduction is like kidnapping: we get abducted, we say goodbye to that part of our body. Adduction is adding the parts of the body together. For the yogi standing in Goddess, with arms and legs spread, the arms are abducted, as are the legs.

This seems simple enough, but again we can hold the limbs still and move the torso. For example, consider the movements when we come into Triangle Pose, as shown in figure 2.10: the top of the pelvis moves down towards the front leg—this is also abduction. Any time the femur and the pelvis come closer together in the frontal plane, abduction occurs, whereas any time they move further apart, adduction is happening. What defines these movements is not only the relationship of the legs to each other, but also their relationship to the pelvis. Either the leg can move in abduction or the pelvis can.

Beyond abduction of the front leg in Triangle Pose, there are other movements in the hip socket, too, such as rotation, but the direction of this rotation depends upon which hip we are looking at. We will examine this in greater detail when we discuss the hip socket and its ranges of movement, but for now, figure 2.10 shows how in Triangle Pose, the front hip joint experiences abduction and a little external rotation, while the back hip joint experiences adduction and some internal rotation.

SIDE FLEXION

Another movement that can occur in the frontal plane is side flexion of the spine. If we move our torso left or right by shifting our pelvis as shown in Triangle (figure 2.10), this is again a form of abduction in the hip socket. However, if we flex only the spine and keep the pelvis still, this is called *side flexion* or *lateral flexion* of the spine. A good example of lateral flexion is the reclining yin yoga posture called Bananasana, or the standard standing Half-Moon Pose (also known as Blown Palm or Ardhachandrasana), shown in figure 2.11.

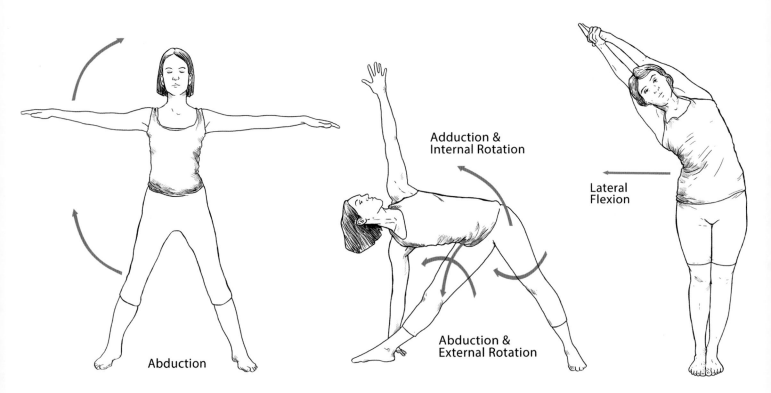

Adduction &
Internal Rotation

Abduction &
External Rotation

Lateral
Flexion

Abduction

FIGURE 2.10 In abduction and adduction, either the legs or the pelvis can move.

FIGURE 2.11 The standing Half-Moon (Ardhachandrasana) involves a lateral flexion of the spine.

HORIZONTAL ABDUCTION

Often, movements occur in more than one plane at a time, which makes it more challenging to understand what is happening biomechanically. Flexion of the leg in the hip socket, combined with abduction, is a common movement in yoga, so a unique name for this movement is used: *horizontal abduction*. We find this in a variety of postures, such as Goddess (see figure 2.12), Tree Pose (Vrksasana) or Straddle Pose (Upavisthakonasana). There are two ways to get to horizontal abduction: by adding abduction to flexion, or by adding external rotation to abduction. Horizontal abduction can happen with the arms in the shoulder joint as well.

PUTTING IT ALL TOGETHER

We have looked at forms of flexion and extension, internal and external rotation, and abduction and adduction in cases where the axis of the body is held still and the limbs move. Now, regard the yogi in Goddess Pose shown in figure 2.12; can you identify all the movements that have occurred here? It is a complicated movement, but when we break it down using the 3D map of the body, we find that there are simple movements in each plane. For both the arms and the legs, we find flexion, abduction and external rotation, all occurring together. Again, we could call this horizontal abduction.

Time for a test to see how well you understand these directions. We will look again at Cowface Pose, as shown in figure 2.13. Now, identify the movements occurring at the hip (A) and the shoulders (B and C). (See the endnote for the answers.[2])

Hopefully, you now understand how your lower body moves, which will be important for understanding what ultimately prevents you from moving further in each of these directions. Technically knowing what we are doing helps us pay attention to what is possible and what limits we have reached.

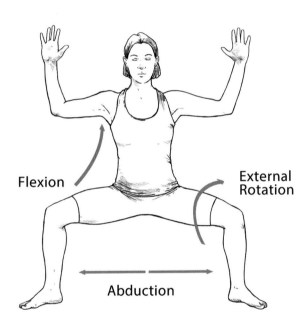

FIGURE 2.12 Goddess is an example of horizontal abduction of the femurs in the hip sockets.

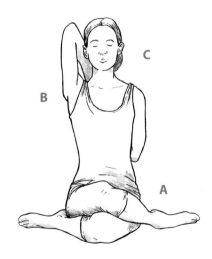

FIGURE 2.13 Cowface: What movements are happening at each joint?

IT'S IMPORTANT: The value of alignment

It makes sense to erect a building starting from the ground up and to work on creating a strong foundation. However, when this idea is applied to our yoga practice, it creates the *fallacy of foundation*. The often taught focus on building your postural foundation from the ground up ignores the simple fact that our body is not a building. We are living systems, not mechanical constructs. In our mother's womb we did not first grow fingers and toes, then feet and hands, then ankles and wrists; we developed from our core outwards. By recognizing the way we grew and developed, we can work towards allowing our postures to manifest in the same fashion—not from the floor up, but from the core out, from proximal to distal.

The positions of the hands and feet are the least important thing happening in a yoga posture, but often they are the most visible part of the pose and thus draw the most attention and modifications. This is not to say that the positions of your hands or feet are unimportant; but these positions are dictated first and foremost by what is happening in your core. A dogmatic assertion that your feet must be parallel and pointing straight ahead ignores the reality of your anatomical uniqueness and the importance of the core, first and foremost. What is happening in your hip sockets is the primary determinant of where your feet will point, followed by the shape of your femur, what is happening at your knees, the shape of your tibia and what is happening at your ankles. To start to structure your posture by beginning with the feet is like the tail wagging the dog: neither efficient nor safe, and greatly annoying to the dog. Unfortunately, it is far easier to see what your extremities are doing than to figure out what is happening in your core. Teachers will spend an inordinate amount of time and attention on the placement of the hands and feet, moving them into some idealized, aesthetically pleasing alignment, without understanding why they were "out of alignment" in the first place. The investigation should actually begin at the core and move outward. Getting this backwards, as many teachers do, risks compromising stability at the core.

There are no universal alignment cues—that is, there are no alignment cues that work for every body. This is not to imply that there are no principles of alignment. However, due to the reality of human variation and your particular anatomical uniqueness, the alignment that works well for one person may not suit you at all. There are *individual* principles of alignment. Our challenge in yoga is to find the alignment that works best for us. As we will soon see, many people need to have their feet pointing outwards in standing yoga postures because their unique biology and biography require this. Forcing these people to look like everyone else will create undue stress in their hips and knees and may make it impossible for them to move through their full, natural range of motion.

Alignment is important! Proper alignment reduces stress in the joints and protects them from dynamically moving into hypermobility, where injury may occur. Good alignment may build architectural stability, minimizing muscular effort and allowing a student to safely linger in a posture. It would be very nice if every posture had alignment cues that worked for every body, and if one medicine would cure every body of cancer. But the reality of human variation teaches us that life is not so idyllic. We are all different, and what works for one person is not guaranteed to work for another. The key question is: What are the alignment cues that work for me?

CHAPTER 2
The Joint Segments of the Lower Body: The Hip Joint

Where should the knee point in standing postures like the Warrior (Virabhadrasana) or in Squats (Malasana)? Where should the feet point? Can everyone do Lotus Pose (Padmasana) safely? Is there always a risk if someone hyperextends the knees or the elbows? We will discover that universal aesthetic cues for alignment fail to protect students from danger in yoga postures. We will also discover that, due to the nature of human variation, an alignment cue that works well for one student may be harmful to another, while another alignment cue thought to be dangerous for all students may be benign or even beneficial for some.

Now, we will begin to investigate the anatomical causes of compression and the consequences of human variation in the lower body, starting from the hip joint, comprised of the pelvis and femur. The pelvis is arguably the body's most complicated set of bones. The hip socket is also located almost exactly in the middle of the body, so the pelvis serves as a great starting place.

It is worth remembering that stress is required for the health of our tissues, including our ligaments and joints. Many aesthetically prohibited alignment positions that look awkward can actually provide healthy stress to a joint. Refraining from those alignments may rob students from healthy stresses. Of course, for some students, too much stress can occur in the same alignment that benefits another student. We have to remain aware of how much stress is occurring and judge wisely whether it is healing or hurting the body.

Form

A joint is a joining of two or more bones, and at the hip joint, the pelvis and femur meet. Technically, the hip joint is referred to as a ball-and-socket joint. The ball of the femur can spin, roll or slide in the cup of the hip socket. Alternatively, if we hold the femur still, the hip socket can move over the ball of the femur. In yoga, we find times when either the pelvis is still and the femur moves or the femur can be held still and the pelvis moves.

To understand the hip joint and its possible ranges of movement, we need to investigate the unique shapes and structures of the pelvis and femur. We can look at these bones separately at first, but eventually we will have to bring them together and see how their shapes affect the function of the hip joint.

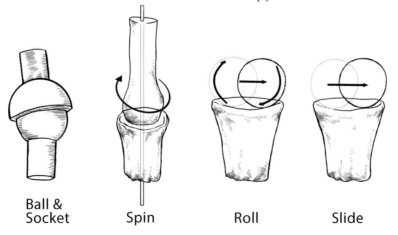

Ball & Socket   Spin   Roll   Slide

FIGURE 2.14 The hip joint is a ball-and-socket joint that allows spin (in flexion and extension), roll and a bit of sliding (in abduction/adduction and external/internal rotation).

THE ARCHITECTURE OF THE HIP JOINT

The word "hip" is problematic from an anatomical perspective. It is sometimes used to refer to the top of the pelvis, where people often rest their "hands on their hips." This "hip bone" is anatomically called the *ilium* (from the Latin for flank or groin: the plural is *ilia*). The top of the ilium is called the *iliac crest* (see figures 2.15 and 2.16.) Sometimes people will feel the greater trochanter of the femur and refer to this as their hip (see figure 2.17). For our purposes, we will define "hip joint" as where the femur and pelvis join at the hip socket. Unless the context obviously refers to the trochanter or the crest of the ilium, anytime we refer to the hips or movement of the hips, we will mean movement at the hip joint or hip socket. Another anatomical term that we will use interchangeably for the hip socket is *acetabulum*.

THE BONES OF THE HIP JOINT

The Pelvis

The word *pelvis* comes from the Latin for a basin or bowl, and that is a great description for this complex bone (see figures 2.15 and 2.16). The top bowl is sometimes referred to as the *greater* (or *false*) *pelvis*, while the bottom bowl is called the *lesser* (or *true*) *pelvis* (see figure 2.18). The function of the pelvis is manifold: it supports, protects and contains our viscera, it provides a broad attachment base for the muscles that move our legs and hips, but even more importantly, it supports the weight of our upper body. The pelvis is actually made up of several bones that have become fused together or joined by ligaments: the sacrum, and the two "hip bones" (also called the *coxal* bones, from the Latin *coxa*, which means hip). Each of the coxal bones in turn consists of three bones fused together—the ilium, pubis and ischium.

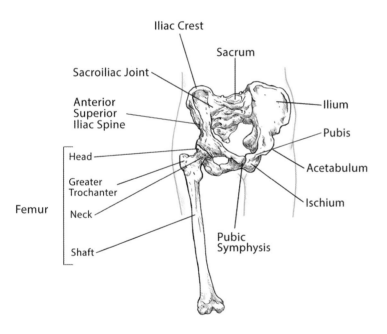

FIGURE 2.15 An oblique view of the pelvis and femur.

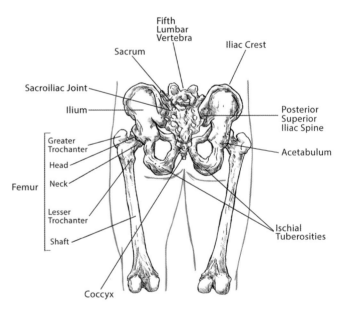

FIGURE 2.16 Posterior view of the pelvis and femur.

In total, seven bones have fused or joined to form the pelvis. At birth, the individual bones are neither fully formed nor fully fused; they are mostly cartilage. By around 15 years of age, their cartilage has ossified into bone, and the fusion of the three bones has been completed. The site of their joining forms the acetabulum (see figure 2.19).[3] In the front of the pelvis, the two coxal bones are connected through the *pubic symphysis*, which is a fibrocartilaginous joint. In the back, the two coxal bones join with the sacrum via the *sacroiliac* joint, which is a slightly articulating, gliding synovial joint. The pubic symphysis, being joined via cartilage, does not allow much movement between the two coxal bones, but some slight motion is possible, especially for women who are approaching the end of a pregnancy; at that time, the cartilage softens, allowing a bit more movement to assist with widening the lower pelvic bowl so that the baby's head can pass through. The sacroiliac joint allows more movement than the pubic symphysis, but the normal range of motion there is small, varying between none to around 15° of nodding.[4] (We look at the movement of the sacrum in *Volume 3: The Axial Body*.)

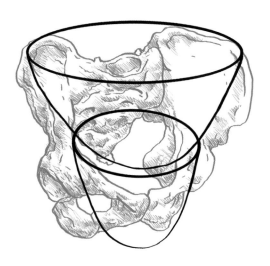

FIGURE 2.18 The pelvic bowls. The pelvis can be viewed as two bowls stacked on top of each other: the greater bowl on top (the false pelvis) and the lesser bowl underneath (the true pelvis).

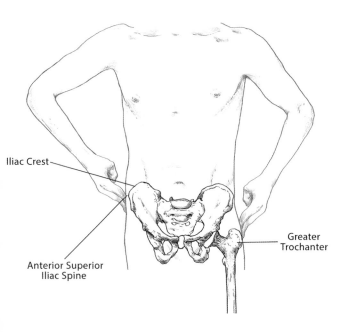

FIGURE 2.17 Palpating the greater trochanter and anterior superior iliac spine

Iliac Crest

Anterior Superior Iliac Spine

Greater Trochanter

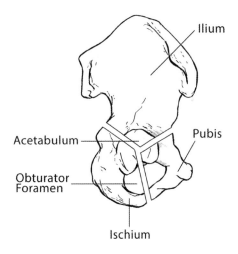

Ilium

Acetabulum

Pubis

Obturator Foramen

Ischium

FIGURE 2.19 The coxal bones. Each is made up of three bones that grow together, forming the hip socket, known as the acetabulum.

Landmarks of the Pelvis

To understand how movement occurs at the hip joint, it is useful to recognize several key anatomical landmarks. While drawings of the pelvis and femur typically show many features, the key points we will refer to constantly are the acetabulum (hip socket), the anterior superior iliac spine (called the ASIS, for short), the head of the femur (sometimes called the ball of the femur), the neck of the femur, and the greater trochanter. Both the greater trochanter and the ASIS can be easily palpated; if you stand with "your hands on your hips," you can feel the ASIS with your forefinger and the posterior superior iliac spine (PSIS) with your thumb. Alternatively, as shown in figure 2.20, you can touch the front and back of your pelvis to find these two landmarks. Sliding your hand slightly down the thigh, you will come to the large boney prominence of the greater trochanter, as shown in figure 2.17. The ischial tuberosities are also easily palpated; they are the famous sitting bones—just reach under your buttocks, towards the anus, and feel the bony prominences there.

The Femur

The femur, the longest and strongest bone in our body, is not nearly as complicated a bone as the pelvis, but it too has unique twists and turns. The twist along the shaft of the femur is called *femoral torsion*,[5] and the turn, occurring between the shaft and the neck of the femur, is called the *femoral neck-shaft angle*, or *neck angle* for short.[6] The femur's torsion and neck angle help determine the ultimate potential range of hip-joint motion for a variety of movements.

In figure 2.22 we see a standard representation of a femur. The key proximal landmarks to note are the head of the femur (which fits into the acetabulum of the pelvis), the neck of the femur, the greater trochanter, the shaft of the femur, and the lesser trochanter. We will look at the distal end of the femur in more detail when we investigate the knee joint. The head of the femur (sometimes called the ball) makes up almost two-thirds of a sphere, but it is slightly ovoid rather than perfectly spherical. It matches the curve of the acetabulum quite closely, allowing the femur head to roll and spin; sometimes, this requires a bit of sliding as well.

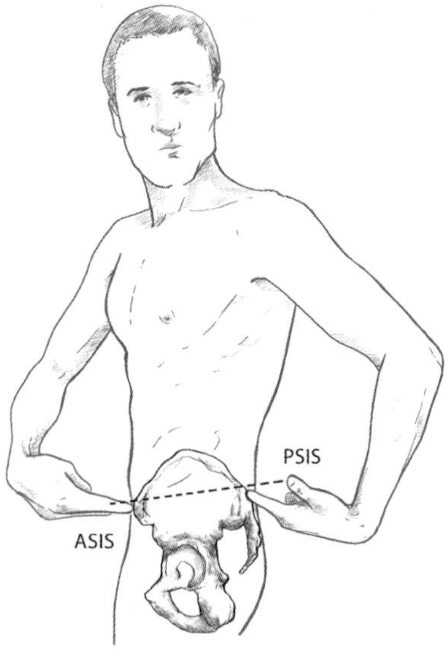

FIGURE 2.20 A side view of the pelvis. Note how the pelvis appears rotated when we are standing; however, this is its natural position. The crest of the ilium is above the ischial tuberosities.

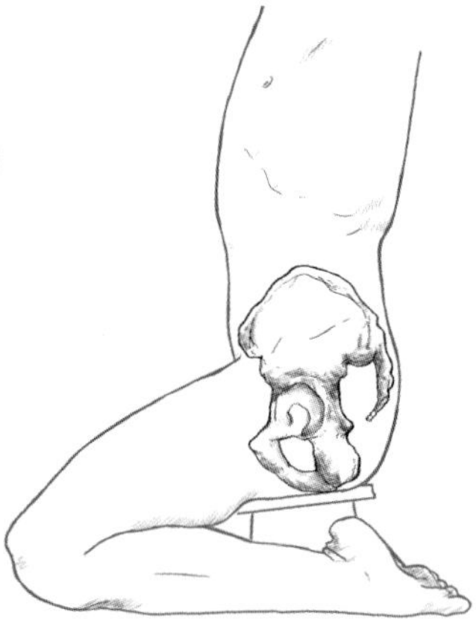

FIGURE 2.21 Side view of the pelvis when sitting. If we are not slouching, the orientation of the pelvis remains vertical.

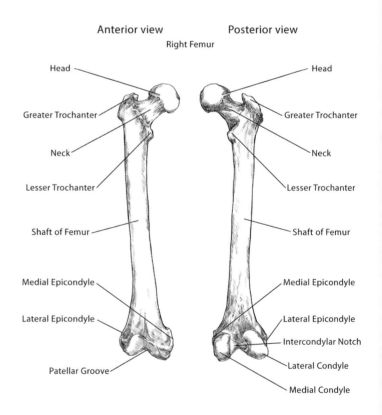

FIGURE 2.22 The femur: a frontal and posterior view.

THE HIP-JOINT CAPSULE AND LIGAMENTS

The femur is bound to the pelvis by five capsular ligaments surrounding and inside the synovial joint capsule of the hip joint. The names of these ligaments come from the bones to which they attach:

- the *iliofemoral* ligament (which joins the femur to the ilium), one of the thickest and strongest ligaments in our body;
- the *ischiofemoral* ligament (which joins the femur to the ischium);
- the *pubofemoral* ligament (which joins the femur to the pubis);
- the *ligamentum* of the femur's head, also called the *ligamentum teres* (which joins the femur to the acetabulum);
- the *transverse ligament of the acetabulum*, which creates a bottom shelf reinforcing the inferior rim of the labrum (not shown in the diagrams, but it is the inferior portion of the joint capsule)

The arrangement of the fibers of the first three ligaments are key in restricting movements (see figure 2.23). They are jointly called the *capsular ligaments* and reinforce the joint capsule in a variety of directions:

- the **iliofemoral** ligament is the strongest of the three. It reinforces the anterior and superior portions of the joint capsule and can limit external rotation and extension. We will often consider it as two ligaments, because the different fibers (superior and anterior) can respond differently to stress;
- the **pubofemoral** ligament reinforces the anterior and inferior part of the capsule, limiting abduction and extension;
- the **ischiofemoral** ligament reinforces the posterior capsule, can limit extension and internal rotation, and—if the hip is flexed—can also limit adduction.[7]

Not surprisingly, not all experts agree upon the individual functions of these ligaments! Some researchers feel that external rotation is not limited by the ligaments at all, while internal rotation is most strongly limited.[8] The role of the ligamentum teres is still being debated;[9] it can contribute a minimal amount of resistance to the movements of adduction, flexion and external rotation, but its main function seems to be as an anchor for the femur into the center of the acetabulum—and, in youth, as a pathway for blood vessels to the head of the femur (see figure 2.24).[10]

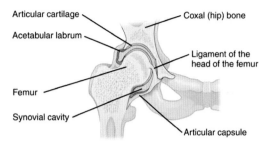

(a) Frontal section through the right hip joint

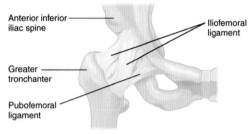

(b) Anterior view of right hip joint, capsule in place

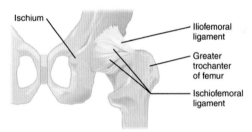

(c) Posterior view of right hip joint, capsule in place

FIGURE 2.23 Ligaments and joint capsule of the hip joint. The most important ligaments in terms of restricting range of movement at the hip are the iliofemoral, ischiofemoral and pubofemoral.

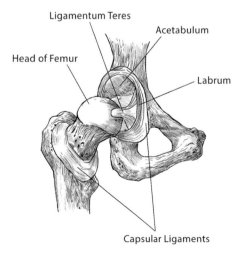

FIGURE 2.24 The ligamentum teres tightens in flexion, adduction and internal rotation but contributes relatively little to the stability of the joint.

THE MUSCLES OF THE HIP

The muscles that create motion at the hip joint are shown in figure 2.25. Flexion is usually caused by the front hip flexors: the psoas, iliacus, rectus femoris, tensor fasciae latae and sartorius. Extension is usually caused by the big buttock muscle and back leg muscles: the gluteus maximus and hamstrings. Abduction is usually caused by the abductor muscles on the outside of the hips: gluteus medius, gluteus minimus and tensor fasciae latae. Adduction is usually caused by the adductor muscles on the inner thigh: adductor magnus, adductor longus, adductor brevis, gracilis, and pectineus. External rotation is usually caused by the obturator internus and externus, gemellus superior and inferior, quadratus femoris, piriformis and gluteus maximus. We are using the term "usually" because it is not always clear which muscles are creating which movements. (See It's Complicated: Which muscles cause which movement can vary.)

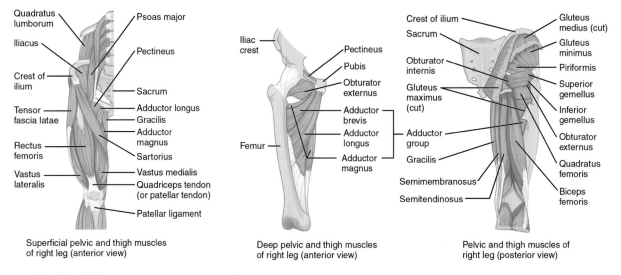

Superficial pelvic and thigh muscles of right leg (anterior view)

Deep pelvic and thigh muscles of right leg (anterior view)

Pelvic and thigh muscles of right leg (posterior view)

FIGURE 2.25 The muscles affecting the hip joint.

IT'S COMPLICATED:
Which muscles cause which movement can vary

We used the word "usually" to describe which muscles cause which movement, but the effect of each muscle can depend upon the orientation of the femur in the acetabulum, the orientation of the body with respect to gravity, the history of the student, and which muscles he habitually uses. One study noted that human variation, which can also affect the proximal and distal attachment sites of the muscles, can change the action of these muscles. For example, the researchers noted that a bigger iliac crest that moves the origin of the gluteus medius anteriorly will create greater internal rotation at the hips.[11] Other anatomists describe muscles that many people do not have; for example, 27% of people have a psoas minor, which assists in flexing the lumbar and side-bending the pelvis, but 73% of people do not have this muscle.[12] Also, when we focus only on the muscles as the cause of movement, we are ignoring the fascia's important role in generating, transmitting and distributing forces. Thus, we cannot make definitive statements that work for all people about which muscles cause which movements. However, we can make a few generalizations about movements occurring from the anatomical position. Please remember, though, that these are simplifying generalizations, and no body works so simply.

THE TYPES AND RANGES OF VARIATIONS

Variations of the Pelvis

All we have to do is look at two people and we can tell that their pelvises are quite different. One person may have a very wide pelvis, while the other has a very slender one. The differences may seem obvious between men and women, but some researchers feel that the data do not support the notion that the average woman's pelvis is wider than the average man's! And of course, within the genders are great ranges of variations for the pelvis and the femur; there are individual cases where men have wider pelvises than women, and vice versa. Several of the differences in pelvises will not affect the range of motion available in one's yoga practice, but a few key differences will have a big effect on whether you can do certain asanas or not. Some differences are so extreme that simple, everyday activities, such as walking or running, are compromised. These extreme variations are usually noticed early in life by a family doctor, and in such cases, some help is typically offered to assist with normalizing the ranges of motion and quality of life. Our investigation will look at the variations that are much more common but still impact how far someone can move in various postures.

TYPICAL GENDER DIFFERENCES

The two pelvises shown in figure 2.26 are noticeably different. The standard differences often pointed out are the widths between the ischial tuberosities (the angle formed is called the *subpubic angle*—see figure 2.27), the verticality of the ilium, the curvature of the coccyx, and the roundness of the pelvic inlet circle. All these features relate to women's ability to bear and birth children. Men's pelvises do not need that particular function, but through our species' evolution, men developed the ability to run, and their pelvises became shaped to enhance running speed and endurance. However, due to natural variations in human anatomy, there are women who have narrower subpubic angles, more like the average man's pelvis, and there are men who have much broader subpubic angles, similar to an average woman's. These variations can have a big impact on, for example, whether a woman has to deliver a baby vaginally or requires a Caesarean section. (See Appendix B: Variations in the Female Pelvis.)

The two pelvises shown in figure 2.26 illustrate average shapes, but no one is exactly average; everyone's pelvis differs from these depictions. Those variations can be trivial or extremely important. For example, the wider the base between the ischial tuberosities, the more stability will be available when we are doing sitting yoga postures, like the Boat Pose (Navasana).

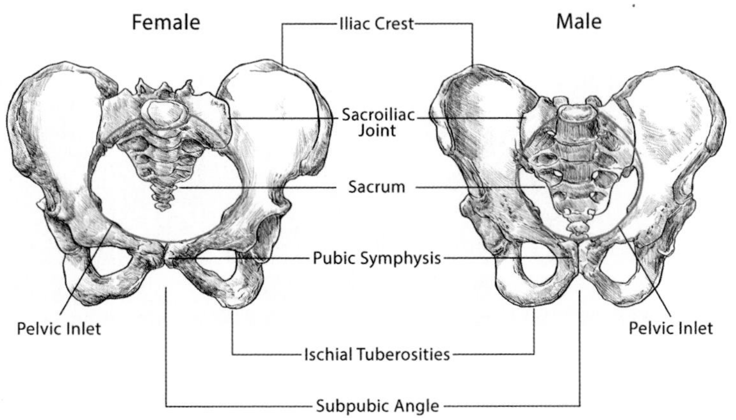

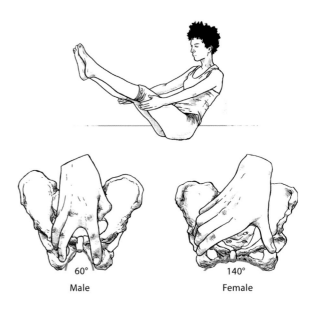

FIGURE 2.27 Subpubic angles. The width between left and right ischial tuberosities (which ranges from 9 to 15 cm)[13] creates the subpubic angle. This angle can vary from 75° to 155° for women (shaped like an inverted margarita glass), and from 50° to 140° in men (shaped more like an inverted martini glass.)[14] The wider the sitting bones, the broader the base, the more stability is provided for sitting postures such as Boat Pose (Navasana).

FIGURE 2.26 Comparing female and male pelvises. Generally, the female pelvis appears broader and shallower than the male pelvis, which appears narrower and taller.

ORIENTATION AND SHAPE OF THE ACETABULUM

The key variations that can affect our mobility and range of motion include (i) the angles of the acetabulum relative to the three planes of the body, (ii) the shape of the acetabulum (including its size, roundness and depth) and (iii) the verticality of the anterior pelvic plane. It is worth pointing out that our bodies are not symmetric: the features found on one side of the pelvis, such as the depth of the acetabulum or its position relative to the rest of the pelvis, are not the same on the other side. Consequently, we do not have the same range of motion in our left and right hip joints.

Note the outline of a pelvis in figure 2.28. The first drawing (a) has a frontal view of the hip joint and illustrates the orientation of the plane of the acetabulum to a horizontal line. This is called the *acetabular angle of abduction* and is here labeled α.[15] The second drawing (b), with a horizontal view of the hip joint from above, shows the angle (labeled β) between the inlet plane of the acetabulum and the side (sagittal) plane of the body. This is called the *version of the acetabulum*.[16] An acetabulum pointing straight out to the side or backwards is referred to as *retroverted*; one pointing forward is called *anteverted*. Both of these angles determine how much range of motion is available in the hip joint. Remember, this is only one pelvis, and yours is probably different.

ACETABULAR ABDUCTION ANGLE

The size of the abduction angle affects our ability to abduct our legs, such as in the side splits. It changes as we grow: from 51° at birth, to 45° by 10 years of age, to 40° as an adult.[18] (Young gymnasts can do the splits more easily than their older colleagues.) By itself this creates the impression that everyone, when they become adults, will have an acetabular abduction of 40°. However, this is deceptive. The statistics cited are averages, and the range of human variation is quite dramatic. So, your value is most likely not the average. (A note to yoga teachers: most of the students in your yoga classes are not average either!) Tables 2.1 and 2.2 show the ranges observed in several studies; these illustrate how studies can vary and thus the danger of taking any one study to be representative of the whole population. Indeed, the average of all these averages is actually 43.5°! While we will stick to an average abduction angle of 40°, please bear in mind that it is very difficult to say what is normal.

TABLE 2.1 Ranges of acetabular abduction.[19]

	MALES	**FEMALES**	**AVERAGE**
Study 1	28–42°	28–42°	37.5°
Study 2	36–43°	37–47°	40.5°
Study 3	48–66°	51–67°	56.5°
Study 4	29–57°	35–45°	39.5°

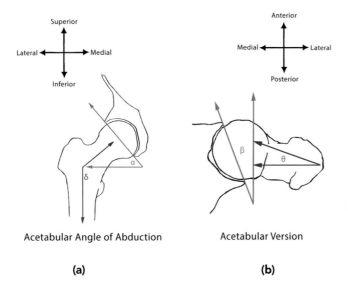

Acetabular Angle of Abduction **(a)**

Acetabular Version **(b)**

FIGURE 2.28 Orientation of the acetabulum. (a) The angle (α) between the acetabular inlet plane and a horizontal line is called the *acetabular angle of abduction*. (b) The angle (β) between the acetabular inlet plane and the side plane of the body, denoted by the sagittal plane, is termed the *acetabular version*. δ is the *femoral neck-shaft angle*, and θ is the *femoral anteversion angle*.

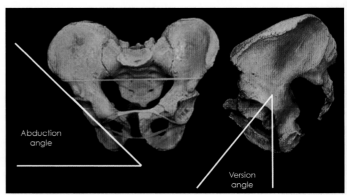

FIGURE 2.29 Abduction and version angles of the acetabula.[17]

Really large variations from the average value can cause problems. Your abduction angle may predispose you to more or less wear and tear in the hip socket. If your abduction angle is 40°, you will have the least amount of wear, but if your angle is over 50°, you will probably have the greatest rate of wear, which may result in *osteolysis*: a wearing away of the hip socket.[20] ("May" does not mean "will": there are many conditions that can increase or decrease bone erosion.) At angles above 50° there is also a tendency for the femur to dislocate and pop out from the acetabulum. On the other hand, angles of less than 30° may lead to impingement problems while flexing the hips. (Note: we will sometime use the term *impingement* when we talk about a bone hitting some part of the body; this is just another example of compression.) To learn more about femoral impingement with the acetabulum, see It's Complicated: Femoral acetabular impingement syndrome, on page 149.

For our purposes, we can use the average value of 40°, but the two standard deviations from these studies give us a range of 31° to 48° for 95% of the population.[21] This means that 5% (or one student out of 20) will be outside this range.

ACETABULAR ANTEVERSION

We have been discussing the acetabular angle of abduction in isolation. When we also consider the version angle of the acetabulum, it can change the consequences of the abduction angle. For example: a 45–55° abduction angle could provide the hip with a better overall range of motion and stability if it were combined with enough acetabular anteversion.[22] The range of version also changes as we age: from 7° at birth to about 21° as an adult, after which there is no change (unless through accidents or pathologies). As we will see, this angle affects our ability to externally or internally rotate the femur in the hip socket.

TABLE 2.2 Ranges of Acetabular Version[23]

MALES	FEMALES	AVERAGE
11–21°	12–24°	17°
13–24°	14–28°	20°
16–28°	18–28°	23°
8.5–32°	14–33°	22°
14–24°	18–29°	21°

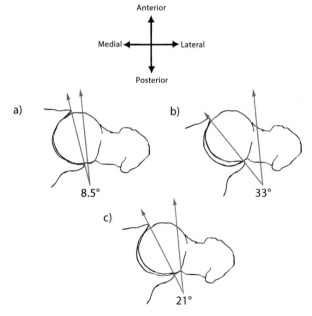

FIGURE 2.31 Acetabular version ranges: (a) is the lowest abduction angle found in Table 2.1; (b) is the highest angle; (c) is an often cited average angle.

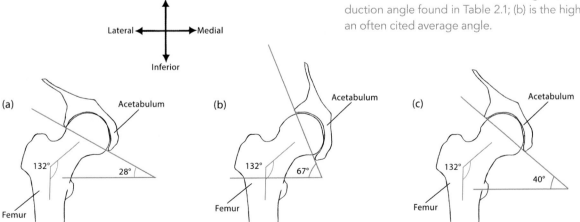

FIGURE 2.30 Abduction angle ranges: (a) is the lowest abduction angle found in Table 2.1; (b) is the highest angle; (c) is an often cited average angle.

Several anatomy textbooks cite a standard average value of 17° for the version angle. However, our examples will use the average of the above five studies, which is 21° with a two standard deviation range of 10° to 33°.[24] Note again, the important point is not which angle is correct; there is too much variation in the studies to dogmatically say "this is the right angle." The important point is that all the studies show a large range of values. That is the reality of human variation. Unfortunately, seeing one drawing in an anatomy book may lock a person into thinking that everyone has that angle: they don't.

Depending upon the orientation of your acetabulum, you may naturally be a good straight-ahead sprinter or you might be better at sports requiring lateral movements. If you have a higher anteversion, meaning your hip sockets face more forward, you are better aligned for sprinting. However, your ability to make quick lateral cuts to the side will be curtailed. If you have a low anteversion, you are better able to externally rotate at the hips (and do Lotus Pose—Padmasana), but at the expense of straight-ahead maximum speed. Hockey players and football middle linebackers require lower anteversion, while cyclists, sprinters and marathoners tend to do better with higher anteversion. There is another benefit to lower anteversion angles: less chance of tearing the ligamentum teres (the ligament that holds the ball of the femur snugly in the acetabulum).[25]

ACETABULAR DEPTH

The depth of the acetabulum is also highly variable and can affect both our range of motion and the degree of wear in the hip socket. While there is some correlation between gender and acetabulum depth, the correlation is mostly an effect of the relationship between total body height and hip socket depth. (We often find that what at first appears to be a distinct gender difference instead turns out to be due more to height or weight than to gender.) The depth can vary from 16 to 24 mm, but as always, there are people outside these reported ranges.[26] This is also reported as a percentage: the depth of the acetabulum divided by its width, times 100. The average ratio in one study was 33.8% for women and 34.8% for men, with one standard deviation of about 3.50%.[27] The degree of shallowness is correlated with osteoarthritis. If the acetabulum is too shallow, the amount of surface that supports the weight of the body is smaller and therefore subject to more stress.[28] However, a deeper hip socket may lead to less arthritis, and it generally yields a more restricted range

of movement.[29] So, those who have shallower acetabula, and thus a greater possible range of motion in the hip socket than people with deeper sockets, will be more likely to develop osteoarthritis in that hip socket. Greater flexibility does not always imply greater health!

We have been considering the bone forming the hip socket purely in isolation. However, the bony ridge that forms the acetabulum is covered by a cartilage lip called a labrum.[30] (See figure 2.93.) It deepens the hip socket, allowing for more solid contact between the femur and the pelvis. The labrum also helps to maintain a vacuum seal between the femur and the pelvis. This extra depth to the acetabulum created by the labrum can also restrict the range of movement available—and sometimes, if the labrum is too thick, it pinches in, causing impingement problems. (We look at this "pincer" in more detail later, in It's Complicated: Femoral acetabular impingement syndrome, on page 149.)

THE ANTERIOR PELVIC PLANE

We often tilt the pelvis when we practice yoga asana. For example, as we move our spine up and down doing Cats (also called Cat-Cow), we rotate our hips from an anterior tilt (in Upward-Facing Cat) to posterior tilt (in Downward-Facing Cat). But what is the neutral position for the pelvis, where it is in neither posterior nor anterior tilt? To answer that, we have to look at the pelvis in the side plane, where the tilting movement occurs.

The anterior pelvic plane, as shown in figure 2.32, is formed by the anterior superior iliac spine (ASIS) and the pubic symphysis. This plane was generally thought to lie within the body's frontal (coronal) plane when we are standing in the anatomical position. It was long believed that every body has a perfectly vertical anterior pelvic plane. However, even here, variations occur: while the range of variation is not related to gender, for 38% of people, the plane is inclined 5° forward of vertical, while 13% of people have a 10° or larger inclination.[31] One study found the anterior pelvic plane averaged 6.9° forward of vertical, with one standard deviation of 9.2; this would mean 95% of people having pelvis angles varying between 25.3° forward (this is called anteversion of the pelvis and means the ASIS juts forward) and 11.5° backwards (called retroversion of the pelvis). The range of total variation was 49.1°.[32]

The anterior pelvic plane is not a reliable indicator of whether or not a pelvis is tucked. Surgeons preparing to perform a hip replacement operation orient the pelvis using the slope of the sacrum, because it is a reliable indicator of pelvic alignment. With the sacrum fixed in this neutral position, many people have a forward projection of the ASIS. This variation, which occurs in almost half of the population, means that the ASIS is projecting forward from a nominally vertical position, which has an important implication for how frequently impingement of the pelvis to the thighs occurs in forward folding. It also makes questionable the instruction to bring one's hips into neutral. If every yoga student aligns her anterior pelvic plane vertically, almost half of the students will have done some degree of pelvic tucking, dropping the sacrum past vertical. If the pelvis is neither tucked nor tilted forward, some students will have their ASIS ahead of their pubic symphysis—and that is the way they are built.

SPOTTING THE IMPORTANT DIFFERENCES IN PELVISES

Now that we know what to look for in evaluating variations of the pelvis, check out the two pelvises in figure 2.33. What differences can you see? Many may catch your eye—such as the width between the ASIS, or the width of the pubic arches—but look at the acetabula. Notice in the top pictures how the pelvis in the frontal view has the left acetabulum rotated more forward than the right. The left and right sides of (a) are not symmetrical: the left is anteverted more than the right. Compare the acetabula in (a) to the those in (b), which are not visible at all! In (b), the acetabula are retroverted. Look now at the side views and what do you see? Again, we could note the differences in the shape and prominence of the iliac spines, how the pubis in (b) is much more forward, the curve and thickness of the sacrum, but focus on the acetabula. In (a), the left acetabulum is anteverted significantly compared to in (b), but from this view we also see that its angle of abduction is much smaller. The acetabulum in (b) is almost pointing horizontally, while (a) has the acetabulum pointing forward and down.

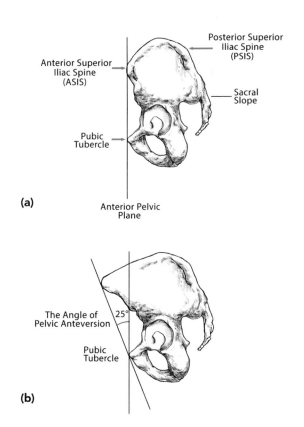

FIGURE 2.32 The anterior pelvic plane is formed by the points of the anterior superior iliac spines and pubic tubercle: (a) shows a vertical plane; (b) shows an anteverted plane.

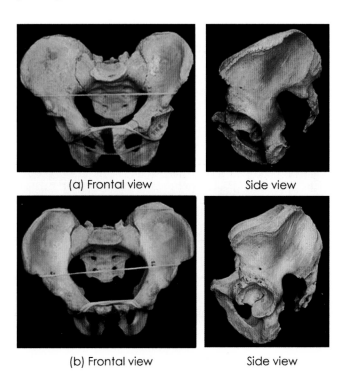

FIGURE 2.33 Comparing two pelvises. Notice the differences and decide which pelvis will allow greater range of motion for external rotation and abduction.

If we assume that the femurs for these two people were exactly the same (which of course they were not), which person would have had the greater potential range of motion for abduction and external rotation? The answer is (b): with the increased angle of abduction of the acetabulum, there is more room to raise the leg out to the side before compression is reached, and with greater retroversion (or less anteversion), there is more room to externally rotate the leg before compression occurs. However, in the opposite directions, (a) would have more potential for internal rotation and adduction than (b).

Variations of the Femur

FEMORAL NECK-SHAFT ANGLE

The angle between the shaft of the femur and its neck (illustrated in figure 2.28) varies considerably by age, ethnic background, and the amount of childhood activity, but not by gender.[33] At birth, the neck of the femur is almost in line with the shaft, usually forming an angle of about 160°.[34] As a child begins to crawl, then walk, stress is placed on the neck of the femur, causing it to bend over time. If the child is very active—for example, at levels often found in developing agrarian societies—the angle becomes sharper. If the child is

raised in a very sedate setting, perhaps spending most of the day sitting at school or in front of a computer screen or television, then the angle will be wider.[35] A relationship has also been noted between the overall length of the femur and the neck angle: the longer the femur, the wider the neck angle, implying that longer-bodied people will have larger femur neck-shaft angles.[36] Despite these findings, the relationship is an average one and may not apply to your body! Various pathologies, such as rickets or polio, can affect the neck-shaft angle. By puberty, this angle is fixed for the rest of your life (barring disease, injury or accident), and yoga is not going to change it.

There is a considerable range for the neck angle (see figure 2.34). For people of European descent living in North America, the angle ranges from 118° to 150°. Only half of this population falls into the narrower range of 130–140°, so there is a 50/50 chance that someone may be outside this range. The two standard deviation range is 120–144° (which means 95% of people are within this range). Many anatomy books cite the average to be around 126°,[37] but one extensive survey found that different cultures had different averages, ranging from 122° to 136°, and normal individuals (i.e., those with no pathology or deformities) were found within the range of 110–150°.[38] So, what is "normal" is not obvious. Despite the indications from this survey, generally if the angle is less than 120°, it is termed *coxa vara*, while if it is

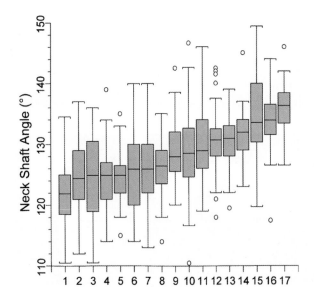

FIGURE 2.34 The range of femoral neck angles by population types. The numbers along the bottom axis represent different populations, from #1 = South Africans to #17 = modern Chinese. Modern North-East Americans of European descent are at #15 and range from 118° to 150°, while 50% of this population is between 130° and 140°.[41] The average is 132°.

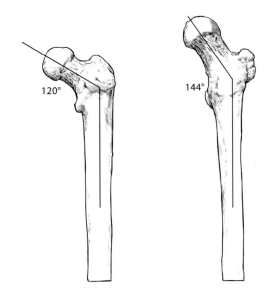

FIGURE 2.35 Femur neck angles can vary greatly depending upon ethnicity and childhood activity. The wider the angle, the greater the potential is for abduction at the hip socket.

above 135° it is sometimes called *coxa valga*; doctors consider both abnormalities, despite how commonly they occur.[39] There is a tendency, even in the medical community, to view variation as abnormality, but sometimes it is natural to be different.[40]

Visually the differences are striking. Figure 2.35 shows two femurs: one with a neck angle of 120°, which is the low value found in North Americans, and the other with an angle of 144°, which is near the high end of the range. We will look later at how the range of abduction of the leg will not be the same for these two people.

Curiously, the study cited above showed that there is no gender variation in the neck angle of the femur! Any sexual differences were small and inconsistent. The researchers did find a range of asymmetry between left and right femurs, but they were unable to determine why; it was not always related to the dominant leg.

It is not unusual for one femur to have an angle of 5° more or less than the other. For yoga teachers, this is an important observation, as it means that you probably can abduct one leg a little more than the other. The femur with the larger neck-shaft angle will be more easily abducted and thus can become your "good side" for demonstrating abduction.

FEMORAL TORSION

The next important variation in our femurs comes from the torsion, or twist, along the shaft. Every long bone in our body has a slight rotation to it. This is noticeable if we place femurs on a table top so that the distal condyles (the "knees") are

sitting flat, and then notice the angle the neck of the femur makes in relation to the table top (or the distance from the table to the ball of the femur). Figure 2.36 shows several femurs with very different degrees of torsion (this is depicted in figure 2.28 by the angle θ). We call this twisting *femoral anteversion*. If there is only a small twist, no twist, or a negative amount of twist, it is called *femoral retroversion*. In general, and all other things being equal, people with less torsion of the femur will find it easier to externally (laterally) rotate their femur in the hip socket (think Lotus Pose—Padmasana), while those with higher torsion will find it harder to externally rotate but easier to internally rotate (think Eagle Pose—Garudasana).

The degree of anteversion (increased angle) or retroversion (decreased angle) will contribute to the natural position of the feet. However, where your feet point is not determined by only one factor; it is far more complicated than that. The degree of version of your acetabula, the torsion in your femurs and the torsion in your tibias all contribute to where your feet "should" point when you are standing in a neutral, relaxed posture. We will look at the proper alignment for the feet in standing yoga postures after we look at the tibia in more detail. But for now, in figure 2.37 we can see that, all other things being equal, the anteversion angles of the acetabulum and femur will tend to cause the feet to either "toe in," pigeon-toed like (called *coxa anteverta*), or "toe out," duck-feet like (called *coxa retroverta*).[42] Again, to really tell where the feet naturally point, we also have to consider what happens at the knee joint, the torsion of the tibia, and the orientation of the ankle, which we will look at in later sections.

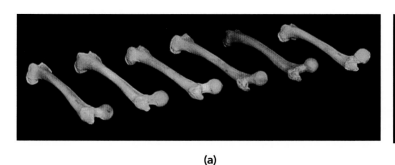

(a)

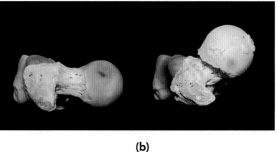

(b)

FIGURE 2.36 Comparing femoral torsion: (a) shows six femurs with varying angles of femoral anteversion; (b) shows the two largest variations: the femur on the left has a negative anteversion of −4° and will find external rotation relatively easy, while the femur on the right has an anteversion of 47° and will find internal rotation relatively easy.

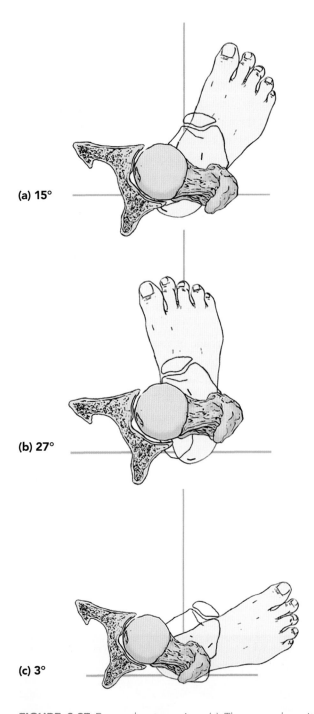

(a) 15°

(b) 27°

(c) 3°

FIGURE 2.37 Femoral anteversion. (a) The normal position of the foot of someone with an average amount of femoral anteversion (15°), in an average hip socket (acetabular anteversion of 21°), with an average amount of tibial torsion (30°). Most people do stand with their feet pointing slightly outwards in a relaxed, anatomical position. (b) Toeing in (*coxa anteverta*) can be caused by a combination of an increase in femoral anteversion to 27°, along with an acetabular version of 33° and only 14° of tibial torsion. (c) Toeing out (*coxa retroverta*) can be caused by a combination of a decrease in femoral anteversion to 3°, along with an acetabular version of 10° and tibial torsion of 45°.

Too large of a femoral anteversion can contribute to pathology in the femoral head due to lack of stress, because the anterior surface of the femur is uncovered. This may also occur if the acetabular anteversion is too large.[43] There is no correlation, however, between the degree of femoral anteversion and the amount of acetabular anteversion.[44] (Having a large version angle in your pelvis does not mean that you will have a small version angle in the femur.) Toeing in caused by femoral anteversion is much more common in children, occurring in about 30% of four-year-olds, but by adulthood this rate has gone down to about 4%.[45] Toeing in and larger femoral anteversion is more common in girls than boys.[46] Along with an increased risk of osteoarthritis in the hip socket, larger femoral anteversion angles (which help us to externally rotate) are also correlated with higher rates of knee problems.

At birth, the range of femoral anteversion is between 30° and 40°; it then starts to lessen. Table 2.3 shows how the angle reduces by about 1.5° per year.[47] As we get older, we may find it easier to sit in Lotus Pose (Padmasana), thanks to more available external rotation due to our decreased femoral anteversion, but when we were young we may have found it easier to sit between our feet (also known as Hero Pose, or Virasana), which requires more internal rotation at the hip socket. Remember, however, that the version angle of the acetabulum also plays a role here and can negate the femoral anteversion.

TABLE 2.3
The amount of femoral anteversion changes with age.

AGE (YEARS)	FEMORAL ANTEVERSION
Birth	36°
2–4	33°
4–6	28°
6–8	26°
8–10	25°
10–12	22°
12–14	21°
14–16	16°
Adult	15°

There is a lot of variability in the average amount of femoral anteversion reported in the literature, but a good estimate for the norm is 15° for adults with a standard deviation of 6°.[48] This means that the two standard deviation range in which 95% of people fall goes from 3° to 27°. As wide as that range is, some studies have found people with values as low as –15°![49] Interestingly, a study of the Indian population found a much smaller average value than the 15° often cited as average in the West: 8°, possibly because Indian children and adults spend more time sitting on the floor, thus encouraging a greater external rotation in their hip joints.[50] This may explain why Indian yoga teachers find it so easy to sit in Lotus Pose while most Westerners struggle to do so. Several studies have noted a difference between men and women, with women having greater anteversion angles than men by up to 6° on average.[51] As mentioned, the amount of femoral torsion and acetabular anteversion/retroversion will affect how easily you can externally or internally rotate your legs at the hip socket, important for postures such as Lotus (Padmasana) and Hero Pose (Virasana). There is a negative correlation between femoral torsion and external rotation: the *more* anteversion of the femur you have, the *less* you will be able to externally rotate your leg.[52]

OTHER VARIATIONS OF THE FEMUR

Look back at figure 2.35 and then at 2.36a. Do you notice any differences in the length of the femurs' necks and the size of their greater trochanters? There are natural ranges in these dimensions as well. Neck length can vary proportionally to body size and body weight, but there is also variability unrelated to either of those factors. For example, there is a correlation between the neck length and the femoral neck-shaft angle: the longer the neck, the greater the neck-shaft angle.[53] Researchers use different definitions for the neck length of the femur, but one summary found the average to be 3.4 cm, with a standard deviation of 0.4 cm. The total range of variations, however, was from 1.8 to 4.2 cm.[54] Another study, using a different definition of neck length, found ethnic variability, with Polynesian women having a larger neck length of 6.82 cm, Chinese and Indian women having shorter neck lengths of 6.1 cm, while those of European descent had lengths averaging 6.6 cm.[55] Again, studies vary, and it is the variability that interests us.

Neck length is a factor in the range of motion available before the greater trochanter squeezes against the side of the pelvis. The longer the neck, the greater the range of motion

possible; a short neck equals limited range. Longer necks also provide greater abduction leverage, making it easier for the gluteus minimus and gluteus medius to abduct the legs. The longer your femoral neck length, the more strongly you can abduct your leg. (See Appendix C: Mechanical Advantage—Pulleys and Levers.) In the general population, femur neck length seems to have been increasing over the last century, possibly due to improved nutrition before puberty. However, longer neck lengths may predispose us to an increased risk of fracture when we are elderly.[56] This makes some sense: if your bones become weaker or osteoporotic over time, then the longer the neck of your femur, the more likely it is to fracture.

While we are looking at the femoral neck, another variability we find is in its cross-sectional shape. The neck is not a perfect cylinder; it is somewhere between a cylinder and a square block.[57] Figure 2.38 shows a cross-section of a femoral neck. Notice how the neck rises up to the superior anterior quadrant. Depending upon how high your neck rises—and, once more, everyone has his or her own unique shape—you may be more or less likely to have your femoral neck come into contact with the acetabulum during flexion, or flexion combined with internal rotation. Studies have found a correlation between the size of the cross-section of the femur and the types of exercise one predominately performs. Also, in general, the thicker the neck, the stronger it is and the less likely to be fractured in a fall.[58]

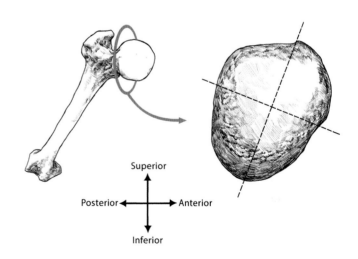

FIGURE 2.38 Femoral neck cross-section.

Another variation that can arise in the neck of the femur, mostly in men, is a *cam*, which refers to a flattened area of the neck instead of the usual concave, saddle shape. If this area of the neck is not as curved as normal, there is a greater likelihood of contact between the neck and the rim of the hip socket, limiting certain movements. We will examine this situation in more detail when we look at internal rotation and a condition called femoral acetabular impingement syndrome (see figure 2.93).

THE GREATER TROCHANTER

The height or thickness of the greater trochanter is also variable, and the range, within one standard deviation, is from 3.3 to 12.7 mm.[59] Again, many studies have used different definitions for the height of the greater trochanter, but they all found significant variations.[60] Some people have a much more pronounced bump on the side of their femurs than others, and this has implications for their range of movement as well. The larger the prominence of the greater trochanter, the sooner compression will be reached in abduction; the lower the greater trochanter, the more room you have before compression occurs.

Other Variations of the Pelvis and Femur

Many yoga teachers frequently tell students to "level the pelvis." Sometimes, instructions are given either to tuck the pelvis (which involves a posterior or backwards rotation of the hips, lessening the lumbar curve in the lower back) or never to tuck the pelvis. These cues are offered to spare the lower back from excessive stress—but how can both tucking and not tucking be best? What does it mean to level the pelvis? One instruction involves palpating the ASIS and the PSIS, keeping the line formed between them parallel to the floor (see figure 2.39). In this way, you can visualize your pelvis being a bowl that is not spilling its contents forwards or backwards.

However, all these instructions are making the unspoken assumption that everyone's pelvises are the same. They are not. The line between the ASIS and PSIS (lets call it the A/PSIS line), which is used to help guide us in knowing when our pelvis is level or not, varies considerably from person to person. Figure 2.39 shows this line to be at an angle of 13° to horizontal, with the ASIS lower than the PSIS, which is the norm for most people. A teachers' intention to

"level the hips" by leveling the A/PSIS line in reality tilts more pelvises than it levels. Most students will need to tuck their pelvis in order to level the A/PSIS line.

Notice the two pelvises shown in figure 2.40. These are the two extreme cases found in a study of only 30 pelvises.[61] There is a distinct difference in the orientation of the A/PSIS lines with respect to horizontal, and yet both of these pelvises are aligned in a neutral position. This study found a range of angles to horizontal of the A/PSIS line from 0° to 23°. The average was 13°, and one standard deviation was 5°. While the study found no gender dependencies, it did notice a distinct and significant difference of up to 11° from side to side. This means that leveling the right hip does not guarantee that the left hip will also be level! Indeed, for about two-thirds of people, it won't be. We are not symmetric, and the attempt to level one hip may end up tilting the other hip. (So, if a yoga teacher asks you to level your hips, ask, "Which one?")

Interestingly, many clinicians and therapists believe that a difference in the two sides of the pelvis is a sign of pathology, and they use the amount of difference from left to right as an indication of scoliosis or leg-length differences. It may be true that the person has uneven leg lengths or scoliosis or sacral pathologies due to an asymmetric pelvis. But in reality, most people have differences in the two sides

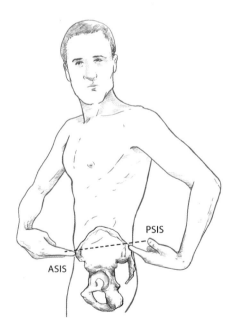

FIGURE 2.39 By palpating the ASIS and the PSIS and keeping the line between them level to the floor, you are "leveling the pelvis." However, the pelvis is no longer in neutral.

of their hips, and this is not always pathology; it can be simply a normal human variation and therefore doesn't need to be fixed.[62]

Imagine the owners of the 30 pelvises involved in this study all showing up in a yoga class. Also imagine the teacher instructing everyone to level their pelvis. Twenty-nine students have to do a pelvic tuck to comply with the instructions, while only one student naturally has her pelvis in neutral when her A/PSIS are level. Figure 2.41(b) shows what is happening to the student with the greatest angle: she has to tuck her pelvis 23° to level her A/PSIS. Notice what

this does to her lumbar spine: it reduces the normal curve considerably. The average person has to tuck their pelvis 13° to bring the A/PSIS to horizontal, which again reduces their normal lordosis.

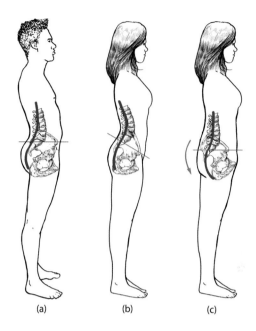

(a)   (b)   (c)

FIGURE 2.41 Leveling the pelvis can reduce the normal lumbar curve. In (a) we see a pelvis with a 0° A/PSIS angle and a neutral lumbar curve. In (b) we see a pelvis with a 21° A/PSIS angle but still a normal lumbar curve. In (c) we see what happens to the lumbar lordosis for the person in (b) when she tries to level the pelvis by doing a pelvic tuck: the lumbar curve straightens out.

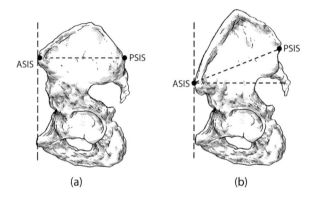

(a)   (b)

FIGURE 2.40 Variations of the A/PSIS line. Both pelvises are in neutral alignment, but the angle of the A/PSIS line to the horizontal is considerably different: for (a) it is 0°, but for (b) it is 21°. Also, notice the difference in the height of the iliac crests.

NOTE TO TEACHERS: Be cautious of creating alignment cues based only on your own experience

We can easily imagine why a teacher decided to ask his students to level their hips. He tried it himself and found that when he leveled his hips, his lower back felt much better. He felt solid and stable in his core. Realizing this, he shared his knowledge with his students. His intentions were good and his logic reasonable, but his ignorance of human variation led him to require his students to put more stress on their spines than he realized. He made the mistake of believing that if something worked for him, it would work for everyone. A better approach would have been to teach his students

to engage in the same process he had followed in getting to know what worked in his body, so that they could find for themselves what worked in their bodies. It is okay to use alignment cues—after all, teachers have to say something. But do not insist that the cues are correct for every body. Avoid dogma. Suggest the cue, but also suggest that the student check out what is happening, to evaluate whether the offered alignment is working for her. If it is not working, be prepared to help the student find a better way.

The researchers concluded that the A/PSIS line angle to horizontal should not be used to assess the orientation of the pelvis.[63] Yoga teachers also should not use this alignment cue. This is not to imply that finding a neutral position for the pelvis is unimportant—it can be very important, especially for people who suffer lower back pain. The point is that the technique of leveling the hips to find the neutral position for the pelvis is flawed. The instruction to level the pelvis will only benefit one person out of 30 but will cause spinal flexion in everyone else, which, ironically, is precisely what the teacher is trying to avoid by suggesting the leveling.

If we cannot use a nice, simple metric like the angle of the ASIS and PSIS to identify the neutral position for the pelvis, what can we do? Follow the advice of Judith Lasater, who suggests training the student to determine the neutral position for herself.[64] She suggests: "feel for any tension in the abdominal wall between the ASIS and symphysis pubis. If you are in neutral, this area will feel soft; if not, it will feel taut." To this we might add, "Also be aware of how your lumbar spine is feeling: if it feels stressed or painful, you may not have found the neutral position for your pelvis."

THE LESSER TROCHANTER

Another factor that affects our ability to move is the length of our muscles, and that can depend upon the distance between the proximal and distal attachment sites. For someone with a high iliac crest, the internal and external oblique muscles of the abdomen are shorter and may have less pulling power than those of someone with a lower crest. However, the tensor fasciae latae, sartorius and iliacus muscles will generate more pulling power in someone with a high crest. (Think of a lever: the longer the lever, the more power we can generate—it is easier to move a stuck screw with a longer wrench than with a short one. A more complete discussion on levers and pulleys and their mechanical advantages is offered in Appendix C.)

The variability in the shape of our bones affects our muscles' power in several ways. With longer or larger bones or varying positions of the muscles' attachment sites, the force of contraction applied through leverage will change. For students whose bump of the lesser trochanter is lower on the femoral shaft, greater leverage can be obtained when flexing the legs (see figures 2.42 and 2.43). This extra power will show its benefits in how strongly the person can flex

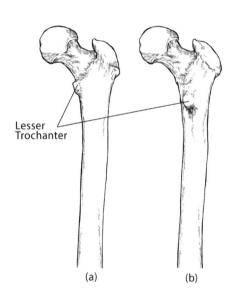

FIGURE 2.42 The lesser trochanter (posterior view). Notice how both the size and the location of the lesser trochanter can vary. In (a), the trochanter is more medially located and higher up the shaft of the femur. In (b), it is lower and more laterally rotated, enhancing external rotation and flexion but slowing down flexion response time.

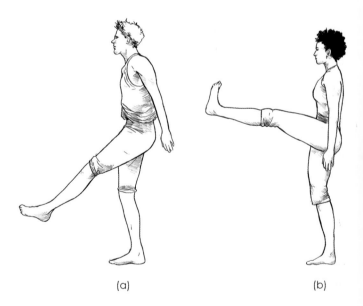

FIGURE 2.43 Mechanical advantage of variations in the pubis and lesser trochanter. The principles of leverage and pulleys combine, thanks to a more distal lesser trochanter in (b) (the lever) and a more pronounced pubis (the pulley), making it easier to lift a leg than in (a), even though the flexor muscles are exerting the same force.

their leg, but the reaction time to do so will be slower. A higher placed lesser trochanter will allow for a quicker response to flexion but with less force of flexion. In addition, if the lesser trochanter is rotated more laterally, engaging the psoas and iliacus not only will flex the hip but will more forcefully externally rotate the leg. A lesser trochanter that is more medially located will result in less external rotation. The degree of medial rotation of the lesser trochanter is quite variable and correlates to the torsion of the femur.[65]

THE THIRD TROCHANTER

Many people have a third noticeable bump on their femur, called the third trochanter (see figure 2.44). Studies vary in their estimation of how frequently this occurs, from as little as 6%[66] to between 17% and 72%![67] There is no consensus as to why some people have a third trochanter, but it is known to be an attachment site for the gluteus maximus. Many mammals have a third trochanter, but not most primates, so perhaps it is part of our evolutionary heritage or something we evolved to help us with walking upright. (Dinosaurs had four trochanters on each femur!) We do not know why we have it, why most people do not have it, or whether it makes the action of the gluteus maximus stronger or more efficient. What this means is that we do not know whether your possessing a third trochanter will make yoga easier or harder for you, but if you feel a third big bump on your femur, you are probably not particularly unusual.

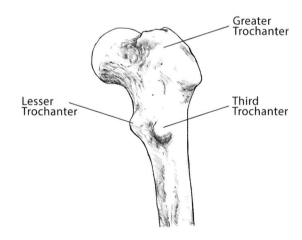

FIGURE 2.44 The third trochanter is an attachment site for the gluteus maximus.

Function: Application in Yoga Postures

We have seen how the architecture and form of the hip joint allow the movements of flexion, extension, abduction, adduction, and internal and external rotation, and we have seen that variations in the shapes of the pelvis and femur can affect these movements. We will now look at the ranges of possible motions for an average person, and for all those yoga students who are not average. In answering our What Stops Me? question, we will also look at the sources of tension and compression and how compression may arise in different places due to natural variations in the bones and joints.

NORMAL RANGES OF MOTION

As we have noted earlier, the hip joint is a ball-in-socket joint, with a relatively deep socket that is extended even further by the labrum. This arrangement allows for a great variety of movement, which can be looked at in three planes: flexion/extension in the side (sagittal) plane, abduction/adduction in the frontal (coronal) plane and internal/external rotation (medial/lateral rotation) in the horizontal (transverse) plane. Together these movements can be combined into circumduction: moving the leg in a circle. (See The Planes of Movement, on pages 91–97, for illustrations of these movements.)

Many texts and studies have tried to quantify the hip's normal ranges of motion, but there is a great deal of variability. Table 2.4 presents some ranges to illustrate both what an average person can do and the human variation around that average. As always, your range of motion is likely to be very different, but this does not necessarily imply any pathology. If you have been doing yoga for several years, you are very likely to have a larger range of motion than the average values shown here.[68]

TABLE 2.4 Average range of motion at the hip joint with one standard deviation, and the ranges of motion for the hip at two standard deviations.

HIP MOTION	25–39 YEARS (1SD)	RANGE (2SD)
Flexion	122° +/– 12°	98–146°
Extension	22° +/– 8°	6–38°
Abduction	44° +/– 11°	22–66°
Adduction	26° +/– 4°	18–34°
Internal (medial) rotation	33° +/– 7°	19–47°
External (lateral) rotation	34° +/– 8°	18–50°

Notice the reference to the ages of the subjects. Several studies have found that range of motion decreases as we age, whereas other studies have not found this relationship. If there is any consensus it is that our range of motion does decline significantly after 80 years of age. One exception seems to be cited most often: our ability to extend the hip can become reduced by an average of 20° between our 20s and 70s.[69]

The ranges shown in table 2.4 are sufficient for us to engage in daily life; the amount of movement needed to walk, for example, is considerably less than the ranges shown. Probably the most challenging activity we do each day is sitting down to tie our shoelaces, with one foot resting on the opposite knee. That requires an average of 115° of flexion, 18° of abduction and 13° of external rotation.[70] This is well within the average person's ability. However, if your vocation or sport requires a greater range of motion, then the question becomes: What's stopping me? What are the limits to the range of motion available to me in my hip joints? This table gives no indication as to *why* the ranges are the way they are. To find that answer, we have to look deeper.

SOURCES OF TENSION

The answer to WSM? falls along a spectrum from tensile resistance at one end to bone-on-bone compression at the other. Tensile resistance to movement in the hip socket can come from the fascia that surrounds the whole area as well as fascial restrictions far from the joint (the so-called anatomy trains), from the muscles that articulate and stabilize the joint, as well as from the ligaments and joint capsule wrapping the joint.

Sources of Tension from the Fascia

TENSILE RESISTANCE	COMPRESSION
Myofascial Meridians	

The myofascial meridians are continuous connections of fascia that envelop the muscles and joint capsules, forming trains of fabric that run around the whole body. The meridians that can impede movement in the hips include the superficial front line, the superficial back line, the spiral lines, the lateral lines, the functional lines, and the deep front line. (See the description of myofascial meridians in Appendix C of Volume 1.) Resistance from the myofascial meridians can generally be sensed as tugging in places remote from the hip joint or remote from the muscular restraints described below. Myofascial resistance is spread out and can appear at any point along the meridians.

Sources of Movement and Tension from the Muscles

TENSILE RESISTANCE	COMPRESSION
Muscles & Tendons	

Tension will arise from the muscles that resist the movement or act to stabilize the joint, as shown in table 2.5. Remember, tension in the muscles has a variety of causes: as described in Volume 1, tension is not simply due to shortness in these muscles.[71]

TABLE 2.5 Muscles causing and restricting hip movement from the anatomical position. Note that the action of the muscles changes as the orientation of the thigh to the pelvis changes, so these muscles may not always produce or resist the movements indicated. (Synergists assist the prime movers.)

HIP MOVEMENT	PRIME MOVERS	SYNERGISTS	RESISTING MUSCLES
Flexion	Psoas major and minor, iliacus, rectus femoris, tensor fasciae latae, sartorius	Pectineus, adductor longus, adductor magnus, gracilis	Semitendinosus, semimembranosus, biceps femoris, gracilis
Extension	Gluteus maximus, hamstrings	Gluteus medius, adductor magnus, piriformis	Rectus femoris, psoas major and minor, iliacus, tensor fasciae latae, sartorius
Abduction	Gluteus medius, gluteus minimus, tensor fasciae latae	Piriformis, sartorius, rectus femoris	Adductor magnus, adductor longus, adductor brevis, gracilis, pectineus, hamstrings
Adduction	Adductor magnus, adductor longus, adductor brevis, gracilis, pectineus	Bicep femoris, gluteus maximus, quadratus femoris, obturator externus	Gluteus medius, gluteus minimus, tensor fasciae latae, piriformis
External (lateral) rotation	Obturator internus and externus, gemellus superior and inferior, quadratus femoris, piriformis, gluteus maximus	Gluteus medius and minimus, sartorius, bicep femoris	Tensor fasciae latae
Internal (medial) rotation	No prime mover	Gluteus medius and minimus, tensor fasciae latae, adductor magnus, longus and brevis	Obturator internus and externus, gemellus superior and inferior, quadratus femoris, piriformis, gluteus maximus

Sources of Tension from the Capsular Ligaments

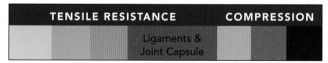

The capsular ligament fibers are oriented diagonally around the joint capsule so that they loosen when the hip is flexed but become taut when the hip is extended to its maximum. Indeed, the passive tension of these three ligaments is the reason extension is so limited. When the hip is fully extended, slightly internally rotated and abducted, it is in its *close-packed* position, which means the joint has its largest degree of stability.[72] These three ligaments effectively "screw down" the femur into the socket at full extension, and there is no "play" or wiggle-room in the joint: it is firmly held (see figure 2.45). Figure 2.46 shows how the capsular ligaments tighten or relax in various movements. Another contributor to joint stability is the relative vacuum in the joint; this suction between the femur and the acetabulum also helps to keep them drawn close together.

Sensing the tension in the hip socket caused by the ligaments is difficult. It is not always obvious why we can't move further. With practice and patient attention, a yoga student may be able to sense that the restriction to movement is happening in the hip socket by noticing a firm, stuck feeling deep in the socket. Determining whether this is caused by the ligaments becoming taut or by compression of the neck of the femur against the acetabular rim is quite challenging, and for some people impossible to know for sure. While this area has a lot of mechanoreceptor nerve endings, these primarily serve a proprioceptive function, helping us to stay balanced when walking, standing or running.[73] It is difficult to consciously sense these tissues; however, nociceptors (pain receptors—see the section in Volume 1 on the nervous system, pages 46–48) are present throughout the labrum and hip capsule and can tell us when something is wrong.[74]

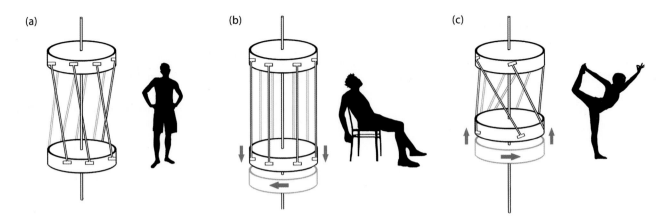

(a)   (b)   (c)

FIGURE 2.45 The capsular ligaments relax or tighten the hip joint. In the standing posture, the three capsular ligaments are orientated diagonally, as shown in the first image (a). With flexion of the leg (b), the ligaments loosen, allowing more range of movement. With extension, however (c), the ligaments tighten up, drawing the femur closer to the acetabulum and thereby restricting movement.

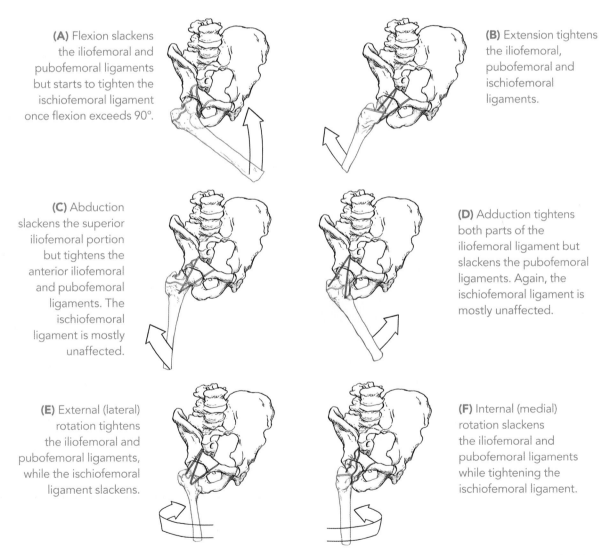

(A) Flexion slackens the iliofemoral and pubofemoral ligaments but starts to tighten the ischiofemoral ligament once flexion exceeds 90°.

(B) Extension tightens the iliofemoral, pubofemoral and ischiofemoral ligaments.

(C) Abduction slackens the superior iliofemoral portion but tightens the anterior iliofemoral and pubofemoral ligaments. The ischiofemoral ligament is mostly unaffected.

(D) Adduction tightens both parts of the iliofemoral ligament but slackens the pubofemoral ligaments. Again, the ischiofemoral ligament is mostly unaffected.

(E) External (lateral) rotation tightens the iliofemoral and pubofemoral ligaments, while the ischiofemoral ligament slackens.

(F) Internal (medial) rotation slackens the iliofemoral and pubofemoral ligaments while tightening the ischiofemoral ligament.

FIGURE 2.46 The effects of movement on capsular ligaments. The red line is the ischiofemoral ligament; the blue lines are the iliofemoral and pubofemoral ligaments.

TABLE 2.6 Tension from ligaments limits movement in the hip socket in a variety of directions.[75]

HIP MOVEMENT	RESISTING LIGAMENTS
Flexion	Inferior joint capsule, >90°, inferior fibers of the ischiofemoral ligament >120°, the ischiofemoral ligament >160°, all three ligaments
Extension	Iliofemoral ligament Pubofemoral ligament Ischiofemoral ligament Anterior joint capsule
Abduction	Pubofemoral ligament Anterior iliofemoral Inferior joint capsule
Adduction	Iliofemoral ligament Iliotibial band
External (lateral) rotation	Anterior iliofemoral ligament Pubofemoral ligament Iliotibial band
Internal (medial) rotation	Ischiofemoral ligament Posterior joint capsule

SOURCES OF COMPRESSION

Once the tensile resistance of the tissues described above has been reduced sufficiently, the next answer to WSM? becomes compression. There are three qualities of compression: soft, medium and hard. Compressive restriction to movement can occur in four areas around or in the hip joint:

- Soft compression from the abdomen or chest hitting the thighs
- Medium compression from tissues caught between the front of the pelvis (the ASIS) and the thigh (which is bone-hitting-flesh compression)
- Medium compression from tissues caught between the greater trochanter and the side of the pelvis (the ilium), which results in two bones trapping flesh between them
- Hard compression, where the neck of the femur impinges upon the labrum of the acetabulum (bone-on-cartilage compression)

As we work through all these sources of compression, please remember: we are assuming that the tensile resistances of the fascia, muscles, ligaments and joint capsules are no longer inhibiting the movement needed to reach compression. Those have either been worked through or were never originally significant enough to limit movement sufficiently to prevent compression.

We will begin our investigation from the acetabulum and move outward.

Compression of the Neck of the Femur against the Rim of the Acetabulum

TENSILE RESISTANCE	COMPRESSION
	HARD: bone on bone

The first possible point of compression to look at occurs when the neck of the femur impinges upon the rim (the labrum) of the acetabulum. For example, if all tensile restrictions of the fascia, muscles and ligaments have been worked so that you can fully abduct the leg while in the anatomical standing position, the point of compression will occur at the superior labrum (see figure 2.47). If we internally rotate the hip, compression can occur at the anterior inferior portion of the labrum. For external rotation, it occurs at the posterior inferior labrum. When we combine internal rotation with flexion, it may occur at the superior anterior labrum. (See It's Complicated: Femoral acetabular impingement syndrome, on page 149.) For some people with normal acetabula, a very deep flexion—of 160° or more—can bring the anterior neck of the femur into compression with the posterior labrum, especially if a little adduction or internal rotation is present. Full flexion with abduction, which often occurs in many postures, such as seated or standing side splits (Upavisthakonasana or Prasarita Padottanasana), can create compression in the posterior superior labrum; however, adding external rotation will spin the neck out of the way so that no compression occurs there. Generally, compression of the neck of the femur against the labrum occurs along an arc following the posterior, superior and anterior rim of the labrum, but only rarely against the inferior portion (see figure 2.49). Exactly where impingement occurs depends upon which combinations of movements have been undertaken and the unique anatomical shapes of the femur and pelvis.

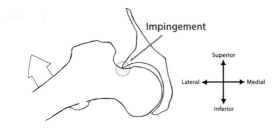

FIGURE 2.47 Abduction can cause impingement of the neck of the femur to the superior rim of the labrum of the acetabulum.

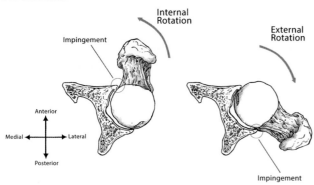

FIGURE 2.48 Internal rotation may lead to impingement of the anterior neck of the femur against the anterior labrum. External rotation may lead to impingement of the posterior neck of the femur against the posterior labrum.

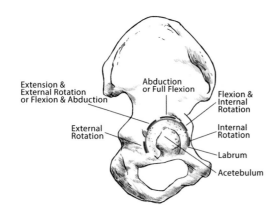

FIGURE 2.49 Compression of the neck of the femur against the acetabulum can occur along a roughly semicircular path on the circumference of the labrum but rarely at the bottom. The red arch shows the possible areas of impingement, while the blue dashes show where certain movements are likely to result in impingement.

Compression of the Greater Trochanter against the Side of the Pelvis

TENSILE RESISTANCE	COMPRESSION
	MEDIUM: bone on flesh

Sometimes, and for some bodies, before impingement can occur between the femur and the hip socket, an earlier point of compression may arise when the muscles and other tissues around the pelvis become caught between the femur and the side of the pelvis. In figure 2.50 we see the greater trochanter rising in abduction, compressing the gluteus medius and gluteus minimus muscles against the ilium. This form of compression, which we are calling medium compression—where tissues are trapped between the femur and the pelvis—can be reached in adduction, external rotation or internal rotation, but rarely is it felt in extension. (The tautness of the capsular ligaments will generally restrict extension before any compression is reached.) The sensation of this form of compression is softer and more superficial than the feeling of the neck of the femur hitting the rim of the hip socket, which feels much harder, deeper and final. When soft tissues, such as muscles, are trapped between two bones, usually a little more compression or range of motion can be generated by outside forces, such as a teacher or therapist pressing forcefully, or through additional force provided by the weight of sandbags.

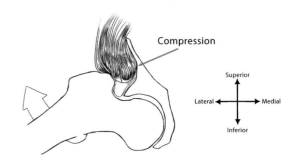

FIGURE 2.50 Abduction can also cause compression of the tissues caught between the greater trochanter of the femur and the side of the pelvis.

Compression of the Pelvis against the Front of the Thigh in Flexion

TENSILE RESISTANCE	COMPRESSION
	MEDIUM: bone on flesh

Moving away from the acetabulum, another instance of medium compression can occur in flexion when muscles and tissues become caught between the ASIS and the flesh of the thighs. Figure 2.51 shows a student in a sitting forward fold (Paschimottanasana) who cannot go any lower due to this form of compression. This has a pinching feel to it, and for many people, the inability to bring their chest to their legs in forward flexions of the hip is due to this uncomfortable sensation at the front of the pelvis. Fortunately, there is a simple solution: abduct the legs enough to go around the points of compression, allowing deeper flexion.

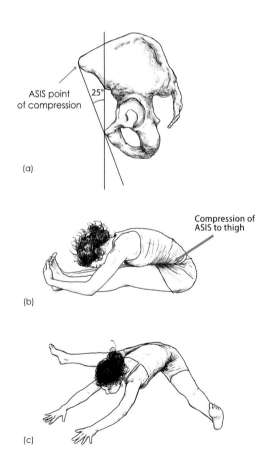

FIGURE 2.51 Compression due to the ASIS (a) coming into contact with the thighs limits flexion (b). However, abducting the femurs (c) allows the ASIS to slip in between the thighs, allowing greater hip flexion.

Compression of the Upper Body on the Lower Body in Flexion

TENSILE RESISTANCE	COMPRESSION
	SOFT: flesh on flesh

If the ASIS does not impinge upon the thigh and the legs remain together, flexion can progress until ultimately, a place of soft compression is reached: the belly or chest comes into direct contact with the legs. At this point the sensations of compression are obvious; however, some residual tension may remain in the back of the body, along the hamstrings or the spine. This is because the remaining tension cannot be stretched out, as the body has no further room to move. But as is the case with compression occurring when the ASIS hits the thigh, abduction here may also allow further flexion! Figure 2.52 shows a limit for flexion when the legs are together but the possibility for further excursions if the legs are abducted.

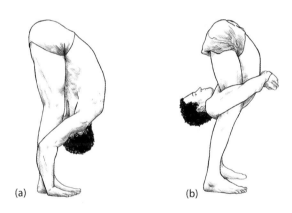

FIGURE 2.52 Flexion in Uttanasana (a) is stopped ultimately by the upper body compressing against the lower body. However, in Tittibhasana B (b), with the legs abducted, further flexion is possible. Eventually, a combination of the capsular ligaments becoming taut, compression of the ribs against each other, and/or compression of the abdominal organs will prevent the student from being able to kiss their own butt. There are no known health benefits of being able to do so.

VARIATIONS IN RANGE OF MOTION

The ultimate range of motion we have, once we have worked through our tensile resistance, is dictated by where and when compression will occur, but that varies considerably due to normal variations in human shapes and sizes.

Variations in Circumduction

Circumduction can be considered a moving combination of internal rotation, adduction, flexion, external rotation, abduction and extension, creating a cone within which the femur rolls around inside the acetabulum. The depth of your acetabulum is one factor that will affect the range of circumduction available to you. With a shallow acetabulum, a greater range of circumduction is available, whereas a deeper hip socket allows less movement. In figure 2.53a, we see an average acetabulum depth of 34% (defined as depth/width x 100); the cone represents the range of circumduction available.[76] Movement outside this cone would result in the neck of the femur impinging upon the labrum. In (b) we see that when the acetabular depth is increased to 41%, the cone of possible movement is reduced: 8° of movement is lost. An acetabular depth of 41% is two standard deviations away from the norm, which means that about 2.5% of the population—one person out of 40—has hip sockets this deep or deeper. In (c) we find that when the depth is only 27% (which may occur in another 2.5% of the population), the range of motion is greatly increased: 20° more movement is available than with an average depth. Thus, between the worst and best acetabular depths in a normal population, we find 28° of variation in range of circumduction.

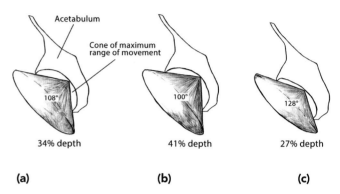

FIGURE 2.53 Circumduction is affected by acetabular depth: (a) normal depth and its associated available range of circumduction; (b) increased depth with less range of motion; (c) decreased depth and increased range of motion.

IT'S COMPLICATED:
Estimating available ranges of motion

In the examples shown, we are not presenting definitive ranges of achievable movements. That is not possible. There are too many variables to model and, since everyone is so different, it would be pointless to try. Rather, we are illustrating that ranges do exist, and we are providing a feel for how large some of the ranges are relative to various factors. For example, when we discuss variations in abduction (see pages 126–130), we show the consequence of differences in the acetabular angle of abduction, the depth of the acetabulum, and the femur neck-shaft angle (see figure 2.54). All of these variations affect how much room we ultimately have to abduct the leg at the hip socket. However, these are not the only factors that determine your range of motion. To make a complete assessment we would have to include the femur neck's length and width, the femur head's size, the width of the acetabulum and its variation from a perfect spherical shape. Even with all this information, the thickness of the soft tissues, fascia and cartilage would also play a part in determining when and where compression would be reached. What is important is that all these factors vary considerably from person to person, and each one has a role in determining your ultimate range of motion.

In some people, the lips of the acetabulum have grown outwards more than average: this over-coverage condition is known as a *pincer*—the edges of the acetabulum "pinch" the neck of the femur more securely, but with negative consequences for range of motion. The blue coloring of the lip of the acetabulum in figure 2.54 shows the pincer extent. The growth of the overhang of the superior and inferior labrum dictates not only the depth of the socket, but also the possible angle of abduction. If the top lip is recessed and shallow, while the bottom lip is extended, the angle of abduction is likely to be higher than if the top lip were prominent and the bottom lip recessed. In some cases, however, the whole rim of the acetabulum has become extended, causing the pincer, which deepens the socket. (See It's Complicated: Femoral acetabular impingement syndrome, on page 149, for more details about pincers.)

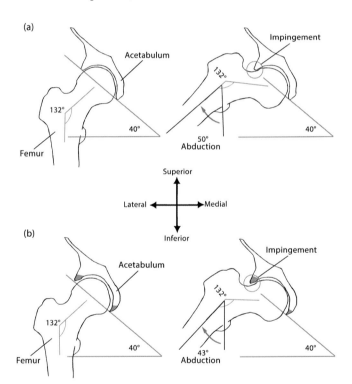

FIGURE 2.54 Abduction can be limited by a pincer. Working with an acetabular abduction angle of 40° and a femoral neck-shaft angle of 132°, (a) has an acetabular depth of 34% and allows 50° of abduction before impingement occurs; (b) has a depth of 41%, thanks to its pincer, and allows only 43° of abduction before impingement occurs.

Several studies have noted the relationship between acetabular depth and the amount of pincer.[77] In the example shown in figure 2.54b, the acetabular angle and the femur neck-shaft angle are 40° and 132°, respectively, but the acetabulum is 20% deeper than normal, thanks to the pincer over-coverage. This small change results in a reduction to the range of motion in abduction from 50° in the first hip to 43° in the second one.

The depth of the acetabulum will affect your ability to move the femur in the hip socket in abduction/adduction as well as in external/internal rotations. What we haven't shown is how the shape of the acetabulum can also affect these ranges of motion. Acetabula are not perfectly circular, and variations in their shape may reduce or increase incidences of impingement of the labrum against the neck of the femur. Variations in the thickness of the neck of the femur (called a *cam* or *pistol grip deformity*) will also affect range of movement. (See page 149.) Yoga will not change any of these factors.

NOTE TO TEACHERS: Yoga is a self-selecting practice

It is natural that students who can move their body through wider ranges of motion will be more likely to continue the practice than students who have more restricted ranges. After a few years, usually the students continuing to practice physical yoga asana are those who have the greater mobility. Those 2.5% who have very restricted mobility tend to quit in frustration. This means that in an average yoga class, you are more likely to find people who have shallower acetabula than people with deeper ones. Knowing this, you can help beginners in the lowest 2.5% of natural range of motion realize that what is normal for them is not the same as what is normal for everyone else; they can continue to do a physical yoga practice without ever having to bring their knees to the floor when sitting cross-legged. How far they can move is not the point—the aim is to move, and to do so within their own natural range.

Variations in Abduction

When tension restricts our ability to abduct at the hips, the commonly cited cause is tension in the adductor muscles. However, tension may also be due to fascial restrictions along the front functional myofascial meridian line, the contra-ipsilateral functional line, the deep front line and the contra-lateral line, indicating a constriction of the superficial and/or deep fascia. The adductor muscles run from the pubis to the inside (medial) aspect of the femur, as shown in figure 2.25 (these are the adductor magnus, adductor longus, adductor brevis, gracilis and pectineus). There are natural variations in the length of people's adductors, their proximal and distal attachments, and indeed their number,[78] but for many people, these muscles are shortened from years of sitting in chairs and therefore never spreading their legs wide apart. However, with time and patience, these tissues can be lengthened until one magical day, the resistance to further abduction is no longer limited by the adductor muscles, or even by the capsular ligaments, but by compression. Some people unfortunately don't have to lengthen their adductors much: compression occurs very quickly due to their unique anatomical structure.

VARIATIONS IN ACETABULAR ANGLE OF ABDUCTION

When we looked at the range in the acetabular angle of abduction, we found an average value of 40°, and two standard deviations gave us a 31–48° range for 95% of the population. What is the difference in the range of abduction of the leg for people with these values? Figure 2.55 shows two examples. In both cases, we have assumed that the femur has a neck-shaft angle of 132° (the average for modern Americans of European descent living in the USA).[79] Compression will occur where the neck of the femur hits the rim of the acetabulum, or when the gluteal muscles get trapped between the greater trochanter and the ilium. In the case of a pelvis with an acetabular abduction angle of 48°, this may happen after 58° of abduction. In the case of a pelvis with an acetabular abduction angle of 31°, the amount of abduction of the leg is 41°—considerably less because the acetabular abduction angle is much smaller.

We find that, all other things being equal (such as acetabular depth, acetabular version, the size and shape of the femur's neck, and its neck-shaft angle), there is an extra range of 17° of abduction of the leg for the hip that has 48° of acetabular abduction, versus the one with only 31°. Consider what this means for someone attempting to spread their

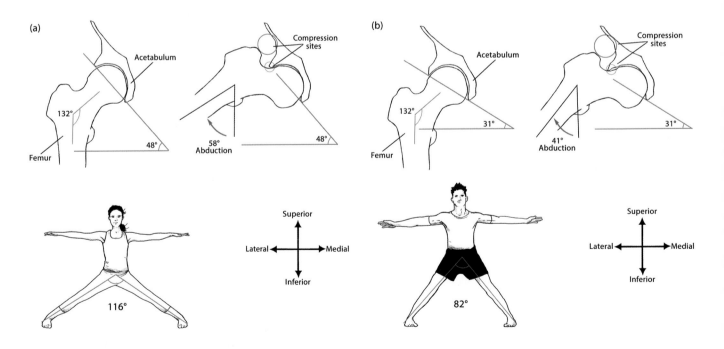

FIGURE 2.55 Limitations to abduction. (a) With an acetabular angle of 48° and a femoral neck angle of 132°, compression may arise after 58° of abduction. (b) With an acetabular angle of 31°, compression may arise after only 41° of abduction. (The larger red circle indicates the amount of space between the femur and pelvis. The smaller circle is the site of bony impingement.)

legs apart while standing: the person with the lower angle of abduction can barely get their legs to 82° separation, while the person with the higher angle of abduction can get to 116°. Notice how challenging the commonly used alignment cue is when you ask these two students to "align your hands over your ankles" when the legs are wide apart. For student (a), this cue will make their stance narrower than it could be, while for (b), their stance will never be that wide. The latter student will be told that they are "tight" and that they will be able to stretch out their adductor muscles in time; but in reality, it is the orientation of their acetabulum that is preventing them from going further, not their adductor muscles. This student will never "stretch out" their adductor muscles enough to allow them to go deeper, and no amount of "just breathe through it and relax" will change this fact. Compression, not tension, is likely to be the limiting factor in this position for this person.

VARIATIONS IN FEMORAL NECK-SHAFT ANGLE

The other consideration for how much range of motion we have to abduct our legs is the shape of the femur. In the above examples, we kept the angle of the femur neck constant. But we have seen that for people living in North America, the most frequent range of this angle is from 120° to 144°. What is the difference in range of abduction of the leg for someone close to these limits? And what happens if someone is at the high end of the acetabular abduction angle (48°) *and* the high end of the neck-shaft angle (144°)? This person will have the best of both worlds. What about the opposite extreme, someone who has the worst of both worlds: an abduction angle of 31° and a neck-shaft angle of 120°? Figures 2.56 and 2.57 show these best and worst cases.

Clearly, one yoga student has a greater range of motion available simply by virtue of the shape of her pelvis and femur. She would still have to do the work required to lengthen the softer tissues, like the adductor muscles, that contribute tension and restrict movement, but her innate capacity for movement is far greater than the second student's. The first student can potentially abduct each leg 70°—and with shallower acetabula, she could do the full 180° splits. The second person's range of motion is so restricted that what stops him likely is neither muscular tension nor tightness of the capsular ligaments, but compression of the femur against the acetabulum. He can only abduct each leg 29°! In total, he will have only 58° of separation available when spreading his legs apart. This will be even worse if he has deep acetabula.

While this is an unusual case, the point is that yoga will not help this person increase his range of motion. This is the guy who, while sitting on the floor cross-legged, has his knees way up by his ears. He is not likely to keep coming back to yoga classes, because of continual embarrassment over his restricted range of motion.

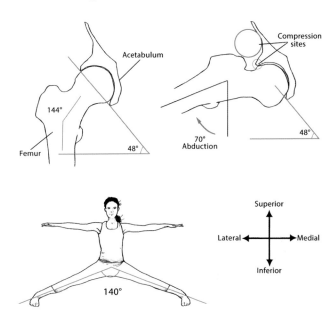

FIGURE 2.56 Abduction with acetabular angle of 48° and femoral neck-shaft angle of 144°. This is a best-of-both-worlds situation.

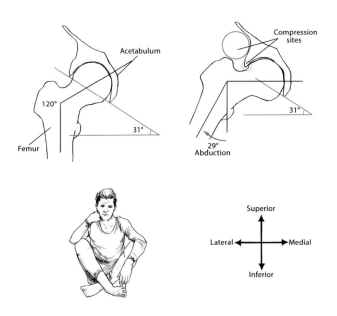

FIGURE 2.57 Abduction with acetabular angle of 31° and femoral neck-shaft angle of 120°. This is a worst-of-both-worlds situation.

OTHER LIMITS TO ABDUCTION

We have been pointing out the limitations when the neck of the femur hits the rim of the acetabulum, but in figures 2.55, 2.56 and 2.57, we also show potential compression sites where the greater trochanter may squeeze tissues against the side of the pelvis. The size of the femur's greater trochanter also plays a role in this situation. If the greater trochanter is larger than those shown, then compression of the gluteal muscles against the ilium may occur before impingement of the neck to the labrum. It can also happen that, even with the same size of greater trochanter, thicker muscles or more fat in this region will cause compression to occur before impingement at the hip socket. In these cases, students may feel a softer sense of compression just above the greater trochanter, rather than the harder feeling of stuckness deep in the hip joint.

Another factor to consider is the length of the neck of the femur. A shorter neck will cause the greater trochanter to compress tissues against the ilium more quickly than a femur with a longer neck. Figure 2.58 shows two femurs: the first (a) has a shorter neck and relatively higher greater trochanter, while the second (b) has a longer neck and a less pronounced greater trochanter. The second is less likely to encounter compression against the pelvis because it is more likely to be stopped first by impingement in the hip socket. The first femur is more likely never to reach acetabular impingement because compression will arise first with the ilium. If compression in one place doesn't stop you, it will happen somewhere else eventually.

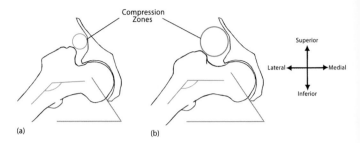

FIGURE 2.58 The zone of compression between the greater trochanter and the ilium will vary depending upon the size of the greater trochanter and the length of the femur neck. In (a), we have a larger greater trochanter and shorter neck. In (b), we have a smaller trochanter and longer neck, creating a larger space between the trochanter and the ilium. (The red circle indicates the amount of space between the femur and pelvis.)

MOVING THE FEMUR OR MOVING THE PELVIS: IT IS STILL ABDUCTION!

Abduction of the hips is required in several yoga poses, and in many of these, the fact that we are abducting the leg in the hip socket is obvious. Think of Goddess (Utkatakonasana) or Warrior 2 (Virabhadrasana II), as was shown in the section The Planes of Movement, on pages 91–98. In the side splits (Samakonasana), we obviously abduct the legs apart. However, in some poses, less obvious abduction occurs. In Triangle pose (Trikonasana), we keep the feet at a set distance apart and then move the pelvis. As was shown in figure 2.10, we tilt the front pelvis towards the femur, which is abduction! (Simultaneously, the back hip moves into adduction.) Students who have any of the discussed variations of their femurs or

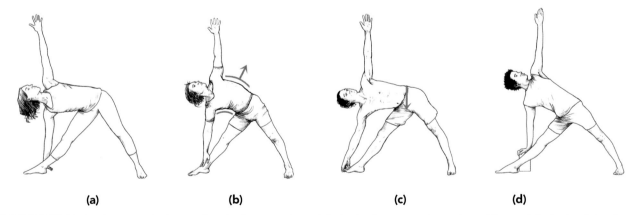

(a)   (b)   (c)   (d)

FIGURE 2.59 Abduction can arise by moving the femur or the pelvis. In the first example, we have (a) a yogini who has lots of room to abduct the hips and can keep her spine straight as she reaches her hand to the floor in Triangle Pose. In (b), we see one strategy for those who cannot abduct the hips as much: lateral flexion of the spine. In (c), we see another strategy: adding flexion at the hips, allowing the pelvis to rotate around the point of compression with the femur. In (d), we see another option: accepting that you cannot abduct very much and resting the hand on the leg or a block.

pelvis that limit their ultimate amount of abduction may reach compression in Triangle pose quickly. Any further movement to the side comes from lateral flexion of the spine.

Students like the yogini in figure 2.59(a), who have a large range of motion for abduction and external rotation due to any of the anatomical variations already discussed, do not need to laterally flex their spine to get their hand to the floor. This is because of their unique anatomical shape. This drawing may not represent your range of movement. You may look more like the second yogi (b), who has reached the limit of his abduction ability and now has to laterally flex the spine if he wants to get his hand lower. Or, like the third yogi (c), you may try to keep your spine long and unbent by going around the point of compression; you do this by adding flexion at the hips, turning your hips to the floor, because, as we will see, flexion allows many students to move away from the points of compression arising in abduction. This strategy is deliberately used in the version of Triangle Pose practiced in Ashtanga yoga, where the shape of the pose involves grabbing the big toe: if you have limited abduction range of motion, your only option then is to let your upper body rotate forward (flexing at the hips). A final Triangle Pose option, shown in (d), is to accept your limitation, keep the spine straight, and rest your hand on the leg or a block.

There is nothing magical about getting the hand to the floor in Triangle Pose. If you can abduct your legs wide enough, you can do it: the wider the legs, the closer your hand is to the floor. Even if the legs are not wide apart, if you can abduct the front hip deeply, you can do it. Some students cannot bring their hand to the floor because of the relative length of their arm to their lower body; if you have short arms in proportion to your legs, this will be your challenge. (In Volume 5, we will look at more examples of how our proportions affect our asana practice.) The reason you cannot bring your hand to the floor in Triangle Pose may have nothing at all to do with tight adductor muscles. But you can still do a great Triangle Pose—it will be *your* triangle.

At times like these, when you see another student or teacher look amazing in a yoga posture and you can't get there, ask yourself what your intentions are. If your intentions are functional as opposed to aesthetic, remind yourself that we don't use the body to get into a pose; we use the pose to get into the body. If it is about function, it is about health and wholeness. Remember your intentions. Remember the truth of skeletal variations and the difference between tension and compression. Once you remember all this, move with awareness towards your edge, and be happy with wherever it happens to be.

HORIZONTAL ABDUCTION

Ultimately, what prevents us from moving deeper into abduction will be compression of the body hitting the body, but there are often ways we can go around an initial point of compression. When you can't abduct your legs further apart in a standing pose, try flexing at the hips or externally rotating the femur. In either case, the orientation of the femur to the acetabulum will change. Figure 2.60 shows a wide-legged sitting posture (Upavisthakonasana) and a standing forward fold (Prasarita Padottanasana A). In the first posture, there is 90° of flexion at the hip, while in the second pose there is almost 160°. In both cases, the femur was fixed and the pelvis moved. With 160° of flexion rotation in the hip socket, the greater trochanter is now further from the side of the pelvis than in 90° of flexion; instead of compressing the gluteal muscles against the ilium, the greater trochanter is actually abducting towards the ischial tuberosities (see figure 2.61). In this orientation, there is much more room on the posterior side of the pelvis for the greater trochanter to move—thus, the femur can now abduct much further. If impingement of the neck of the femur against the acetabulum is the source of compression, flexion will also change this dramatically. Since the acetabulum is angled downward in the frontal plane (remember, this is called its abduction angle), when the hips are flexed and abducted, the neck of the femur moves towards the posterior rim of the acetabulum, which is further away from the neck of the femur than the superior rim, again allowing more room for abduction.

For these reasons, you may find that you can abduct more and find a wider distance between your legs when you flex at the hips, if compression was previously stopping your progress. The greater the flexion, the greater the horizontal abduction available.

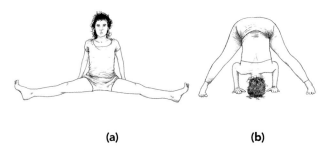

(a)   **(b)**

FIGURE 2.60 Horizontal abduction. The wide-legged sitting posture (Upavisthakonasana) (a) and the standing forward fold (Prasarita Padottanasana A) (b) use flexion in the hip sockets to allow a student to go around the points of compression that commonly stop vertical abduction, thus allowing a wider abduction of the legs.

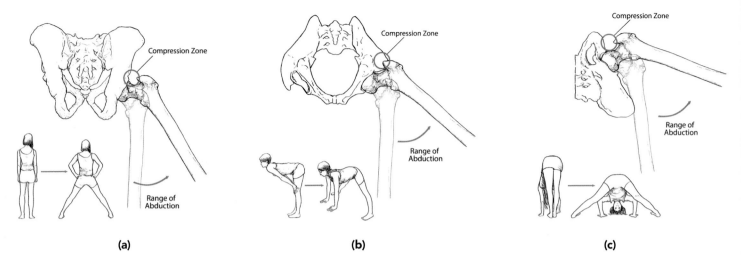

FIGURE 2.61 The range of abduction available varies by the amount of flexion of the pelvis. In (a), we see the pelvis from the back (posterior) side and the amount of abduction available at the right femur. In (b), with 90° of pelvic flexion, the range of abduction is increased. We now see the pelvis from the inferior (floor) view. In (c), with 180° of flexion, the range is increased even further before compression arises; we now see the anterior side of the pelvis.

The other way to achieve horizontal abduction is to externally (laterally) rotate the leg and then add the abduction. This again has the effect of revolving the greater trochanter out of the way of the superior labrum or the superior part of the ilium. We do this in Triangle Pose (Trikonasana): we externally rotate the front leg in the hip socket and then perform abduction there (which we see in figure 2.59). If we kept the front foot facing forward, there is no way we could abduct in the hip joint as deeply to the side. Try it yourself—try a Triangle Pose with the front foot facing forward, in the same direction as your belly button (which is simple abduction), and then try it with the leg externally rotated so the foot points out to the side (which creates horizontal abduction at the hip joint). Notice the difference? Adding the external rotation in the hip socket allows you to go around the point of compression, at least until a new point of compression is reached.

Even with flexion or external rotation at the hips, horizontal abduction has its natural limits, albeit in different places than we find in simple abduction. Whether we flex and abduct or externally rotate and abduct at the hip joint, in either case, we end up in horizontal abduction, and the point of compression will be either the superior neck of the femur impinging on the posterior rim of the acetabulum or the top of the greater trochanter compressing the gluteal muscles against the same part of the pelvis. To complete our understanding of horizontal abduction, and the implications of its inherent limitations, we also need to understand hip-joint external rotation and its limitations, which we look at in the next section.

Variations in External (Lateral) Rotation

The muscles generally given credit for causing external (lateral) rotation, either of the femur rotating in the hip socket or of the pelvis rotating around the femur, are the gluteal muscles and the six deep rotators, comprised of the obturator internus and externus, gemellus superior and inferior, quadratus femoris, and piriformis (see figure 2.25). Within the gluteal group, the gluteus maximus does most of the work, but the medius and minimus assist as synergists, as do the sartorius and bicep femoris. As always, which muscle plays a dominant role depends greatly on the position of the femur in the hip socket. The gluteus minimus and medius will act as external rotators if the hip is extended, but in the anatomical position their action is purely abduction, not rotation. Resisting movement from the muscular perspective is the tensor fasciae latae and, if the hip is flexed to 90°, the gluteus minimus and medius; at that angle, they become internal rotators. In the anatomical position, there is really no strong primary internal rotator muscle that will resist external rotation. The action of the tensor fasciae latae is mostly involved in tensing the iliotibial band and supporting the smaller gluteal muscles in abduction, although it can also assist with flexing the hip.

All this means that there really is no one muscle that resists external rotation of the hip. So, why is it so challenging to externally rotate the hips? The pubofemoral ligament and the anterior iliofemoral ligament can limit external rotation, but compression quite quickly becomes a limiting factor in how much people can externally rotate. Where and when compression arises will depend on your unique anatomy.

External rotation is one of the classic movements in yoga; it is required to sit in Lotus Pose (Padmasana) comfortably and to do all the really cool, advanced postures like Dwipadasirsasana, which is the two-feet-behind-the-head pose. External rotation is also required in many sports and dance styles: in ballet, it is required for first, second and third positions; in hockey, basketball and football, it is required to make quick lateral cuts; in golf, it is required to load up tension in the front hip at the top of the backswing, just before the downward swing; and in swimming, it is required to do the frog stroke.

When we looked at the range of version of the acetabulum and the torsion of the femur, we found considerable variations. At birth, the acetabulum has a small version angle (around 7°), causing the hip sockets to face laterally out to the side, but as we approach puberty, this angle moves more forward. An average version angle of the acetabulum for adults is 21°, but the normal range of angles is between 10° and 33°. Women have been observed to have 5° more anteversion than men, on average,[80] probably due to the more rounded pelvic inlet plane, which pushes the acetabulum further forward, but some studies have found no gender differences.[81] Again, what is important is not the average value but that there is a range of values.

Similarly, the twisting torsion of the shaft of the femur creates an anteversion angle between the neck of the femur and its lower condyles. The average value varies depending upon which study is cited, but a usable figure is 15°. Again, the important thing is the range of values, which for two standard deviations goes from 3° to 27°.[82] Once more, several studies have noted a difference between men and women, with women having greater average anteversion angles than men by up to 6°.[83] The version angles of the femur and acetabulum have a significant effect on our ability to externally rotate the femur or pelvis at the hip socket, and thus on how well we can do certain yoga postures or perform in certain sports. What ultimately constrains the amount of external rotation is impingement of the neck of the femur against the labrum of the acetabulum. As shown in figure 2.62, the normal angle of the femur into the acetabulum is from behind, in the anatomical position. We show the femur in this position so that the knees point straight ahead and the feet point slightly outward, which is how we define the anatomical position. (Why the feet do not normally point in exactly the same direction as the knees is due to tibial torsion, which will be explained when we look at the tibia.)

In figures 2.63 and 2.64 we see what happens when an average person externally rotates the femur from the anatomical position shown in figure 2.62: the posterior portion of the femur neck eventually comes into contact with the posterior-inferior lip of the acetabulum (assuming, as always, that what little tensile resistances existed have been worked through). Once impingement occurs, no further external rotation can happen unless we flex the hip, which we will look at shortly. In the case shown in figure 2.63, an average person's foot was already pointing outward at a 30° angle due to tibial torsion, but by adding external rotation, the femur comes to a compression limit after 25° of femoral rotation; this means that the foot has a total turnout of 55°.

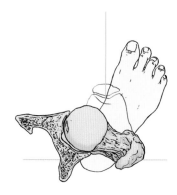

FIGURE 2.62 The femur's torsion causes it to come into the hip socket from behind the frontal plane, in order to keep the knee pointing forward.

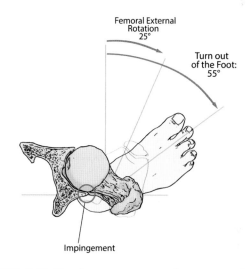

FIGURE 2.63 The femur can externally rotate until it compresses its neck against the acetabulum. In this example, compression will occur at 25° of external rotation by the femur. (The femur has a torsion of 15°, the acetabulum has an anteversion of 21°, and tibial torsion is the norm of 30°.) The foot's total turnout angle is 55°.

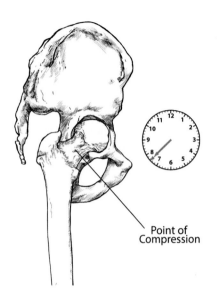

FIGURE 2.64 Femoral impingement in external rotation, as seen from the side view. Depending on the femur's neck-shaft angle, the point of impingement may be lower or higher along the back (posterior) side of the labrum. In this case, we find compression occurring at the inferior posterior labrum (at about the 7:30 o'clock position). The impingement cannot actually be seen in this view, as it is behind the neck of the femur.

There is no correlation between the acetabular version angle and the femur version angle.[84] There are people who have large acetabular angles but low femur angles, and vice versa. In these cases, the two variations tend to cancel out. However, there are also people who have a large version angle for both the femur and the acetabulum, and people who have smaller angles for both. Let's look at a worst case and a best case in terms of maximizing external rotation at the hip joint. In the worst case, we have an unfortunate soul who has considerable anteversions of both the acetabulum and the femur. They have very little room to externally rotate their foot because simply pointing the foot forward takes up most of their available room to move. In the best case, we have someone with very little acetabular anteversion (sometimes this is called retroversion) and very little torsion in the femur. In the anatomical position, this person's foot is already quite externally rotated. This person has the best of both worlds and can easily externally rotate the foot out to the side. Again, we are not citing extreme occurrences here but rather using the ranges that represent about 5% of the population.

As we see in figure 2.65, the person with the worst case can hardly externally rotate the femur in the hip socket. His foot points out only 32°. The person in figure 2.66, the

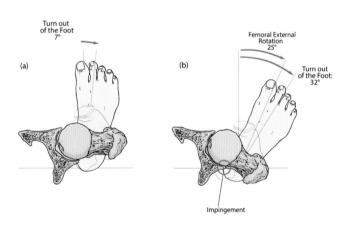

FIGURE 2.65 Worst-case scenario. If someone has 27° of anteversion for the femur and 33° for the acetabulum, they may not be able to externally rotate their leg much. Notice how in (a), their foot is pointing almost straight ahead (a turn-out angle of 7°) in the anatomical position. But in (b), with their maximum amount of femoral external rotation, the foot can only turn out 32° after a 25° external rotation of the femur.

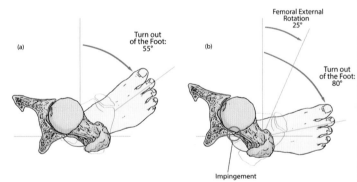

FIGURE 2.66 Best-case scenario. If someone has 3° of anteversion for the femur and 10° for the acetabulum, they may be able to externally rotate the foot from an initial 55° turnout (a) to 80° in total (b).

best case, can easily externally rotate their leg (but internal rotation may be a challenge). When we add the 30° of torsion available from the tibia (again, this is explained in detail in the section on the tibia), this creates an ability to turn out the foot 80°. In figure 2.67 we see a ballerina in first position with this amount of turnout. She clearly has the bones to achieve this important position.

In all these cases, we are ignoring the effect of acetabular depth and femur neck length and width. As we saw with abduction, these factors also have a big impact on range of motion. The person with the best external rotation may have even more range than shown here if she has a shallow acetabulum, and even more if she has a narrower and longer femoral neck. That person may easily be able to have her feet completely turned out 180° in first position. These people do exist, although they are rare, but dancers who cannot get close to the magical 180° position do not last long in ballet.[85] At the other end of the spectrum, a thicker and shorter neck or deeper hip socket will serve to reduce the range of external or internal rotation. It is unlikely, but possible, that the size of the greater trochanter will affect external rotation when there is no flexion to the hip joint.

EXTERNAL ROTATION WITH HORIZONTAL ABDUCTION

The site of compression varies with horizontal abduction. This is very important to realize and understand because it often occurs in movement. Figure 2.68 shows the dancer we saw in figure 2.67, but because she has added horizontal abduction, she can now point her feet 180° away from each other. We may be greatly restricted in our range of external rotation in the hip joint by compression while we are standing in the anatomical position, but by flexing and abducting the hip, our range of external rotation increases, sometimes dramatically. Since the acetabulum is angled anteriorly, medially and inferiorly, there is more room for the neck of the femur when we combine abduction and external rotation. With the femur horizontally abducted 90°, the place where the neck of the femur may potentially compress against the acetabulum has rotated 90°, making the impingement area the inferior rim. However, compression could arise due to the posterior side of the femur and, perhaps, the lesser trochanter trapping the adductor muscles between the femur and the pelvis.

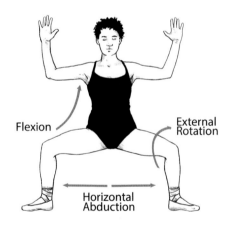

FIGURE 2.68 The Goddess (Utkatakonasana). The same person who could not fully externally rotate her feet finds that once she horizontal abducts the hips, extra rotation is available to point her feet straight out to the sides.

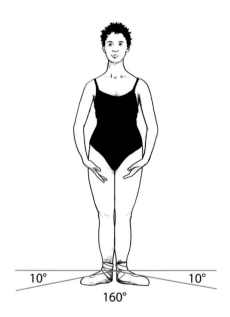

FIGURE 2.67 Ballet's first position. This dancer shows us what the best-case scenario of acetabular and femoral version would look like. She is not completely turned out; for that she would need either a shallower hip socket and longer femur neck, more turnout from her knees, tibia and ankles, or less version of her femur and acetabulum.

EXTERNAL ROTATION WITH FLEXION

Most students will feel that what stops their external rotation when the hips are flexed is not compression at all, but rather a restriction around the hip socket itself. This is caused by the iliofemoral ligaments becoming taut and restricting further rotation (see figure 2.69). The key observation is that external rotation is quickly stopped by bony compression when the hip is in the anatomical position, but most often by ligamentous tension when the hip is flexed. However, once flexion is well past 90°, compression may again arise, this time between the posterior neck of the femur and the anterior rim of the acetabulum (see figure 2.70).

We now understand why there is greater external rotation available when the hip is flexed than when it is in the anatomical position. The anterior iliofemoral ligament is taut with external rotation and about 90° flexion. For many students, these fibers loosen a bit when they move deeper into flexion, so they can externally rotate their legs more easily when folding forward in Lotus Pose (Padmasana), Cow-face Pose (Gomukhasana) or Butterfly (Baddhakonasana). While the superior fibers of the iliofemoral ligament remain taut in deeper flexion, their tension does not increase. The ultimate limit again becomes compression, this time of the posterior neck of the femur against the anterior rim of the hip socket. Students who feel a strain in the knees when externally rotating their legs in Lotus Pose may find the pain lessens when they flex the pelvis more and fold forward. This also explains why many students who practice Ashtanga find that the preparatory position of Ardhabaddha Padmottanasana is hard on the bent knee but less stressful when folding forward (see figure 2.71). When we are standing, the hip is in the anatomical position, so external rotation may be limited by compression, and grabbing the foot and binding may be impossible; but upon folding forward, we achieve greater external rotation and can easily maintain the binding.

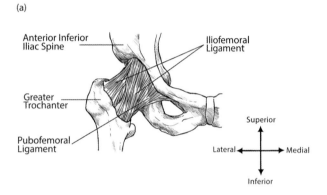

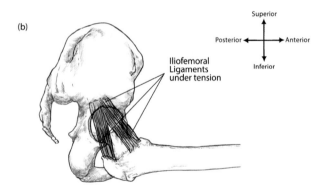

FIGURE 2.69 With flexion and external rotation, the neck of the femur moves away from compression with the labrum. Now the restriction to further movement may be due to tension in the iliofemoral ligaments. In (a) we see the ligaments in their anatomical, unstressed position. In (b) we see them elongated due to external rotation and flexion of the femur.

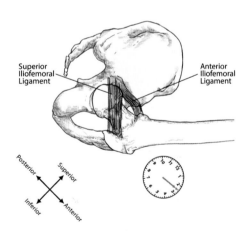

FIGURE 2.70 With deep flexion, the anterior iliofemoral ligament slackens, allowing greater external rotation. The superior iliofemoral ligament remains taut, but restriction to further rotation is again mostly due to compression of the neck of the femur against the superior or anterior rim of the acetabulum around the three o'clock position.

Variations in Flexion

For the great majority of the world, the resistance to flexion in the hip socket is tension in the hamstrings. The hamstrings run from the ischial tuberosities (our sitting bones), along the back of the thighs to below the knee. Thus, they are two-joint muscles: they can extend the hips and flex the knees (see figure 2.25). When the leg is extended at the knee and the pelvis is flexed, the hamstrings are fully stretched; however, with the knee bent, more flexion is available at the pelvis. There are natural variations in the length of people's hamstrings, but these variations can also occur through habitual use. Athletes, for example, require taut hamstrings to provide the spring for jumping and sprinting; for athletes, the hamstrings are their *hamsprings*, and they should be very careful about stretching them to make them longer, lest they lose their springs. Homo sapiens is the jumping primate—no other primate can run or jump like we can, and this is due to the springs of our hamstrings and Achilles tendons, and the arches of our feet[86] (see figure 2.72). With years of training, athletes' hamstrings become stronger and shorter, the springs stiffer. There is a tradeoff for these individuals: flexion is limited by tight or stiff hamstrings. This is not a bad thing, as their sport requires some degree of stiffness in the hamstrings, and stretching them out may cause reduced performance. However, you can have too much of a good thing, and some athletes' hamstrings are overly tight, restricting daily functional movement.

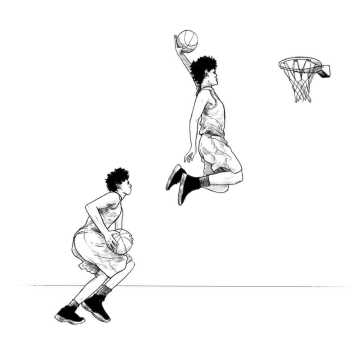

FIGURE 2.72 The "hamsprings." Stiffness in the hamstrings and Achilles tendons allows athletes to leap high and run fast.

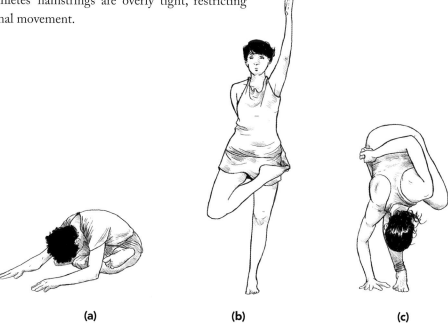

(a)   **(b)**   **(c)**

FIGURE 2.71 (a) Padmasana, (b) Ardhabaddha Padmottanasana (preparatory) and (c) final position. Flexion may allow deeper external rotation in the hip socket, making challenging postures more accessible.

Due to the orientation of the capsular ligaments, flexion at the hip joint slackens the ligaments that bind the femur to the pelvis. For this reason, hip flexion allows the largest range of motion of the femur in the acetabulum. An average person can flex the hip 122° when their knee is bent. (When the leg is straight, that range decreases to about 80°, on average.)[87] The variation in maximum hip flexion ranges from 110° to 134°, mostly due to hamstring tension.[88] It is possible that, at flexion greater than 120°, the ischiofemoral ligament will become taut, restricting further flexion (see figure 2.74). Indeed, at some point, all the capsular fibers will become taut—the ball cannot rotate forever.[89] But it is a very rare person who can move so deeply into hip flexion that their capsular ligaments are what stop them (see again Tittibhasana B in figure 2.52b).

As always, the amount of flexion varies from person to person. Hip flexion occurs by the head of the femur rotating in the acetabulum, or by the acetabulum rotating over the head of the femur. Such motion does not usually cause any impingement of the neck of the femur on the rim of the acetabulum. (There are rare cases where it can happen— see Appendix D: Flexion-Caused Impingement at the Hip Joint.)

While impingement of the femur neck and the acetabulum is rare, compression can arise in flexion by the upper body coming into contact with the lower body, as was shown in figure 2.51. However, there is a more mysterious source of compression that many people feel but do not understand: compression of the ASIS against the thigh. Recall that the ASIS is the easily palpated point on the front of your hips (see figure 2.20). The degree to which the ASIS juts out varies (see figure 2.32) from –11.5° (a retroversion of the pelvis) to 25.3° (an anteversion of the pelvis).[90] The other factor that comes into play is the distance between the left and right ASIS; for people with wider pelvises, the likelihood of compression occurring is greater than for those who have narrower distances between the two ASIS. The latter do not need to abduct their legs to go around the point of compression here because their legs are already outside the width of the two ASIS. Another factor is simply the size of the thighs: people with more flesh on the top of their femurs will more readily compress the thigh to the ASIS. Anyone who feels stopped in lunges or Child's Pose due to

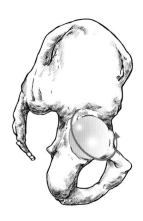

FIGURE 2.73 The "ball" of the femur simply spins in the hip socket during flexion.

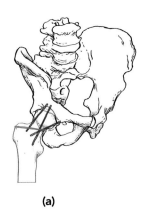 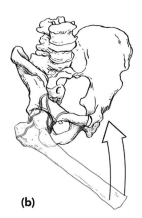 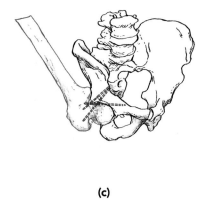

(a)   (b)   (c)

FIGURE 2.74 Flexion in the hip slackens the capsular ligaments up to 90° but tightens the ischiofemoral ligament once flexion exceeds 120°. (a) With no flexion, the ligaments are neither taut nor slack; (b) with 90° of flexion, all the ligaments are lax; (c) with 180° of flexion, all the ligaments are once more taut, especially the pubofemoral and ischiofemoral ligaments. (In blue are the iliofemoral and pubofemoral ligaments. In red is the ischiofemoral ligament.)

uncomfortable pinching in the front of the ASIS needs to abduct the legs to go further into flexion.

Unfortunately, many yoga students are given the following alignment cues:

- In Child's Pose (Balasana), the knees must be together (see figure 2.75a).
- In reclining Knees-to-Chest Pose (Apanasana), the knees are held together (see figure 2.75c).
- In Low Lunges (Anjaneyasana) and all its variations, the front thigh, knee and foot must point straight ahead (see figure 2.75e).
- In Happy Baby (Ananda Balasana), keep the knees in towards the sides of the body.

- In Noose Pose, the twisting squat of Second Series Ashtanga (Pashasana), keep the feet and legs together.
- In all forward folds (Paschimottasana and Uttasana), keep the legs together.

Try as they might, many students cannot comply with these instructions because of an uncomfortable or painful pinching sensation at the top of their pelvis. Compression is preventing them from getting the full experience that these poses have to offer (see figure 2.75). However, there is a simple solution: allowing the leg(s) to abduct slightly takes the ASIS away from the thigh, permitting greater depth in the posture. It is okay for your knees not to be together or pointing straight ahead in the postures listed above!

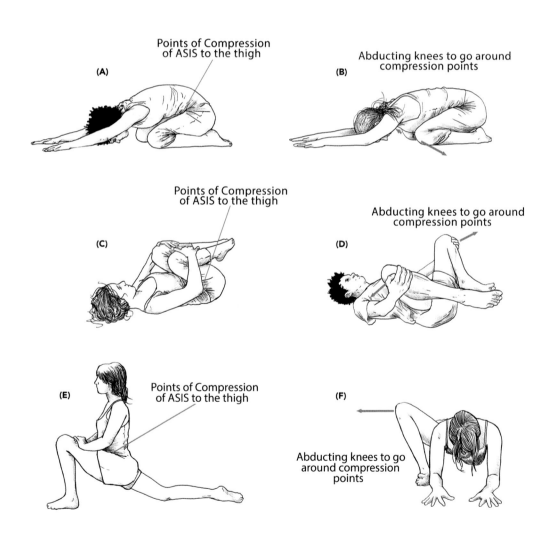

FIGURE 2.75 Compression of the ASIS and the femur can occur anytime flexion is attempted, but fortunately, there is a simple way around the point of impingement: abduct the legs.

Compression in flexion does not have to be the end of the story; going around the point of compression is often possible, at least until enough tensile resistance has been worked through so that the next point of compression appears. Winging a knee out to the side is not a bad option in a lunge—in fact, we ask for this in lunge variations where we come onto our elbows with both arms inside the front foot. Some winging out is allowed in Happy Baby (Ananda Balasana), indeed it is required, but some students require much more winging than others. It is not wrong to allow some abduction in any of the above postures; actually, for many students it is necessary if they are to reach a tension edge and not hang out in painful pinching.

FLEXION WITH INTERNAL ROTATION

In hip flexion, the head of the femur (the ball) simply rotates in the acetabulum or the acetabulum rotates around the head of the femur. However, when we start to add other movements, the story becomes more complicated. We have already seen how flexion can make external rotation more available. This same effect occurs with abduction; pure abduction can be stopped through compression of the greater trochanter against the gluteal muscles, but with flexion, the greater trochanter swings more towards the back of the pelvis, allowing more abduction space before compression occurs. Where abduction, adduction or external rotation are assisted by flexion, when we internally rotate the femur and add flexion we have a different story: we start to bring the neck of the femur closer to the acetabulum. Depending upon the shape and orientation of the acetabulum, the depth of the socket, and the thickness of the neck of the femur and its orientation, impingement can occur when we internally rotate and flex the hip. This is looked at in greater detail in It's Complicated: Femoral acetabular impingement syndrome, on page 149. It is important to understand that impingement is rarely caused by flexion all by itself but instead by the combination of flexion and internal rotation.

FLEXION WITH ABDUCTION

Just as a little bit of hip flexion can help with abduction, a little bit of abduction can help with flexion, and not just by avoiding compression. When flexion is stopped due to tightness in the hamstrings, a little bit of abduction not only moves away the possible impingement points already described, but it also brings the proximal attachment of the hamstrings closer to the distal attachments, shortening the

hamstrings, thus allowing more flexion (see figure 2.76). For example, flexing at the hip sockets in a seated forward fold (Paschimottanasana—see figure 2.77a), where both legs are straight and together, is more challenging than in Head-to-Knee Pose (Janusirsasana—see figure 2.77b), where one knee is bent and that leg is angled away from the straight leg. In Head-to-Knee Pose, the pelvis is not square to the straight leg, and thus there is abduction in the hip socket, allowing more flexion than is available when the hips are square.

Too much abduction, however, makes flexion difficult once more (see figure 2.77c). Which muscles resisting abduction will change as we increase the angle of abduction. We can consider a range of tightness, varying between the hamstrings and the adductors. With legs together, pure flexion puts a lot of stress on the hamstrings. With about 45° of abduction, the length of the hamstrings needed is less, making flexion easier. However, once we pass the 45° mark, the resistance is more keenly experienced in the adductor muscles, which until now were silent. As we abduct wider and wider, the hamstrings no longer feel the dominant stress—the adductors do. Since the adductors and hamstrings both attach to the pelvis below the hip socket (the adductor magnus attaches close to the hamstrings on

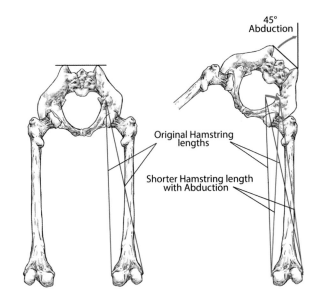

FIGURE 2.76 Viewing the hamstrings in flexion with abduction, when sitting with hips flexed. From the ground perspective, we can see how abducting the leg shortens the distance the hamstring has to span, which allows greater flexion. The red lines, representing the hamstrings' length in abduction, are shorter than the purple lines, which represent the hamstrings' length in adduction.

the ischium, while the other adductors attach near or on the pubic ramus),[91] tension in either set of muscles tends to have the same effect: they pull the sitting bones underneath us, forcing us to sit more upright, reducing flexion in the hip socket and often requiring more flexion from the spine—see figure 2.77c. (We will be looking in Volume 3 at the implications, for the spine, of flexion at the hip joint.)

Variations in Adduction

Stand with your legs together, then adduct your legs more together. What's stopping you? Obviously, your legs! Adduction seems very simple to understand when we think about both legs moving closer together. But a deeper definition involves the movement of the femur in the acetabulum, and once we realize this, our initial confidence in understanding this movement starts to fade. We have seen what abduction means: the greater trochanter of the femur moves up towards the ilium. Adduction is the opposite: the greater trochanter moves down and away from the ilium (or the ilium moves up and away from the greater trochanter).

Not surprisingly, the movement of adduction is created by the adductor muscles, specifically the adductor magnus, adductor longus, adductor brevis, as well as the gracilis and pectineus. Supporting adduction are the bicep femoris gluteus maximus, quadratus femoris and obturator externus. The classic cause of tension, if it is causing resistance to adduction, is found in the abductor muscles. The abductors, as shown in figure 2.25, are the gluteus medius and minimus and the tensor fasciae latae, and occasionally the piriformis. Additionally, tension may be present along the spiral and

lateral myofascial meridian lines, indicating a constriction of the superficial and/or deep fascia.

It is easier to understand adduction if we start from a supine position, as shown in figure 2.78: lying down on the floor with the legs straight.

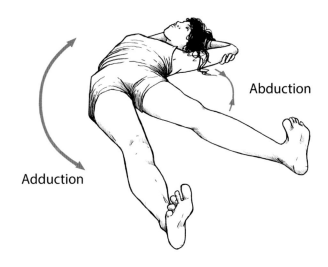

FIGURE 2.78 Bananasana: Adduction and abduction in a supine position.

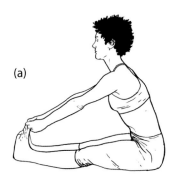 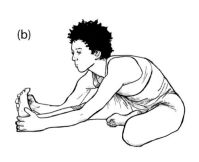 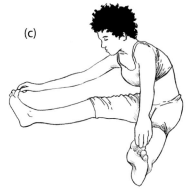

(a)   (b)   (c)

FIGURE 2.77 The effect of abduction and flexion combined. With pure flexion, there is often a limited range of folding forward available, as shown in (a) Seated Forward Fold (Paschimottanasana). Similarly, in (c) Wide-Legged Forward Fold (Upavisthakonasana), we see that with lots of abduction, folding forward is also restricted. However, in (b) Head-to-Knee Pose (Janusirsasana), we find that a bit of both flexion and abduction allows the greatest depth in forward folding.

With the left leg abducted as far away as it can go, it no longer blocks the movement of the right leg, which is free to adduct further to the left. Now what is stopping you? Why can't you adduct the right leg further? The answer is no longer that one leg is hitting the other leg; there may be tension on the right side of the body. The tension story is pretty simple: short or tight abductor muscles. The gluteus medius, gluteus minimus, tensor fasciae latae, and even the piriformis can all experience tension and reduce our range of adduction. It is also possible that the capsular ligaments will restrict you, specifically the iliofemoral ligament. (Some studies claim the ligamentum teres will also resist adduction, while other studies say such restriction is minimal.)[92] For some students, tension is felt in the top of the iliotibial band, but this is usually because of tension in the tensor fasciae latae muscle.

If you have stretched out the restraining muscles and fascia, and the ligaments are not taut, then you may have reached the point where compression is stopping you. This can occur in a couple of places: rarely, the neck of the femur may impinge upon the bottom of the acetabular rim (the transverse ligament), or, more likely, the shaft of the femur

is compressing the adductor muscles against the ischial tuberosity. The difference between tension and compression is quite noticeable: tension will be felt along the outside of the adducted hip where the muscles attach to or near the greater trochanter, while compression will be felt near the inner groin. Tension can be worked on, but compression will not change with time or practice.

Anatomical factors and human variations can affect how far you can go before you reach compression. Since, in adduction, the shaft and neck of the femur may compress tissues against the ischial tuberosities, the narrower your pubic arch, the more room you have to adduct before compression is reached (see figure 2.79). Obviously then, people with a wider pubic arch will have less room to adduct. Some women have a pubic arch of 140°—this is a very large margarita glass and would decrease the amount of adduction available. Some men have very narrow pubic arches, only 60°—the narrowest martini glass, in which case adduction can be much deeper. Remember, not all women have a 140° pubic arch; some have a much narrow of arch of only 90°, and some men have an arch around 90° as well (see figure 2.27).

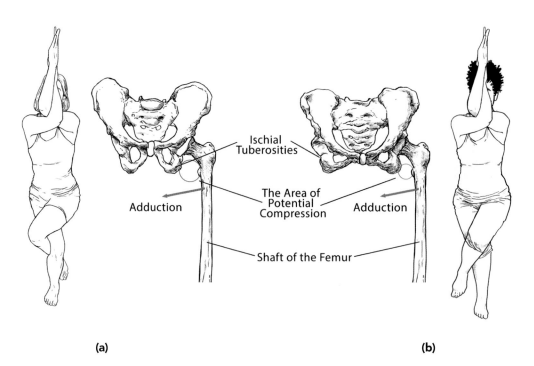

(a)   (b)

FIGURE 2.79 Adduction can be limited due to compression of the tissues between the shaft of the femur and the ischial tuberosities. The narrower pubic arch (a) allows more potential adduction space; this student can easily wrap her legs in Eagle Pose (Garudasana). If the pubic arch is wider (b), there is less room for adduction, and the student cannot wrap her legs as easily.

If your acetabular angle of abduction is over 50°, which means the side of the pelvis is more vertical, you are also likely to reach compression earlier than someone with an abduction angle of 30° or less. A lower angle means that the acetabulum is angling downward, creating more room for adduction; a higher angle means the acetabulum is angling more upwards, limiting adduction (see figure 2.28). The femoral neck-shaft angle also affects how quickly compression is reached. If you have a large angle, this increases your range of abduction but will lessen your range of adduction. If you have a smaller angle, you may be able to adduct more easily but at the potential cost of having less available room for abduction (see figure 2.35). A final factor to consider is the depth of the acetabulum and the length of the femur neck, because these can also change the amount of adduction available before compression is reached; shallower depth and longer necks increase the range of adduction.

As is usually the case, there may be a way to go around the point of compression: if the leg is extended backwards, the femur is no longer in direct opposition with the ischium. See figure 2.80 for an example where a dancer has both legs adducted, but one leg is extended behind her (called fourth position, in ballet). She may have more room to adduct that back leg than the front leg.

ADDUCTION WITH FLEXION

Another option to increase the range of adduction, one more commonly used in yoga asana practice, is to flex the hip. A little bit of flexion does not help, as it may bring the lesser trochanter into opposition with the ischium, but flexion of 30° or more allows greater adduction, because the ischial tuberosities are diagonally angled medially/anteriorly away from the femur's shaft. This is why coming into Eagle Pose (Garudasana) is easier if the hips are more flexed: that may allow for enough adduction and internal rotation to hook the foot behind the standing leg (see figure 2.81). As you flex the hip and add internal rotation, you may find that the ischiofemoral ligament becomes a restricting factor.

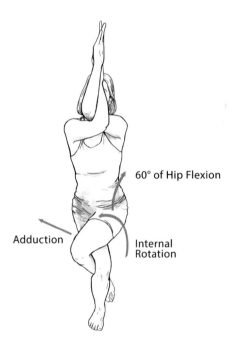

FIGURE 2.81 Eagle Pose (Garudasana) requires adduction and internal rotation, and these are easier to achieve with a deeper flexion of the hips.

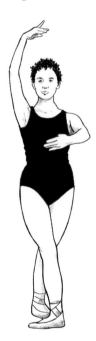

FIGURE 2.80 Adduction is easier if the hip is in extension or flexion. In ballet's fourth position, both feet are adducted. In the closed fourth position shown here, the back heel lines up with the front foot's toes. Not everyone has the range of external rotation to do this with their front foot.

When flexion approaches 90°, we have maximized the amount of adduction available by minimizing the opportunities for compression. We can call this *horizontal adduction* (comparable to horizontal abduction, but in the other direction). Some students find that they can more easily adduct their thighs when they sit in Cow Face Pose (Gomukhasana) than when they are in Eagle Pose (see figure 2.82). This is because there is more flexion occurring at the hip sockets.

When flexion continues, however, to around 120° or more, the neck of the femur is now more likely to impinge on the superior anterior acetabular rim when the leg is adducted. This is because the acetabulum is diagonally inclined in the frontal plane; the higher the femur rises, the more lateral the rim of the hip socket is, so the rim is more likely to come into contact with the femur, limiting adduction. This can occur to some students in Cowface Pose when they start

NOTE TO TEACHERS: Explore from the core outwards

It is very easy to see what is happening at the extremities, but more important is what is happening closer to the core. Teachers can readily see where the hands and feet are and what the limbs are doing, but it takes a keener eye to note what is going on closer to the axis of the body. Figure 2.84 shows two students in the same posture. Student A appears to be doing a beautiful, one-knee reclining twist (Jatharaparivartanasana), but student B struggles to get her knee to the floor. If the intention of this pose is to twist the spine, then many teachers will automatically go help the second student. But look closer. Both students have the same amount of twist to their spines, as indicated by the angle of the pelvis to the floor. The height of the knee off the floor is a measure of the student's ability to *adduct* the leg, not of how deep the twist is. The second student cannot adduct her leg as much, so her knee is floating. If your intention as a teacher is to help the second student stay in the posture and avoid rolling backwards, then extending her leg may provide the leverage she needs to counterbalance her hips. This is shown in the third drawing. In all three cases, the amount of twist to the spine is the same! Both students have the same twisting abilities, but they differ in their ability to adduct in the hip socket. Be careful what you focus on and try to adjust; look first at what is happening at the core, then work your way out to the extremities.

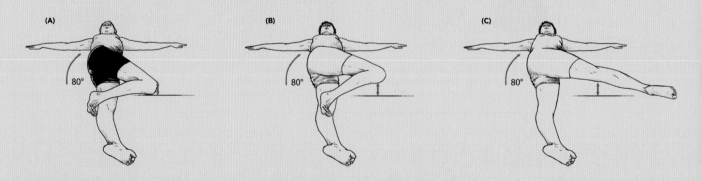

FIGURE 2.84 Focus on the core first. The two students shown in (a) and (b) are in a reclining twist (Jatharaparivartanasana). In (a), her knee is on the floor. The second student's knee is floating (b). But in both cases, the amount of twist, indicated by the angle of the pelvis to the floor, is the same. In (c), the second student has extended her leg to help balance the weight of her pelvis, but she has not changed the amount of twist to her spine.

to fold forward, deepening the flexion at their hips, which may cause the legs to move apart; with the deeper flexion, less adduction is available.

This can also occur in seated twists where one knee is close to the chest. For many students, this posture is challenging, not because they don't have the range of motion required to twist their torso, but because they cannot adduct their thigh sufficiently. Figure 2.83 shows two very different students with the same amount of spinal rotation; however, due to variations in their ability to adduct their leg, one student easily binds her hands behind her back while the other cannot. If you were unaware of the limitation to adduction, you might falsely assume that failure to bind the hands behind the back was due to insufficient spinal twisting. For this student, a lack of adduction creates her limitation, and in this case it is due to compression of the neck of the femur against the superior anterior acetabular rim. (We are again assuming all other tensile resistances to adduction have been worked through.)

Variations in Internal (Medial) Rotation of the Hip Joint

There is no primary internal (medial) rotator muscle in the anatomical position. The tensor fasciae latae can provide some internal rotation, but it is mostly involved in tensing the iliotibial band and supporting the smaller gluteal muscles in abduction. The tensor fasciae latae can also assist with flexing the hip. Once the hip is flexed, many muscles become able to strongly create internal rotation. The list includes the gluteus minimus and medius, the anterior fibers of the gluteus maximus, the adductor longus and brevis, the pectineus and the medial hamstrings (semitendinosus and semimembranosus); see figure 2.25. Surprisingly, even the normally externally rotating piriformis becomes an internal rotator when the hip is flexed 90°.[93]

A minimal amount of internal rotation is needed for walking or running. In sports that involve more lateral movements, there is a greater need to internally rotate the pelvis, but not too many yoga postures require active internal rotation. Eagle Pose (Garudasana) is one. A few passive postures in yoga do require internal rotation, such as Reclining Hero Pose (Suptavirasana), as shown in figure 2.88. In some standing postures, such as Triangle Pose (Trikonasana), the back leg is slightly internally rotated. However, many teachers prefer an alignment where the back leg in Triangle and Warrior Two (Virabhadrasana II) is not rotated internally or externally at all; instead, the foot is turned 90° and thus points in the same direction as the belly. Unfortunately, this is not a good cue: the position of the foot is not an accurate guide for determining whether the leg is rotated. Due to other factors (such as tibial rotation), having the foot pointing in a particular direction may not guarantee that the thigh is internally or externally rotated.

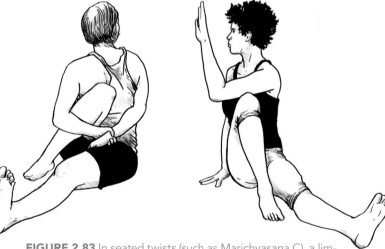

FIGURE 2.83 In seated twists (such as Marichyasana C), a limiting factor that prevents wrapping the arm behind the back and binding the hands together is the amount of adduction of the leg available. The student on the right cannot adduct her leg enough to allow her to reach her arm around it. The student on the left easily adducts the bent leg across her body and binds. In both cases, the amount of spinal twist is similar.

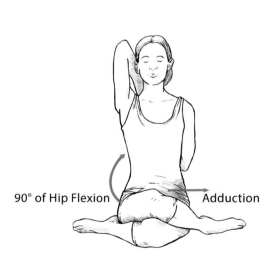

90° of Hip Flexion — Adduction

FIGURE 2.82 Cow Face (Gomukhasana) provides enough flexion of the hips to allow maximum adduction of the legs.

In the beginning of our yoga practice, for many people, our ability to internally rotate our leg is limited by the tension in our external rotator muscles; these are the obturator internus and externus, gemellus superior and inferior, quadratus femoris, piriformis, gluteus maximus—with some resistance by the gluteus medius and minimus—sartorius and bicep femoris (see figure 2.25). With 90° of flexion at the hips, some of these muscles change their role, as noted above, but some remain resistant to internal rotation. The biggest resistance comes from the posterior fibers of the gluteus maximus, the obturator externus and the quadratus femoris.[94] If these muscles are short or tight, they will resist the inward rotation of the femur. Once these tissues have been lengthened through practice, the next most common cause of restriction will be the capsular ligaments, specifically the ischiofemoral ligament and the superior iliofemoral ligament. If the ligaments are lax enough to allow further rotation, the next cause of restriction will be compression: either impingement of the neck of the femur to the acetabulum or the squeezing of tissues between the greater trochanter and the pubis or the ischium. Note that this progression is not always the case—in some people, their range of motion is so limited by the shape of their bones that they reach compression very easily and quickly, and their muscular or ligamentous flexibility is never given a chance to be a limiting factor. These students may feel a pinching sensation in the inside of the hip joint when attempting internal rotation and never feel a tension on the lateral side of the hip.

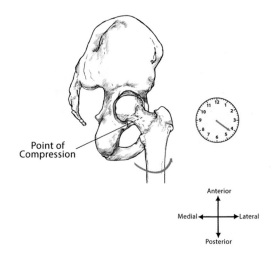

Point of Compression

Anterior

Medial ← → Lateral

Posterior

FIGURE 2.85 Femoral impingement in internal rotation, as seen from the side view. The impingement site is between the femur and pelvis and on average occurs about the 4:00 o'clock position.

As was shown in figure 2.62, the angle of the femur into the acetabulum is from behind, in the anatomical position. Figure 2.85 shows what happens when we are flexible enough to fully internally rotate the femur from the anatomical position: the anterior portion of the femur neck comes into contact with the anterior inferior lip of the acetabulum. Exactly where this impingement occurs depends upon the femur neck angle. If the neck angle is close to 120°, the point of impingement will rise up towards the 3:30 o'clock position; if the neck angle is closer to 144°, the point of impingement will be lower, towards the 5:00 o'clock position. The odds are that at least one person out of 20 will have either of these extremes. For the average femur, the point of impingement will be around the 4:00 o'clock position.

Just as variations in the orientation and angle of the acetabulum and the femur affect the amount of external rotation available to us, these same factors affect our ability to internally rotate the leg. However, because the acetabulum is angled anteriorly and medially (called its anteversion), its anterior rim is angled away from the neck of the femur, allowing a greater range of internal rotation than is offered in external rotation. Unfortunately, femoral torsion (its anteversion) can, for some people, cancel the benefits of having a large acetabular anteversion. For others, the arrangement of the femur and acetabulum can lead either towards a greater range of internal rotation or to an extremely short range. If the acetabular version is high and the femur is also highly anteverted, these factors combine to allow a great range of internal rotation—perhaps too great of a range, since many pathologies can arise if internal rotation is too extreme.[95] However, if the acetabular version is low and the femoral torsion is low, little internal rotation is possible, no matter how much a person stretches his external rotators. In this latter situation, tension is quickly worked through, and the compression of the neck of the femur to the acetabulum is the governing limitation.

The range of internal rotation possible in these two situations is illustrated in figures 2.86 and 2.87. (Once more, we are assuming a normal acetabular depth and normal femoral neck width and length, but these could easily vary as well, which would affect the ranges of motions available.) Again, we are not using the extreme variations that can be present in rare individuals; we are presenting what is likely to appear in at least one student in a yoga class of 20 students or more.

In the very best case, a student can turn her foot in 98°! That is an extreme amount of rotation potentially available, but for some people, the rotation would be stopped sooner by capsular ligament tension or compression caused by the greater trochanter squishing tissues between it and the pubis. However, there are people who can turn their feet inward so much that their toes touch and their heels point 180° away from each other. You can try the following experiment yourself; it will challenge your balance. Stand up and rotate your feet internally until your toes touch, then try to point your heels in the opposite direction. You may even be someone who can rotate your feet backwards, as shown in figure 2.86. Now the question becomes: WSM? Why can't you rotate even further? Do you feel an area of compression in the hip socket or tension along the outside of the hips?

In the very worst case, a student can only inwardly turn her foot 50° before impingement occurs. With such little rotation, it is unlikely that tension of the capsular ligament or muscles or compression between the greater trochanter and the pubis will be the cause of restricted movement. For these people, their inability to internally rotate is due primarily to the shapes of their bones, and there is nothing they can do about those—they might as well simply enjoy the range of motion they have and not break their hips trying to get more. Striving for more internal rotation than is easily available can create problems; many studies, for example, have linked lessened internal rotation ability with higher occurrences of osteoarthritis. We can begin to understand this correlation by considering that with lessened internal rotation, impingement is more likely to occur, which, over time and with ongoing stress to the labrum, can break down the protective cartilage in the acetabulum.[96] People with larger ranges of motion for internal rotation are less likely to suffer osteoarthritis in the hip socket.

INTERNAL ROTATION WITH FLEXION

When we add flexion to internal rotation, tension may arise in the posterior fibers of the gluteus maximus, the obturator externus and the quadratus femoris.[97] On the other hand, the restrictions may be due to impingement, which can arise more quickly than with internal rotation alone. The superior rim of the labrum moves forward and downward in flexion on top of the internally rotating neck of the femur. Another contributing factor is the cross-sectional shape of the neck of the femur; as was shown in figure 2.38, the neck of the femur is angled upwards (superior anteriorly), which makes contact with the acetabular rim more likely when we add flexion. This can lead to a condition known as *femoral acetabular impingement syndrome* (FAIS). Sometimes, the impingement arising here is incorrectly blamed on flexion; it mostly occurs when *both* flexion and internal rotation are combined—for example, when we come into a reclining one-knee twist. Impingement by itself is not a problem, but if it occurs too often and with too much stress, it can lead to pathology. This pathology seems to arise only in people who have an underlying morphological predisposition to it; women with thicker, overhanging labra and men with thicker femoral necks tend to

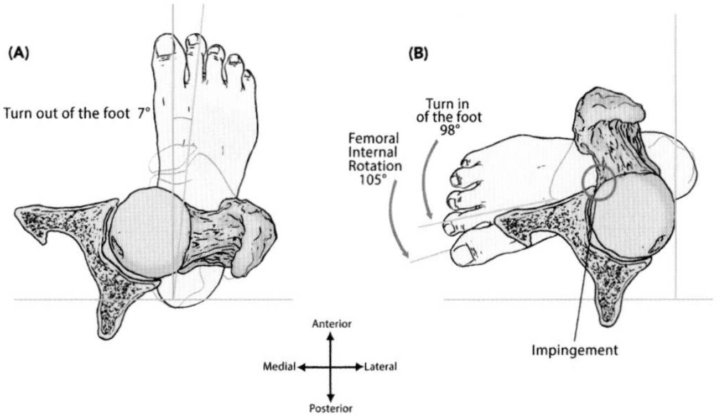

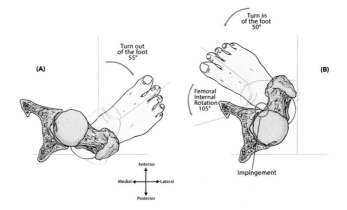

FIGURE 2.86 Best case scenario: someone with 27° of version for the femur and 33° for the acetabulum may be able to internally rotate 105°! Notice how in the anatomical position (a), their foot is pointing almost straight ahead (with a turnout angle of 7°). But in (b), with the maximum amount of internal rotation, the foot turns inward at 98°.

FIGURE 2.87 Worst case scenario: someone with 3° of version for the femur and 10° for the acetabulum may be able to go only from the neutral anatomical position (a), which has the foot turned out 55°, to an internally rotated position (b), with the foot turned in 50°.

experience FAIS far more often than people who do not have these anatomical anomalies. (See It's Complicated: Femoral acetabular impingement syndrome, on page 149, for references and a deeper discussion.)

A common posture that combines internal rotation with flexion is Hero Pose (Virasana). Here, with sufficient internal rotation, a student sits between the heels, allowing the feet to move out to the side (see figure 2.88). Students with insufficient internal rotation when their hips are flexed cannot do this; at best, they can sit on their feet but not between them. What is often preventing these students from moving their feet apart and sitting lower is the added flexion of the hips to the internal rotation: these students may be compressing the neck of the femur into the labrum. However, if they subtract the flexion in this pose and come into the Reclining Hero (Suptavirasana) version, they may find that more internal rotation is available, and thus they are able to move their feet apart enough to lie down between them. Often, students cannot get to the reclining version of this pose because they have been guided into the posture from the sitting version. They get stopped there and can't go further, even though they could do the reclining version. However, if they try coming into the posture from already lying down, they won't have to pass through the compression point of flexion. (This can be done by adopting a supine "windshield wipers" position of the legs—feet wide apart and knees dropped to one side—and drawing the internally rotated leg's foot up beside the hip, then trying the same thing with the other leg.)

INTERNAL ROTATION WITH ADDUCTION

When we combine adduction (which on its own can be limited by the iliofemoral ligament or by the shaft of the femur compressing against the ischium) with internal rotation, which is restrained initially by the ischiofemoral ligament, we arrive at the situation where both of these capsular ligaments become very taut. Additionally, internal rotation on its own can begin to compress the flesh between the greater trochanter and the pubis, and when we add adduction, the squishing intensifies. Plus, when adduction is added to internal rotation, there is a greater potential for impingement of the neck of the femur against the inferior anterior acetabulum (more specifically, the transverse ligament of the acetabulum). There is not a lot of range of motion available for most people when these two movements are combined, unless you add flexion to the equation to minimize the compression caused in adduction. (The problem of internal rotation with flexion remains, however. The addition of flexion is only helping to minimize the adduction restrictions.)

You can try the following experiment. Stand on one leg and with no flexion at the hips, then try to wrap the other leg around you, as we do in Eagle Pose (Garudasana). Most likely, you won't be able to tuck the foot behind the opposite calf. However, try the Eagle Pose again, but this time flex your hips and sit down a little (see figure 2.81). When we add flexion at the hip joint, we begin to "unwind" the capsular ligaments: they are no longer taut and don't restrict us. Also, as we add flexion, we allow more room to adduct the leg in front of us because flexion moves the

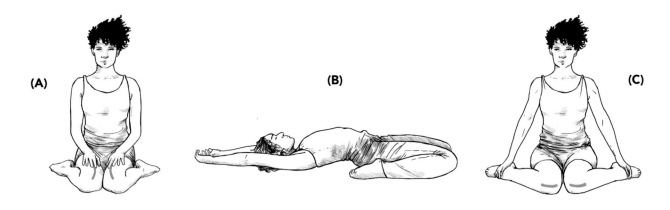

FIGURE 2.88 Hero Pose (Virasana) and Reclining Hero Pose (Suptavirasana). Due to the addition of flexion to internal rotation, many students cannot sit between their legs like the student in (a) but when they take away the flexion (b), they find they can lie down between their feet. The student in (c) has more room for internal rotation and can move her feet further apart.

ischial tuberosities further away from the shaft of the femur, reducing possible compression. Flexing the hips beyond 30° allows for enough internal rotation and adduction for many people to be able to hook their foot behind the calf. If the student flexes further (by sitting down lower into the pose), they will find they can adduct and internally rotate further as well. This works well to about 45° of flexion, but going past there, compression will raise its inevitable head: you will feel your legs hitting each other, or the inferior neck of the femur will impinge on the anterior acetabulum, and no further adduction or internal rotation will be available.

There is a special breed of people who can both adduct and internally rotate at their hips sockets a lot, and they are required to do so by their profession: hockey goalies. When goalies drop to their knees in their version of a butterfly, they are strongly internally rotating their legs so that they can spread their shins along the ice, covering as much territory as possible. This requires a highly unique hip architecture, and very few people can do this. Curiously, this internal orientation of the hips sockets and neck of the femur makes it very difficult for hockey goalies to also be strong skaters; the best hockey skaters are those who have a good range of external rotation, because skating requires strong lateral (external) push with the legs. It is not, therefore, surprising that hockey goalies choose their position at a young age—they were never destined to be the fastest skaters on their team, but they were able to do what most players could not: the hockey butterfly pose. There is a similar pose in yoga, the X-Pose, which is basically a reclining hockey goalie butterfly position (see figure 2.89b).

INTERNAL ROTATION WITH ABDUCTION

Combining internal rotation with abduction does not seem to help increase either internal rotation or abduction. If a student's abduction is restricted by the capsular ligaments, specifically the pubofemoral ligament and the ischiofemoral ligament, then if we add internal rotation, we shorten the pubofemoral ligament, making it more lax, but we tighten and stress the ischiofemoral ligament more. If the ischiofemoral ligament is already taut, due to the abduction, it will resist adding internal rotation. If abduction is restricted not due to the capsular ligaments but due to compression of tissues between the rising greater trochanter and the ilium (specifically the anterior inferior iliac spine—AIIS), when we add internal rotation to the game, we rotate the greater trochanter forward, in front of the AIIS, thus reducing the amount of compression. Eventually, we will compress tissues against the pubis, but we will have gained a few extra degrees of abduction because of our internal rotation. There are not too many postures in yoga where we need to combine abduction with internal rotation, but one example is simply standing with your legs as wide apart as possible (see figure 2.55). If you can't move your legs any further apart, trying internally rotating: point your toes more inward, and see whether this allows you a few more degrees of abduction. One reason we are not taught this in yoga classes is because we can achieve the same thing, only deeper, by flexing and externally rotating the hips, as was discussed in the section on horizontal abduction (see page 97).

Abduction with a little bit of internal rotation is found in the martial arts. A Bruce Lee-style kick does involve

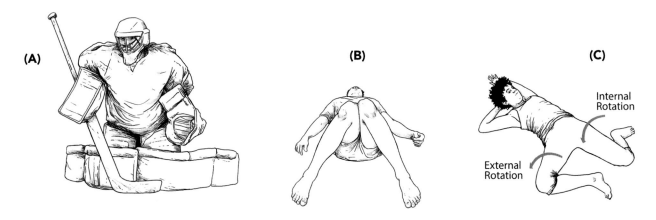

(A)   **(B)**   **(C)**

Internal Rotation

External Rotation

FIGURE 2.89 Modern hockey goalies' butterfly pose (a) requires 90° of internal rotation of the femur and adduction. The Reclining X-Pose (b) is close to the goalie's pose. The Reclining Windshield Wiper (c) is internal rotation and adduction of the femur on one side, with external rotation and abduction on the other.

some internal rotation with abduction, but not much (see figure 2.90). As in our yoga practice, martial artists need to be aware of the consequences of their unique body structure. One orthopedic surgeon and karate champion aptly warns: "Listening to one's body is important. Some people's hips are not designed for high kicks [FAI can occur], and you can stretch all you want, but a bony impingement will remain."[98]

INTERNAL ROTATION WITH FLEXION AND ABDUCTION

While adding flexion to internal rotation may cause impingement more quickly than internal rotation alone, if we add abduction to the mix, we get more room to internally rotate. Check out figure 2.91. Sitting between the heels in Hero Pose (Virasana) requires internal rotation at the hip socket, but for many students, due to the flexion at the hips, the anterior neck of the femur impinges upon the superior acetabulum. However, if we abduct the knees apart, there is now more space for further internal rotation! The common alignment cue "keep the knees together" in this posture makes it impossible for some people to ever sit between their feet. But even a little abduction makes the pose possible.

Notice in figure 2.91 that there is no stress to the knees in Hero Pose (Virasana) if we can internally rotate the femur. If we look carefully, we will see that the femur has rotated, not the tibia. In this case, the student has a large range of internal rotation available, and there is no discomfort or pain in the knees while staying here. For her, this is perfectly safe, but not for everybody. If internal rotation is not available, then twisting in the knee has to happen in order to sit between the feet. As we will see when we look at the knee-joint segment, for some students, that is perfectly okay! They have the laxity in the knee ligaments to accommodate the twist at the knee. For other students, however, who don't have the necessary laxity in the knee ligaments, trying to sit between their feet will wreak havoc, death and destruction upon the knee.

The cue to keep the knees together in Hero Pose, or to never move the feet apart, is good advice for some students, but for others it is unhelpful and for yet others unnecessary. The only way to know which camp you are in is to pay attention to what your body allows and not force it into a pose. B.K.S. Iyengar offers beginners the option of allowing the knees to be apart in Reclining Hero Pose (Suptavirasana),[99] but his labeling this a "beginner's" option ignores the fact that many experienced yogis will also need to keep their knees apart, due to their unique anatomical shape. For them, trying to bring the knees together is not a good idea.

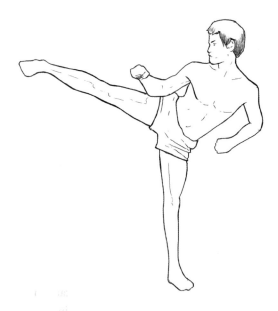

FIGURE 2.90 A martial arts kick. Abduction is combined with a slight internal rotation for the lifted leg, but with external rotation for the standing leg.

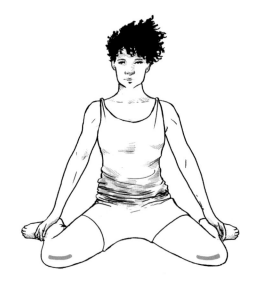

FIGURE 2.91 Hero Pose (Virasana) with knees abducted may allow a greater range of internal rotation at the hips, with no stress on the knees. Note that here, the femur (indicated by the colored lines) has rotated, and there is no twist at the knee.

IT'S COMPLICATED:
Femoral acetabular impingement syndrome

Femoral acetabular impingement syndrome (FAIS) can arise when we constantly compress the neck of the femur against the labrum of the acetabulum. FAIS most commonly occurs in the superior anterior portion of the labrum.[100] Pure flexion alone rarely causes impingement to this area, but when flexion is accompanied by internal rotation of the femur, then impingement is more likely here.

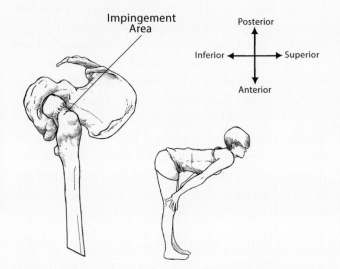

FIGURE 2.92 Flexion with a little internal rotation can create an impingement at the superior anterior labrum, but only in some people.

Fortunately, FAIS is almost always accompanied by some underlying morphologic uniqueness in the shape of either the acetabulum or the femur, usually due to a congenital cause or a developmental issue during childhood.[101] For people with an average-shaped femur or acetabulum, FAIS is rare. But if your labrum is thicker and more extensive, creating more coverage of the head of the femur, then the femoral neck is more likely to hit the labrum when movement occurs. This condition, which occurs in 27% of women and 17% of men, is known as a *pincer* of the labrum; think of the labrum "pinching" in towards the neck of the femur, effectively deepening the hip socket.[102] If the femoral neck is thicker than normal, occurring in about 24% of men but in almost no women,[103] then this too increases the likelihood of impingement during movement, a condition known as a *cam* or *pistol grip*. In this situation, the shape of the neck of the femur is more "cam-like" (and looks like the grip of a handgun) and thus closer

to the labrum (see figure 2.93). The extra width is 90% of the time on the superior anterior side of the neck.[104] One study has found that acetabula with cam femurs are shallower than normal hip sockets, while pincer acetabula, not including the labrum, are deeper than normal ones.[105]

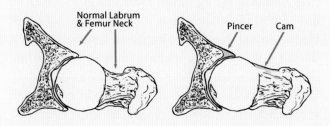

FIGURE 2.93 Pincer and cam.

Sometimes the labrum grows closer to the femoral neck or the femoral neck grows closer to the labrum; rarely, both conditions happen together.[106] In any case, movement involving internal rotation is what brings these two body parts together. If you suffer from FAIS, then it's a good idea to externally rotate your thighs as you come into forward folds (standing or sitting), and thus move the neck of the femur away from the anterior superior labrum.[107] Of course, due to your uniqueness, FAIS can happen in other parts of the labrum. Pay attention and notice which movements create discomfort and pain, then mindfully adjust your practice to suit your body.

The common yoga cue of standing in Mountain Pose (Tadasana) with your big toes touching and the heels slightly apart requires, for most students, a slight internal rotation at the hip sockets. Some students, however, to achieve this position need a great deal of internal rotation (often due to a large tibial torsion, but for many other reasons as well). Now, with the request to fold forward into a Standing Forward Fold Pose (Uttanasana), flexion is added to the internal rotation applied. For most people, this will never be a problem, but for some, especially those predisposed to FAIS, adding internal rotation before commencing Uttanasana is not a good idea. How will you know if this warning applies to you? Pay attention. What do you feel when you fold forward? If there is pain in the hip, try allowing your feet to point outward before folding forward, and see whether that makes a difference.

Variations in Extension

Our range of extension is the only movement in the hip socket that definitely correlates with age; the older we get, the less we are able to extend.[108] Extension is resisted by the hip flexor muscles, specifically the rectus femoris, psoas major and minor, iliacus, tensor fasciae latae and sartorius (see figure 2.25). Tightness along the superficial front line and ipsilateral functional line myofascial meridian may also restrain our movement into extension. For many students beginning a yoga practice, these are the obvious culprits stopping them from extending the leg further behind them. However, for many other students, these muscles and fascia are sufficiently lengthened and therefore no longer the limiting factor. For the vast majority of yoga students, extension is finally limited by the capsular ligaments wrapping the hip socket. All three ligaments become taut after about 20–30° of extension, effectively "screwing down" the head of the femur into the acetabulum. The "close-packed" position of the hip joint occurs

IT'S IMPORTANT: Remember, compression can be good!

When we hear terms like femoral acetabular impingement syndrome, it is easy to jump to the conclusion that this must be bad, but contact between the bones and their cartilage is not unhealthy per se. Too much or too frequent stress can be bad and result in osteoarthritis. But if we run away from stress out of fear, we may easily suffer effects from the opposite extreme. No stress at all in a joint leads to osteoporosis—a dangerous weakening of the bones—and contracture, which is a shrink-wrapping and tightening of the joint capsule. Bones and cartilage need stress to stay strong. Joints, too, need stress to remain healthy. This means that the bones have to press into each other. Femoral acetabular impingement, simply because the femur and the acetabulum are touching, is not always a problem. Too much stress is not good, but some is absolutely necessary. Tissue compression is problematic only when it happens too often, with too much force and without enough recovery time between stresses.

when extension is combined with a little bit of internal rotation and abduction, causing all three ligaments to be maximally taut.[109] A few students' ligaments will be long enough or lax enough to allow compression between the neck of the femur and the acetabulum. This is likely to occur only if the acetabulum has a high version and low angle of abduction, and the femur has a shorter neck with a high neck-shaft angle and low torsion. Given this rare combination of conditions, when the femur extends, the posterior neck of the femur may impinge upon the posterior rim of the acetabulum.

The limitations to extension show up in many yoga postures, such as King Dancer (Natarajasana), Wheel Pose (Dhanurasana) and the front splits, known as the Monkey Pose (Hanumanasana). The last is very challenging for most students because they cannot extend the back leg very far, which causes the pelvis to flex forward, putting more stress on the front leg's hamstrings. In figure 2.94 we find three students with very different monkeys. The first (a) has tightness in her hip flexors, preventing her from extending her back leg and lowering her hips. The second (b) has worked through the muscular tension and reached 30° of extension in the hip socket of the back leg, close to virtually everybody's maximum. Notice that her pelvis is at a 45° angle to vertical. For her torso to be completely vertical, she must extend her spine the additional 45°. (Note: other, less flexible, students may have their torso vertical in this pose as well, but only because they are creating a deep extension in their spine, not at their hip socket. Their inability to extend the back leg means that their pelvis is tilted much more forward, which requires a deeper extension angle in their lumbar spine to bring their torso upright.)

Since no one can extend the back leg a full 90°, a choice has to be made: (i) square up the hips and allow the pelvis to be off the ground, a little or a lot (perhaps by supporting the sitting bones on a block or having the hands on the floor), or (ii) lean to the front leg side, tilting the pelvis until the front leg's sitting bone is on the ground. This tilting lifts the back leg's hip more off the floor, but at least the front leg's hip is down.

For this pose, and for many others that require hip extension, the less extension that is available in the hips, the more the spine will need to extend to reach the vertical position for the torso. The trade-off then is between low hips and much more spinal extension, or higher hips and less spinal extension. In figure 2.94a, the student is not extending her spine because to do so she would have to take her hands off the floor. She could do this if she had blocks under her pelvis.

EXTENSION WITH ABDUCTION AND EXTERNAL (LATERAL) ROTATION

There is an urge to abduct and externally rotate the legs to get around the restriction of the capsular ligaments in hip extension. This shows up in postures requiring hip extension, like the Supported Bridge Pose (Setubandhasarvangasana) and the Wheel Pose (Dhanurasana). Examine the back leg of the student in figure 2.94c. She has her pelvis angled and her back leg externally rotated. She does not quite have the range of motion to get either sitting bone onto the floor, so she is keeping her hands on the floor for support. The abduction of the pelvis helps to deepen the extension of the back leg.

The reason that external rotation and abduction may help increase extension relates to the capsular ligaments, but it is complicated—and if your eyes have already glazed over, you may wish to skip the rest of this paragraph! In the close-packed position, where the femur is locked down into the acetabulum, no further extension is possible. The capsular ligaments are maximally taut. However, for some students, if they add external rotation, they shorten the ischiofemoral and, more importantly, the iliofemoral ligaments, the latter being the strongest of the capsular ligaments. Unfortunately, external rotation stretches the pubofemoral ligament even more, but abduction shortens the pubofemoral ligament again, as well as the iliofemoral ligaments. The combination of abduction with external rotation provides more room to extend the leg before the capsular ligaments again become taut.

Many yoga teachers believe that the tendency to externally rotate an extended leg is due to the action of the main extensor muscle, the gluteus maximus, which is also a strong rotator. This can happen; if the main power for extending the back leg or the pelvis is coming from the gluteus maximus, such as in the Wheel Pose or Bridge Pose, this will cause external rotation and abduction in the hip joint. In the case of the Monkey Pose, however, the gluteus maximus is not working hard, so it is not responsible for the external rotation seen here.[110]

Some teachers warn that allowing external rotation in the back hip socket in the Monkey Pose can overstress the adductors and create too much twisting stress into the sacroiliac joint on that side. And yet, in Warrior 1 Pose (Virabhadrasana I), this is exactly the alignment cue often given: the back leg is extended and externally rotated. In figure 2.95, we see a student in a Warrior 1 Pose with the front thigh parallel to the floor, displaying 30° of pelvic extension for the back leg at the hip socket. It is not clear why teachers will not allow external rotation in the Monkey, Wheel or Bridge poses to assist with hip extension but will require external rotation of the back leg in Warrior 1 to achieve the desired extension.

From a functional yoga point of view, we don't care how the leg looks; we care about the sensations being created, and we adjust or not depending on the quality of those sensations. The reality is that many students need to allow some external rotation and abduction of the back leg to reach their maximum range of hip extension.

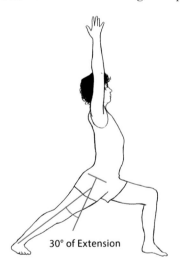

FIGURE 2.95 Warrior 1 Pose (Virabhadrasana I) requires extension of the back leg and is taught with external rotation and a little bit of abduction. In this example, with the front thigh parallel to the floor, the back hip is extended 30°.

30° of Extension

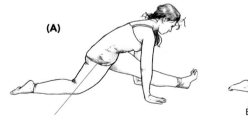 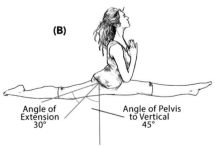 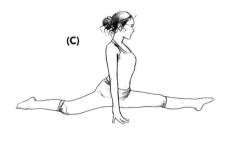

(A) (B) (C)

Angle of Extension 30° Angle of Pelvis to Vertical 45°

FIGURE 2.94 Forward splits, aka Monkey Pose (Hanumanasana). For beginners (a), tension in the hip flexors will prevent significant extension of the back leg, but in time (b), when that muscular tension has been worked through, tension in the capsular ligaments may stop further progress. For intermediate students (c), when the hips are almost on the ground, extension restrictions may cause the back leg to externally rotate and abduct.

Hip-Joint Summary

We can employ the WSM? spectrum to summarize what may stop you from greater ranges of motion in your hip sockets. Table 2.7 shows the spectrum applied to each of the main movements possible in the hip joint. As we start from the left end of the spectrum, progress in working through tension is relatively easy, but as we get closer to the right, it becomes progressively harder (ligaments are difficult to stretch), and at the far right, the game is over: no further progress in that direction for that pose will ever happen once one bone hits another. Asking "What stops me?" helps to locate where you are along this spectrum, and thus you will know whether it is wise to try to go further. Remember, due to the reality of human variation, the shape and orientation of some people's bones mean that they will move very quickly to the right, while others have a very large range of motion available before reaching their final edge.

Warning: This table does not indicate *why* the tension may have arisen. As we saw in Volume 1, tension has many causes other than short muscles, including emotions, nervous system interactions, hydration, or pathologies. Scar tissue or inflammation can cause tension, and compression can arise from a torn labrum. The limitations suggested in the table are indicators of possibilities, not static facts. The table is for general guidance rather than specific evaluation. Everyone has to answer for themselves: "What stops me?"

TABLE 2.7 The WSM? spectrum for the hip joint

MOVEMENT IN THE HIP JOINT	TENSILE RESISTANCE				COMPRESSION		
	SURFACE TENSION	MYOFASCIAL MERIDIANS*	MUSCLES & TENDONS	LIGAMENTS & JOINT CAPSULE	SOFT: FLESH ON FLESH	MEDIUM: BONE ON FLESH	HARD: BONE ON BONE
FLEXION	Buttocks; back; back of legs	Superficial back lines	Hamstrings: semitendinosus, semimembranosus, biceps femoris; gluteus maximus; gracilis	Past 90° of flexion, the ischiofemoral ligament; inferior joint capsule. Past 160° of flexion, all capsular ligaments, possibly the ligamentum teres.	Chest hitting the thigh	ASIS hitting the thigh	Superior acetabulum impinging upon the superior anterior neck of the femur. Past 160° of flexion, the superior acetabulum impinging on the inferior neck of the femur.
FLEXION WITH INTERNAL ROTATION	Buttocks; back; back of legs and outside of hip	Superficial back lines and the spiral lines	Hamstrings: semitendinosus, semimembranosus, biceps femoris; gluteus maximus; gracilis; some external rotators (minimal)	Past 160° of flexion, all capsular ligaments	Chest hitting the thigh	ASIS hitting thigh	Superior acetabulum impinging upon the superior anterior neck of the femur

MOVEMENT IN THE HIP JOINT	TENSILE RESISTANCE				COMPRESSION		
	SURFACE TENSION	MYOFASCIAL MERIDIANS*	MUSCLES & TENDONS	LIGAMENTS & JOINT CAPSULE	SOFT: FLESH ON FLESH	MEDIUM: BONE ON FLESH	HARD: BONE ON BONE
FLEXION WITH ABDUCTION	Buttocks; back; the back of the legs and inner groin	Superficial back lines and the lateral lines	Past 45° of abduction: the adductor muscles. With 180° of flexion and full abduction, also the piriformis, gluteus maximus, obturator externus, quadratus femoris, gracilis, semitendinosus and semimembranosus	Pubofemoral ligament		At 180° of flexion, the greater trochanter squeezes various tissues against the ischium	At 90° of flexion, the posterior acetabulum impinges on the superior neck of the femur. Past 90° of flexion, the inferior rim against the superior neck of the femur.
EXTENSION	Lower belly, front of pelvis and front of thigh	Superficial front line and ipsilateral functional line	Hip flexors: rectus femoris, psoas major and minor, iliacus, tensor fasciae latae and sartorius	Iliofemoral, pubofemoral and ischiofemoral ligaments become taut after about 20–30° of extension	Minimal compression of buttocks to back of thigh		The superior posterior neck of the femur and the superior posterior acetabulum may impinge. This is only likely to occur if the acetabulum has a high version and low angle of abduction and if the femur has a high neck angle and low torsion.
EXTERNAL ROTATION	Minimal resistance. If any, it may be felt in the inner groin.	Minimal resistance. If any, it may be from the spiral lines	Tensor fasciae latae minimally	Pubofemoral ligament and anterior iliofemoral ligament, iliotibial band, possibly the ligamentum teres			Posterior inferior acetabulum with posterior neck of femur

THE HIP JOINT

MOVEMENT IN THE HIP JOINT	TENSILE RESISTANCE				COMPRESSION		
	SURFACE TENSION	MYOFASCIAL MERIDIANS*	MUSCLES & TENDONS	LIGAMENTS & JOINT CAPSULE	SOFT: FLESH ON FLESH	MEDIUM: BONE ON FLESH	HARD: BONE ON BONE
EXTERNAL ROTATION WITH FLEXION	Minimal resistance. If any, it may be felt in the inner groin.	Minimal resistance. If any, it may be from the superficial back lines.	With 90° of flexion, the gluteus minimus and medius, the anterior fibers of the gluteus maximus	With 90° of flexion, the pubofemoral ligament and iliofemoral ligaments are taut; over 90°, the anterior iliofemoral and pubofemoral ligaments may shorten; the superior iliofemoral ligament lengthens.		With 90° of flexion, the lesser trochanter may trap the adductor muscles between the femur and the pelvis. With 180° of flexion, the greater trochanter compresses flesh against the pubis.	With 90° of flexion, the anterior inferior rim of the acetabulum impinges upon the posterior neck of the femur. With 180° of flexion, the anterior superior rim is against the posterior neck.
INTERNAL ROTATION	Minimal resistance. If any, it may be felt in the outside of the legs/hip.	Minimal resistance. If any, it may be from the spiral lines.	Obturator internus and externus, gemellus superior and inferior, quadratus femoris, piriformis, gluteus maximus, with some assistance from the gluteus medius and minimus, sartorius, bicep femoris	The ischiofemoral ligament and the superior iliofemoral ligament, posterior joint capsule		Tissues between the greater trochanter and the pubis or the ischium	Anterior inferior acetabulum with anterior neck of femur
INTERNAL ROTATION WITH FLEXION	Minimal resistance. If any, it may be felt in the outside of the hip and buttocks.	Minimal resistance. If any, it may be from the spiral lines and superficial back lines.	Obturator externus, quadratus femoris, posterior fibers of the gluteus maximus, gemellus superior and inferior	With 90° of flexion, the ischiofemoral ligament is taut.			With 90° of flexion, the anterior superior rim of the acetabulum impinges upon the anterior neck of the femur.
INTERNAL ROTATION WITH ADDUCTION	Minimal resistance. If any, it may be felt in the outside of the legs/hip	Minimal resistance. If any, it may be from the spiral lines and lateral lines.	Posterior fibers of the gluteus maximus, medius and minimus	Iliofemoral and ischiofemoral ligaments are taut.		Tissues between the greater trochanter and the pubis or the ischium	Impingement of anterior neck of the femur against the transverse ligament of the acetabulum

MOVEMENT IN THE HIP JOINT	TENSILE RESISTANCE				COMPRESSION		
	SURFACE TENSION	MYOFASCIAL MERIDIANS*	MUSCLES & TENDONS	LIGAMENTS & JOINT CAPSULE	SOFT: FLESH ON FLESH	MEDIUM: BONE ON FLESH	HARD: BONE ON BONE
ABDUCTION	Inner groin	Front functional lines, contra-ipsilateral functional line, deep front line, and contra-lateral line	Adductors: adductor magnus, longus, brevis; gracilis; pectineus	Pubofemoral ligament, ischiofemoral ligament, inferior joint capsule		Greater trochanter squeezing gluteus medius and minimus against ilium	Impingement of superior acetabulum and superior neck of the femur
HORIZONTAL ABDUCTION	Inner groin	Front functional lines, deep front lines, superficial back lines	Quadratus femoris; gemelli; obturator externus; adductor magnus, minimus, longus and brevis; gracilis; pectineus. Hamstrings: semitendinosus, semimembranosus, biceps femoris	Pubofemoral ligament becomes very tight		Greater trochanter compresses the gluteus muscles against the back of the pelvis.	Superior neck of the femur impinges on the posterior rim of the acetabulum.
ADDUCTION	Outer hips	Spiral lines and lateral lines	Posterior fibers of the gluteus minimus and medius and tensor fasciae latae	Iliofemoral ligament; possibly the ligamentum teres; iliotibial band and ligamentum teres	The inner thighs collide.	The medial shaft and neck of the femur compress tissues against the ischial tuberosities.	
ADDUCTION WITH FLEXION	Outer hips and buttocks	Spiral lines, lateral lines and superficial back lines	Gluteus maximus, posterior fibers of the gluteus minimus and medius, piriformis, quadratus femoris, obturator internus, tensor fasciae latae	Ischiofemoral ligament	The inner thighs collide.	The medial shaft of the femur and lesser trochanter compress tissues against the pubis.	The inferior neck of the femur may impinge on the anterior acetabulum.

* See Volume 1, pages 71–74 for a description of the myofascial meridians.

Table 2.8 shows the particular parameters of the pelvis' and femur's shape, size and orientations that play a significant role in determining our available range of motion. Each parameter is a morphological variation of the bone. Shown are how frequently it appears on average, along with the total observed range found in certain studies already cited. Also provided are the standard deviations found in the studies, and the range in which 95% of people will likely fall (the two standard deviation limits). The latter range shows that we are likely to find such variations in a class of 20 yoga students. This also means that one student in 20 will be outside the two standard deviation range.

TABLE 2.8 Variations of the pelvis and femur

BONE	TYPE OF VARIATION	AVERAGE VALUE	1 STANDARD DEVIATION (67% OF PEOPLE)	2 STANDARD DEVIATION RANGE (95% OF PEOPLE)	TOTAL RANGE OBSERVED
Pelvis	Acetabular angle of abduction	39.7°	4.3°	31.1–48.3°	29.4–57°
Pelvis	Acetabular version	21.3°	5.8°	9.7–32.9°	(12.9)–40.5°
Pelvis	Acetabular depth	34.2%	3.5%	27.2–41.2%	27–43%
Pelvis	Version of the anterior pelvic plane	6.9°	9.2°	25.3–(11.5)°	31.4–(17.6)°
Pelvis	Angle of ASIS/PSIS line to horizontal	13°	5°	3–23°	0–23°
Femur	Femoral torsion	15°	6°	3–27°	(15)–33°
Femur	Femoral neck-shaft angle	132°	6.1°	120–144°	110–150°
Femur	Neck length	3.41 cm	0.43 cm	2.55–4.27 cm	1.84–4.16 cm
Femur	Greater trochanter height	8 mm	4.7 mm	0–16.7 mm	Not Available
Tibia	Tibial torsion	29.6°	7.7°	14.2–45°	2–82°

Negative values are in parentheses.

CHAPTER 3
The Joint Segments of the Lower Body:
The Knee Joint

As we move from our core to the floor, we must pass through the biggest synovial joint in our body: the knee. We have not finished looking at all the implications that variations in our pelvis and femur have for our range of movements, but to understand the consequences we have not yet investigated, we need to look at other areas of the lower body and see how they are impacted by our individual uniqueness. We will next look at the distal portion of the femur, the proximal tibia and the knee joint.

As with most lower body joints, stability is more important than mobility,[111] and the knee is a good example of this. We can look at the knee as a mechanism that resists movement and transmits loads from above to below. Obviously, however, the knee does move, and within our yoga practice there are four major concerns that have dictated a variety of alignment cues:

- Where should the knee be in full extension (and do we need to "microbend" the knee to avoid hyperextension)?
- What should be the alignment of the knee with respect to the pelvis when the knee is flexed, as in standing poses like Warrior Two (Virabhadrasana II)?
- What should be the alignment of the foot/ankle with respect to the knee when the knee is flexed, again applicable to standing postures like the Warriors (Virabhadrasana) or the Triangle (Trikonasana)?
- Should we attempt postures that may be risky for the knees, such as Lotus (Padmasana), Pigeon (Kapotasana) and Hero (Suptavirasana)?

To understand why these concerns may be important or unimportant, we must first grasp the architecture and mechanics of the knee, its ranges of motion, the ranges of human variations in this part of the body, and typical pathologies that can arise.

Form

The knee is the largest joint in the body and one of the most complex. Unlike most joints, there is no bony stop to limit movement; instead, ligaments, tendons, muscles and fascia combine to resist hypermobility. Sometimes the knee joint is called a hinge joint because its primary action is flexion and extension, like a door swinging on its hinges.[112] Sometimes it is called a *condyloid* joint, referring to the "knuckles" found at the distal end of the femur. Sometimes it is called an *ellipsoid* joint, referring to the shape of the condyles. It is all of these.

THE ARCHITECTURE OF THE KNEE JOINT

As shown in figure 2.100, four bones come together around the knee-joint segment: the femur, kneecap (patella), tibia and fibula. Together they make up four separate joints, which we simply call the knee. The four joinings are:

- the patella and the femur, called the *patellofemoral* joint
- the fibula and the tibia, called the *tibiofibular* joint
- the medial condyle of the femur with the tibia
- the lateral condyle of the femur with the tibia

There are a couple of notes worth making right at the start: the patella only articulates with the femur and never touches the tibia; and, for most people, there is very little movement available between the fibula and the tibia. The fibula serves as a supporting strut to the tibia and as an attachment site for the biceps femoris and the lateral collateral ligament. The little bit of movement that does happen here is important for ankle mobility, which we will look at later.

Due to the shapes of the femoral condyles at the distal end of the femur and the tibial condyles at the top or proximal surface of the tibia, the fit between the femur and tibia is not exact. To help improve the contact, there are two

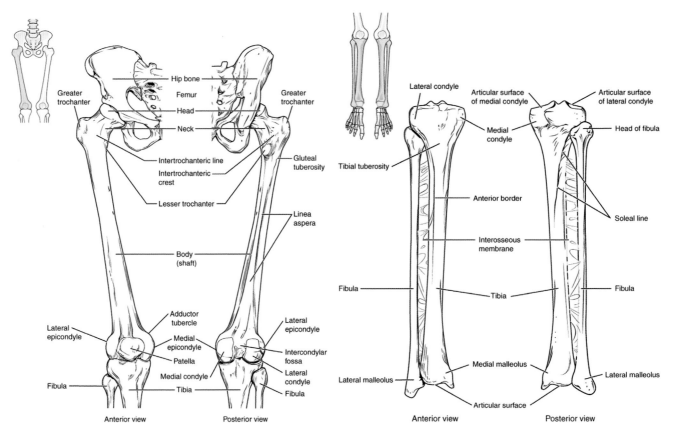

FIGURE 2.100 The four bones of the knee-joint segment: the femur, patella, tibia and fibula.

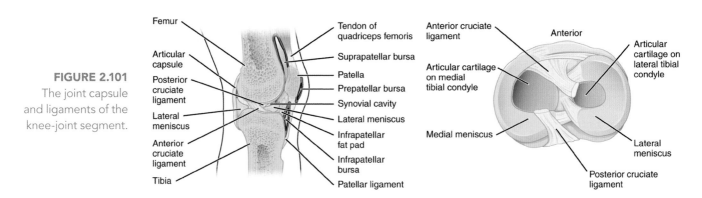

FIGURE 2.101 The joint capsule and ligaments of the knee-joint segment.

C-shaped pads made of cartilage, called menisci (the singular is meniscus, from the Greek for a "small moon," thus, a crescent shape). As mentioned, the knee is inherently unstable, having no bony stops as are found in the elbow joint, for example; stability is provided by the soft tissues of the joint capsule, ligaments, tendons, muscles and superficial fascia. Figure 2.101 illustrates the extent of the support from the ligaments and capsule, and figure 2.102 shows the muscles crossing the knee that help to create or resist movement. Not shown are most of the 14 bursae[113] that are scattered throughout the knee and provide friction-reducing support for the tendons and ligaments.

While the knee is one femur's length from the pelvis, movement of the pelvis can affect the range of motion at the knee due to several muscles that cross both joints. The rectus femoris, which flexes the hip, can extend the knee, and the hamstrings that extend the hip can flex the knee. Tension in these muscles arising from movement of the hips can reduce the range of motion in the knees, and vice versa. For example, when the knees are extended, it is harder to flex the hips. Thanks to the fascial continuity throughout the body, muscles that are not normally considered factors in knee movement can affect the knee even though they act mainly on the hip, such as the gluteus maximus; it can assist with knee extension because of its pull on the iliotibial band. Again, we find that answering the WSM? question is not simple.

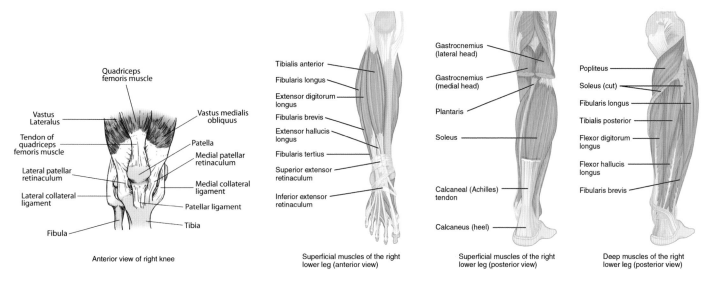

FIGURE 2.102 The thigh muscles crossing the knee-joint segment, and the muscles of the lower leg.

THE BONES OF THE KNEE

To investigate the form and function of the knee, we really only need to examine the femur, tibia and patella. We can leave the fibula for when we reach the ankle.

The Femur

The distal (bottom) end of the femur (see figure 2.103) broadens out to form the *condyles*. The lateral condyle protrudes more anteriorly than the medial condyle and provides a greater ridge of support for the patella, preventing it from slipping while moving. However, the medial condyle projects more inferiorly than the lateral, helping to make the base of the two condyles more horizontal. This is necessary because the femur is angled slightly to the vertical compared to the tibia (see the later discussion of the Q-angle, on pages 167–168). Between the two condyles are two valleys called the *intercondylar notch* (sometimes referred to as the *intercondylar fossa*) and the *patellar groove* (sometimes called the *intercondylar groove* or the *trochlea*). The patella articulates with the femur and glides up and down the patellar groove, while the cruciate ligaments find their home within the intercondylar notch. The distal ends of the femur are relatively flat, allowing for a wide base to distribute the weight of the upper body onto the tibial plateau when we are standing, but the anterior and posterior shapes of the condyles are curved like the bottom of a rocking chair, to allow easy flexion and extension of the knee.

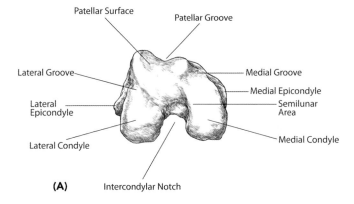

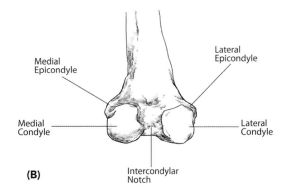

FIGURE 2.103 The distal end of a right femur: (a) distal view, (b) posterior view.

The Tibia

The tibia, the longest bone in the body after the femur, broadens its proximal (top) end from a narrow triangular shaft into a wide plateau, which provides a nice, wide base of support for the femur. While the two condyles of the femur are convex, the tibial plateau has one slightly concave surface on the medial side to receive the femoral medial condyle; however, the lateral surface of the tibial plateau is flat to slightly convex.[114] This means that the tibial condyles are not exact matches to the femur condyles. Fortunately, in between the two bones we have the menisci, which help to make the congruence between the femur and tibia more secure. The medial tibial condyle is larger than the lateral due its role in supporting the larger medial femoral condyle, but this extra support means that osteoarthritis is much more common on this side of the tibia. Just as the femoral condyles have a notch between them, the tibial condyles have a slight ridge between them called the *intercondylar eminence* (see figure 2.104). On the front of the proximal tibia is a raised prominence called the *tibial tuberosity*; this bump provides a large surface for the attachment of the patellar tendon, which, in turn, is the distal portion of the quadriceps tendon.

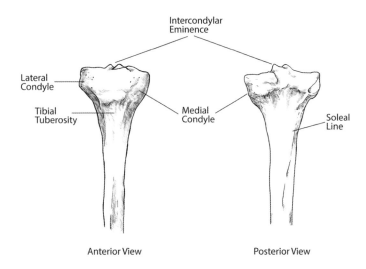

FIGURE 2.104 The shape of the tibia, anterior and posterior views.

The Patella

When a tendon is subjected to friction, it may develop calcium deposits to stiffen it, and these deposits may develop into a sesamoid bone.[115] The sesamoid bone will help to increase the lever arm of the muscle and/or, as in the case of the patella, will act as a pulley to change the direction of the force. The patella (which is Latin for "small plate") is a sesamoid bone—the largest one we have—that floats in the tendon of the quadriceps and slides up and down along the distal femur (see figure 2.105). The underside (posterior) of the patella is covered in thick articulating cartilage, which helps to distribute compressive forces when the patella is pressed against the femur.

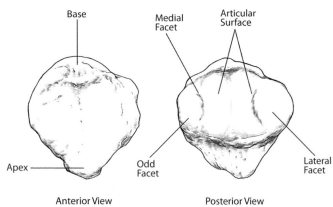

FIGURE 2.105 The patella, anterior and posterior views.

THE KNEE-JOINT CAPSULE AND LIGAMENTS

As mentioned, because the knee joint is not constrained by any bony stops, restrictions to movement ultimately come from the surrounding soft tissues. The ligaments and joint capsule are the biggest but not the only contributors to knee stability. While we can simplify the role of the various ligaments, the reality is much more complex than providing a list of which ligament provides stability in which directions. Movements of the body are rarely in just one of the three possible planes. To maintain stability and control, the knee requires many ligaments and other soft tissues, including co-contraction of opposing muscles, to work together. The roles performed by the ligaments given in this section are not meant to be viewed in isolation: please keep in mind that many tissues cooperate to produce mobility and stability.

The Fascia Lata

It is normal for anatomists to divide tissues into layers and structures, but always remember that the body is not actually like that. The layers are integrated, and the structures morph into other structures. We find this illustrated nicely around the knee joint. There is a fascial body stocking wrapping the lower body like a pant leg; it is three-dimensional and goes from the superficial level to deep inside the leg. In the thigh, it is called the *fascia lata*. The fascia lata varies in thickness; it is quite thin around the inside and back of the leg but thickens considerably on the outside, about where a seam would be in a pair of blue jeans. This thickening, which is due to constant stress on this length of the fascia from the gluteus muscles and the tensor fasciae latae, is the infamous *iliotibial band* (the IT band). It is often shown spanning the top of the iliac crest to the lateral condyle of the tibia, but the IT band does not actually exist as a separate entity in the body. Anatomists who want to illustrate this tough segment of ligamentous tissue sculpt an IT band out of the fascia lata. In reality, the IT band is contiguous with the fascia lata, which in turn is contiguous with the tendons of the quadriceps and the retinaculum that joins with the patellar tendon. Via a septa that divides the quadriceps from the hamstrings, the fascia lata dives deep down to merge with the femur bone. As the body stocking of fascia continues down the leg, its name changes to the *crural fascia*. The crural fascia is continuous with the patella and the tendons of the hamstrings, sartorius, gracilis and popliteus and covers the muscles of the calf. It also sends septa down deep to merge with the tibia and fibula.

The fascia lata surrounding the leg is connected to or merges with the tendons of the quadricep muscles, which in turn become part of the retinaculum of the knee (see figure 2.106). Like the IT band, a *retinaculum* (from the Latin for a cable or halter that retains or "holds back") does not really exist as a separate structure within the body, but rather is a thickening of fascia around the body, under which tendons grouped together from various muscles can stay together and slide with minimal resistance.[116] We have retinacula around our wrists, ankles and knees. The tendons of the big thigh muscles, the vastus lateralis and vastus medialis, send off fibers that become the lateral and medial retinacula, which in turn become the *patellar ligament*. We are often shown drawings of the patella embedded within the quadricep femoris tendon, but not always shown are the connections laterally and medially via the retinacula to the fascial bag surrounding the leg and to the vasti muscles, all of which help to support and stabilize the patella.

This superficial layer of fascia is just the first of three conceptual levels of fascia investing the knee joint. The next layer consists of the knee's ligaments and tendons, and the deepest layer is the joint capsule. While the knee is designed to allow a great deal of flexion and extension, lateral movements (valgus and varus) are primarily prevented by the medial and lateral collateral ligaments (except when the knee is flexed) and by the cruciate ligaments. Twisting of the knee while the leg is straight is prevented by the same ligaments. Anterior or posterior displacement of the tibia relative to the femur is prevented primarily by the anterior cruciate ligament and the posterior cruciate ligament, respectively, although the collateral ligaments also assist.

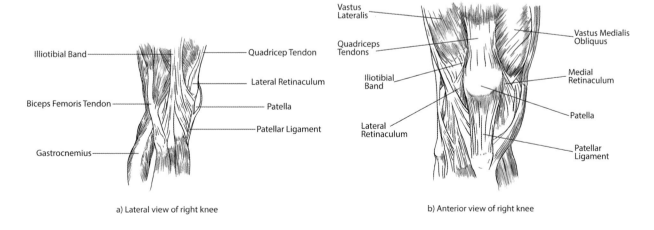

a) Lateral view of right knee

b) Anterior view of right knee

FIGURE 2.106 The fascia of the knee is continuous with the ligaments and tendons.

The Cruciate Ligaments

The two cruciate ligaments are hidden away within the intercondylar notch of the femur and run from the tibial plateau to the inner notch of the femur. (Cruciate is the Greek word for "cross-shaped," and that is what these two ligaments do—they cross over each other). The names refer to their position on the tibial plateau: the anterior cruciate ligament (ACL) runs from the anterior tibia, just lateral to the medial meniscus, to the medial side of the lateral femoral condylar notch (see figures 2.101 and 2.107); the posterior cruciate ligament (PCL), the thicker and stronger of the two,[117] runs from the posterior tibia to the lateral side of the medial femoral condylar notch.

The ACL is one of the most commonly injured ligaments in the body, and most ACL injuries are caused by high-speed stress on the knee when the foot is planted or fixed. Either an extreme inward and sideways stress (valgus) or hyperextension of the knee, combined with the femur attempting to externally rotate over the tibia, creates a high stretching stress on the ACL, which can rupture it. Jumping and landing with knees flexed and slightly internally rotated can also cause ACL problems, especially in women who have greater valgus angles than the norm.[118] Women have a two to eight times higher risk of ACL injury than men.[119] The exact causes of predilections to injury are not agreed upon; contributing factors include anatomical, hormonal and neuromuscular variables.[120] A smaller intercondylar notch has been correlated with a weaker and smaller ACL; women do have narrower notches than men, on average.[121] Too much estrogen is also thought to weaken the ACL,

making injury more likely.[122] Landing after a jump without feet plantar flexed (thus landing on the heels or with feet flat) or with too much flexion in the hips can increase the stress on the knees and may be a contributing factor to some athletes' ACL problems.[123] Frequently, ACL tears are combined with medial meniscal and medial collateral ligament tears—the so-called "unhappy triad."

The posterior cruciate ligament (PCL) displays a range of variation.[124] In 69% of people, the PCL has a separate slip of ligament connecting it to the menisci, adding a little bit more stability to the knee.[125] Injuries to the PCL usually occur with injuries to other parts of the knee as well, most often the ACL. These injuries are commonly caused by either extreme and sudden hyperextension of the knee (such as falling over an already hyperextended knee), hyperflexion of the knee or pretibial trauma (such as can occur in an auto accident when the dashboard of the car pushes the tibia forcefully backwards relative to the femur).[126]

The Collateral Ligaments

On the two sides of the joint capsule are long ligaments that support the capsule and provide lateral and medial stability to the knee. As shown in figures 2.101 and 2.107, the medial collateral ligament (MCL) is a flat band arising from the medial (inner) epicondyle of the femur, running downward and slightly from back to front and attaching to the posterior medial tibia. It is often shown as a separate band, but in reality it is contiguous with the medial patellar retinaculum. The posterior distal fibers of the MCL are also contiguous with the posterior medial joint capsule, the medial meniscus and the tendon of the semimembranosus muscle. The lateral

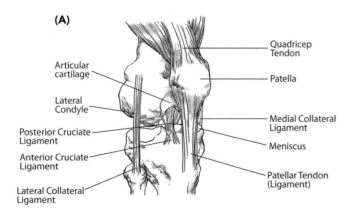

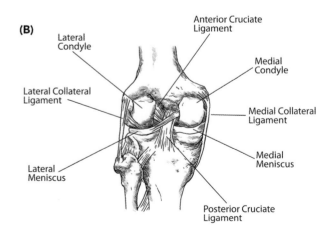

FIGURE 2.107 The ligaments of the knee: (a) anterior/lateral oblique view (right knee); (b) posterior view (left knee).

collateral ligament (LCL) is wrapped up into a strong cord running almost vertically from the lateral (outer) epicondyle of the femur down to the proximal head of the fibula, where it becomes part of the tendon of the bicep femoris muscle. Unlike the MCL, the LCL is not connected to a meniscus.

The Joint Capsule

The knee's joint capsule forms the largest and most complicated synovial capsule in the body.[127] While the capsule envelops the bottom of the femur and the top of the tibia, it folds around the cruciate ligaments and the menisci (which stay outside the joint capsule)[128] and runs superiorly along the anterior femur, creating a pouch underneath the patella and the quadriceps femoris. This pouch, also called the *suprapatellar bursa*, changes shape and size as the knee flexes and extends. It cushions the patella and allows it to slide smoothly against the patellar groove. Too much pressure or irritation of the suprapatellar bursa can lead to inflammation and swelling under the kneecap, a condition known as "clergyman's knees"—so called because it frequently afflicted people who spent a long time kneeling.[129]

The Menisci

The distal femur has two very rounded condyles; the proximal tibia is relatively flat. These two surfaces are not very congruent, and articulation would be risky if it were not for the presence of the menisci (see figure 2.101). The exact function of the menisci is not certain, but they probably act as shock absorbers, and they help to make the two irregular endings of the bones fit better.[130] They are thicker at the outer edges than in the middle, which helps to create a bowl shape in which the rounded femoral condyles fit. As a shock absorber, the meniscus flattens out when a load bears down upon it, distributing the stress radially. The composition of its collagen fibers and their orientation help to distribute the multidirectional forces to which the knee is subjected. The menisci may also help to reduce the amount of sliding that the femur can do across the top of the tibia. In addition, menisci help spread lubrication within the joint, spread weight over a broader surface and protect the edges of the bones' cartilage.

When we walk, our knees are subjected to compressive forces equal to three times our body's weight; when we run, this can become four to eight times our weight. The menisci bear 40–70% of this stress.[131] How much the meniscus can handle depends upon its size, shape and thickness, which

is, not surprisingly, quite variable and can change as we age. Exercise can make it thicker and stronger, but too much stress can make it thinner.

As we age, we lose blood flow to the inside of the menisci.[132] Due to the lack of vascularization within the knee joint and their position outside of the joint capsule, damage to the menisci is very hard to heal. Close to the outer edge of the menisci there is blood flow to them, but by the time we are adults, the inner two-thirds of the menisci have no vascularization at all.[133] If the inner cartilage is torn or ruptured, sometimes the only recourse is surgery to snip out the damaged portion; however, most doctors prefer to wait a while before opting for surgery. Range of motion enhancement and gentle stresses are often recommended (such as cycling), but full weight bearing is delayed until the acute phase of the injury has been resolved. After this stage, some rehabilitation has been achieved by stressing the knees passively through periods of sitting on the heels (in yoga, this is called Hero Pose—Vajrasana), or by placing dowelling or rolled up washcloths behind the knees while sitting on the heels.[134] As always, for any injury, a student should seek medical advice from her health-care team, not from a yoga teacher (unless the teacher is appropriately qualified). Recent advances in regrowing cartilage through stem cells seeded into artificial scaffolds hold out the hope that one day, replacement menisci may be grown for transplant within the knee.[135]

Both menisci are connected to the tibia by *coronal ligaments*, to each other by the by the *transverse ligament*[136] and to the patella by the *patellomeniscal ligaments*.[137] The medial meniscus is connected to the medial collateral ligament, to both the anterior and posterior cruciate ligament, and to the semimembranosus hamstring muscle. Unlike the medial meniscus, the lateral meniscus is not connected to a collateral ligament and thus has more mobility. It is also larger than the medial meniscus. The lateral meniscus is joined to the medial femoral condyle by a *posterior meniscofemoral ligament* and is also connected to the popliteal tendon.

When the knee flexes, the menisci slide backwards, pushed by the femoral condyles and pulled by the attached tendons and ligaments.[138] When the knee extends, they slide forward. In rotation, the menisci also move but in opposite directions: in external (lateral) rotation of the tibia, the lateral meniscus moves forward as the lateral femoral condyle slides forward over the tibia; in internal (medial) rotation, the medial meniscus moves forward. The lateral meniscus is better able to slide out of the way of strong shearing forces than the medial meniscus, which is more fixed in position and thus more often torn. This is one reason that yoga students who have forced their knees in the Lotus Pose (Padmasana) may have torn their medial meniscus; it wasn't able to slide out of the way and was crushed between the medial femoral condyle and medial tibial condyle. Any hint of pain in the inner knee in any externally rotated hip posture is a sign to back off and not continue the pose—or risk tearing the medial meniscus. Since the menisci effectively triple the surface area of the tibia to help distribute the weight of the femur, if they are damaged, or have to be surgically removed, the stress on the tibia can increase by over 200%.[139] Over time, this can lead to degeneration of the articulating cartilage and to osteoarthritis.

THE MUSCLES OF THE KNEE

Many muscles cross the knee (see figures 2.25 and 2.102), and several of these cross other joints as well, making their actions complicated. The quadriceps femoris and sartorius help to extend the knee but also assist in flexing the hips. The hamstrings flex the knee but likewise can extend the hips. The hamstrings can also rotate the tibia when the knee is flexed. The gastrocnemius, the most famous of our calf muscles, also helps to flex the knee and plantar flex the foot. If the quadriceps femoris is tight, when it contracts to extend the knee, it may begin to flex the hip. If the hamstrings are tight, when they shorten and contract to flex the knee, they may begin to extend the hip. In the other direction, when people with tight hamstrings flex the hip, they tend to flex the knees too.

The Quadriceps

The four main quadriceps include the *rectus femoris* (also called the *quadriceps femoris*) and the three vasti: the *vastus lateralis* (on the outside of the thigh), *vastus medialis* (on the inside of the thigh) and *vastus intermedius* (which hides underneath the rectus femoris). These all merge into one tendon just above the kneecap, called the *quadriceps tendon*, which in turn envelops the patella and becomes the *patellar tendon* (also called the *patellar ligament*), which in turn merges with the tibial tuberosity. All four muscles in concentric activation extend the leg when it is flexed, or through isometric activation resist further flexion, or through eccentric activation slow down the rate of flexion. However, one slight variation

to the quadriceps is important when we consider stresses on the knee: the *vastus medialis obliquus*. This consists of the lowest (distal) fibers of the vastus medialis. These fibers run almost horizontally to the patella and assist in keeping the patella tracking in the intercondylar groove.

The Hamstrings

There are two palpable sides to the knee, indicating the route of the hamstrings. If you palpate your outer (lateral) knee, you will feel the tendon of the bicep femoris, which merges with the top of the fibula. However, you may feel two tendons, one slightly anterior to the other. The more anterior tendon is probably your vastus lateralis. Notice how it ends more to the side of the patella, while the more posterior bicep femoris tendon continues down to the head of the fibula. Perhaps, though, you are palpating the iliotibial band, which follows a similar path to the vastus lateralis but runs more distally than the kneecap and curves in towards the tibial tuberosity.

On the inner (medial) knee, just below the joint, you will feel several tendons: those of the semis—the semimembranosus and semitendinosus—and the sartorius and gracilis. The semimembranosus tendon is hard to palpate; it runs deeper than the others and joins the medial condyle of the tibia. The semitendinosus, sartorius and gracilis come together to form an extended tendon that merges at a point called the *pes anserinus* (Latin for goose's foot, because their union looks a bit like one). The pes anserinus merges with the medial tibia just distal to the semimembranosus tendon.

The Popliteus and Gastrocnemius

The popliteus, "the key that unlocks the knee,"[140] supports the back of the knee yet is an underappreciated muscle. It runs from the inside (medial) tibia, just below the condyle, diagonally upwards to the outside (lateral) femoral condyle. The popliteus has several functions: it helps to initiate flexion of the knee, but it also assists with internally (medially) rotating the tibia, unlocking it from its closed position in full extension.

The gastrocnemius (from the Greek for "belly of the leg"), like the hamstrings, has two heads that connect on either side of the back of the knee; however, they merge with the thigh above the joint (see figure 2.216), while the hamstrings merge with the leg below the joint. At the distal end, the gastrocnemius becomes the Achilles tendon (also called the *calcaneal tendon*), which allows it to plantar flex the foot.

THE TYPES AND RANGES OF VARIATIONS

Variations in the Femur

Like the proximal end of the femur, the distal end has its range of variations, which can affect our ability and ease in flexing and extending the knee. Figure 2.103 shows the patellar groove and intercondylar notch. The depths of the groove and notch, as well as the condyles' sizes and the width between them, are highly variable; one study found the average width between the condyles to be 5.0 cm, but one standard deviation was 1.3 cm, which means two-thirds of the population have widths between 3.7 and 6.3 cm.[141] Some have speculated that this broad range is one reason why certain people never develop knee problems while others do.[142] Individuals with a narrower intercondylar notch may be predisposed to cruciate ligament problems.[143] There are also variations in the angles of the trochlea—the sides of the patellar groove—that may cause kneecap tracking problems (see figure 2.110).

Variations in the Tibia

There are considerable variations in the size and shape of the tibia, which can affect its functionality,[144] but undoubtedly the most interesting aspect of the tibia in terms of alignment in our yoga practice is its twist, known as *tibial torsion*. The bone itself has a twist along its length, so the relatively flat top of the tibia is not oriented the same as the bottom. The average amount of tibial torsion we have depends greatly upon which study you choose to quote. Cited averages range from 23° to 38°.[145] For our purposes, we will work with 30° as an average, with a standard deviation of 8°; this assumes that 95% of people have a tibial torsion somewhere between 14° and 46°. About one person in 20 will be outside this range, and the total range is quite dramatic: from as little as 2° to as large as 80°![146] Typically, the dominant leg has about 2° more torsion than the other leg, but not always. Usually, no differences are apparent based on gender, but again, not always. There are great differences, however, due to ethnicity, with Indian and Japanese populations having far less tibial torsion than Caucasians. It is speculated that the differences arise primarily from habitual sitting practices. As babies, we have very little tibial torsion, but by the age of eight, we will have obtained a twist comparable to our ultimate adult value.[147] This minimal tibial rotation as children is one reason that many young children have a pronounced toe-in posture, which they eventually outgrow.

Figure 2.108 shows two tibias. Notice the significant differences in the orientation of the distal end, where the foot attaches. The amount of tibial torsion on the right is 14°, compared with 46° on the left. Out of 20 students in a yoga class, 19 will have ranges of tibial torsion between these two extremes, but one student may be outside even these amounts. As we will see, this greatly determines where the foot will point in many yoga postures. If we insist that the foot must always point straight ahead in standing postures or lunges, students with high tibial torsion will have to accomplish this directive by pronating the foot or by internally rotating the leg either from the hip or at the knee—or by doing all three movements. Indeed, since the average amount of tibial torsion is 30°, almost everyone has to perform some sort of internal rotation of the thigh or leg to align the feet parallel, which may not always be the best alignment for their knees or hips.

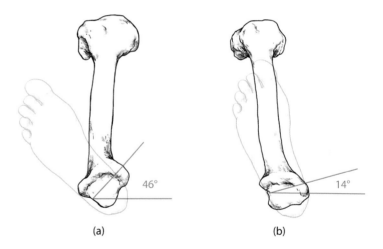

(a)   (b)

FIGURE 2.108 Tibial torsion within two standard deviations of the norm. A right tibia with (a) 46° of torsion, (b) 14° of torsion; 95% of the population is within this range.

Another potentially interesting source of variability in the tibias is the slope of the plateau. In the side plane, the tibial plateau is generally angled backwards and downwards. This slope is about 11° on average from front to back; however, the angle varies from about 1° to 19°.[148] There is no consensus on whether this posterior tibial slope predisposes us to more or fewer injuries.[149]

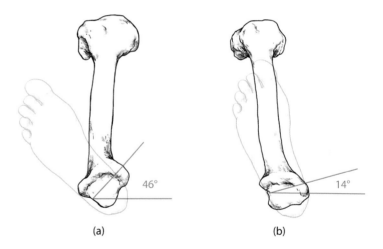

THE KNEE JOINT

Variations in the Patella

The rounded shape of the patella is highly variable. Its shape may lead to tracking problems and a noisy slippage of the kneecap back into the patellar groove (the click many people hear in their knees as they slightly bend or straighten the leg may be due to this inexact tracking). In about two percent of people, the patella consists of more than one bone, which is called a bipartite patella (see figure 2.109). This may be because two or three bones failed to fuse, but rarely does this variation cause any problems.[150]

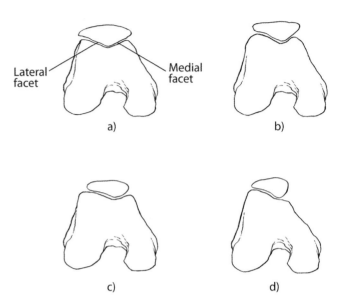

FIGURE 2.110 Variations in the cross-section of the patella and the femoral patellar groove.

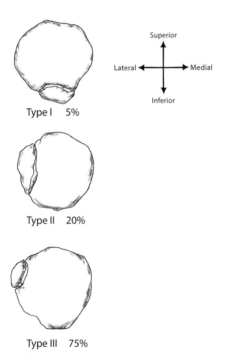

FIGURE 2.109 Three main variations in the shape of bipartite patellae, with their frequency of occurrence.[151]

The patella can be 2 to 3 cm thick, not including the articular cartilage, which is some of the thickest cartilage in the body, and these variations in thickness determine its surface shape.[152] The cross-sectional shape is also quite variable, as shown in figure 2.110; here we can see that just as the patella comes in different shapes, so does the trochlea of the femur, which forms the valley within which the patella moves (the patellar groove). Normally, the high lateral edge of the trochlea keeps the patella inside the valley of the patellar groove. In some cases, however, the two shapes do not allow for a nice confinement of the patella to the patellar groove, and this can lead to instability in the knee, dislocation of the kneecap and patellofemoral pain.

Other Variations of the Knee

UNIQUE BONES

We have looked at the bones normally forming the knee that one would come across in an anatomy text: the femur, tibia and patella. But remember, these books present an average view, whereas the real world is not so cut and dried. Some people have extra bits of bone floating around in their fascia. These auxiliary or "supernumerary" (exceeding the normal number) bones may serve no function and not be a problem, or they can be functional, or they are sometimes pathological.[153] One interesting example, occurring in around 20% of the population, is a second kneecap, called the *fabella*[154] (from the Latin for "little bean"). One in every five people has a second kneecap—perhaps you do! This kneecap occurs *behind* the knee, in the lateral tendon of the gastrocnemius. It is a sesamoid bone, like the patella, but much smaller—on the order of 0.4 to 2.2 cm.[155] The presence of a fabella may be a cause of lower leg and knee pain, restrictions in the range of flexion or at the end of the range of extension, and restrictions in a student's ability to sit with legs crossed.[156] But for most people, the presence of their fabella is unremarkable and causes no problems; they don't even know they have it.

THE Q-ANGLE, VARUM AND VALGUM

The pelvis is wider than the distance between the knees, which means the femur has to follow a line angled inward from pelvis to knees. This results in an angle between the axis of the femur and the axis of the tibia, called the *Q-angle* (see figure 2.111).[157] The Q-angle is measured as the angle between the line from the anterior superior iliac spine of the pelvis to the middle of the patella, and the line rising from the center of the tibial tuberosity and the center of the patella. Clearly, people with wider pelvises and/or shorter femurs will tend to have larger Q-angles. The common statement that women have greater Q-angles than men simply represents the fact that women are, on average, shorter than men; when women are matched to men of equal height, their Q-angles are similar.[158]

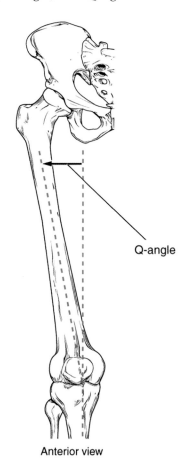

Q-angle

Anterior view

FIGURE 2.111 The Q-angle is roughly the angle between the line of the femur and a vertical line through the patella.

One study[159] of 150 men and women found average Q-angles of 14° for men and 17° for women, with one standard deviation of 3°. Again, these researchers did not adjust their findings to compensate for the variations in height between the genders. The standard deviation means that some

women had a Q-angle of only 11°, while some men had an angle of 20°; thus, some men do have larger Q-angles than women.

The relative positioning of the knees is determined by the Q-angle. If the angle is large, the knees tend to bend in towards each other (see figure 2.132). If the angle is greater than 15°, this knock-kneed condition is called *genu valgum*, or *valgum* for short[160] (genu is Latin for "knee" and is found in the word genuflect, which is to bend one knee to the ground). This makes the person unable to bring their feet together when standing (again, see figure 2.132): the knees knock into each other. Because of this, some yoga students will never be able to stand with their feet together, due to the shape of their bones. If the Q-angle is 0° or less, the knees bow away from each other.[161] This bow-leg condition is called *genu varum*, or *varum* for short.

The Q-angle is affected by a number of factors, including the femoral neck-shaft angle, the acetabular abduction angle, femoral anteversion, the positioning of the tibial tuberosity, and tibial torsion.[162] These factors are not subject to change through a yoga practice because they are characteristics of the bones. The Q-angle does change as we age; babies are quite bowlegged at about six months old, then their legs straighten out by around 18 months, but they keep changing and become quite knock-kneed by four years of age. Fortunately, they start to correct again until they reach the normal, slightly genu valgum state around 11.[163] Unfortunately, pathologies such as osteoarthritis can affect the Q-angle, so it may change even when we are adults.

It was long thought that if the Q-angle is too high or too low, certain pathologies can develop. The reason for this belief is that extreme genu valgum may place a great deal of stress on the medial side of the knee. It was thought that this could lead to weakness in the medial ligaments and excessive compression of the lateral condyles, causing osteoarthritis. On the other side, extreme genu varum could excessively stress the lateral ligaments and increase compression of the medial condyles, again resulting in weakness in the joint and osteoarthritis. It was believed that, along with osteoarthritis, these misalignments of the knee could result in deterioration of the menisci, the subchondral bone and the ligaments. However, having these misalignments does not *automatically* result in problems! One study found that 25% of the healthy knees studied had varus alignment, and 36% had valgus alignment.[164] Many people have varus and valgus alignments but suffer no problems at all. It was also believed that extreme valgus could lead to patellofemoral problems because the kneecap could be pulled off track by a large Q-angle; however, this concern has diminished due to a lack of correlation between Q-angles and patellofemoral problems. This non-correlation has led many clinicians to ignore the Q-angle.[165]

There is no known cure for genu varum or genu valgum, short of surgery. Sometimes children are given braces to guide the direction of growth of the bones, but the results are mixed.[166] While there is no cure, there are exercises that can help people deal with the effects of genu valgum. We will look at some examples later when we examine the valgus and varus movements of the knee.

Is the Q-angle something yoga teachers or students should worry about? As always, the answer depends upon the individual. If a student has a significant variation in Q-angle from the norm *and* if the student is suffering from knee pain, it makes sense to consider strengthening the muscles supporting the knee joint and to experiment with different knee alignments in various postures to ensure the condition does not get worse. But remember, abnormality is not necessarily pathology. Many people are quite knocked-kneed or bow-legged but will not suffer any problems because of those variations.

Function: Application in Yoga Postures

We have seen how the architecture and form of the knee joint allows the movements of flexion and extension. We will now look at the ranges of possible motions for an average person, and for all those yoga students who are not average. We will discover that other movements at the knee are possible, including a certain amount of twisting. In answering our WSM? question, we will also look at the sources of tension and compression.

MOVEMENTS OF THE KNEE JOINT

The knee moves predominantly in flexion and extension, which is why it is often called a hinge joint. However, when the knee is flexed, other directions of movement are possible, which is why it is often referred to by more complex names such as a condyloid or ellipsoid joint. Several muscles can act to cause internal (medial) and external (lateral) rotation of the tibia, but no muscles can actively cause the knees to draw inward to each other (valgus) or move outward away from each other (varus). While valgus (abduction) and varus (adduction) are not caused by muscular action, these movement may occur as the result of other movements or stresses, such as abduction or adduction at the hips with feet planted on the ground.[167]

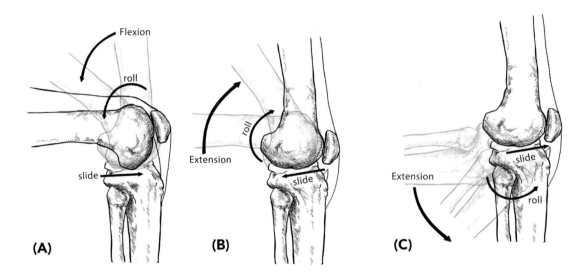

FIGURE 2.112 The knee joint utilizes both sliding and rolling in flexion and extension. We can view movement as either the femur moving over a stationary tibia (a and b) or the tibia moving under a stationary femur (c).

The illustrations in figure 2.112 were shown in Volume 1, Appendix F, on the biomechanics of joint motion. When the knee flexes, the femur both rotates downwards and slides forward along the tibial surface (shown in 2.112a). In extension, the opposite happens (2.112b): the femur rotates upward and slides backwards on the tibial surface. The other possibility is to have the tibia move under a stationary femur (2.112c). In this case, the tibia slides and rolls in the same direction; the rounded shapes of the femoral condyles assist in the rolling action, while the relatively flat surface of the tibia assists in the sliding action.

When conditions are right, the knee can permit a moderate amount of rotation between the tibia and the femur. This twist is allowable when the knee is flexed, which loosens up ligaments that restrain rotational movements when the knee is fully extended. How much rotation is available without harm depends upon the length and laxity of the person's ligaments.

NORMAL RANGES OF MOTION

What is the normal range of motion of the knee for adults? As always, the answer is: it depends!

Flexion

A 1965 study showed that the average range of flexion was about 135°, but a 1984 study indicated much more: 150°.[168] Table 2.9 shows the results of another study, which showed that we lose a tiny amount of flexion as we age, but the overall range is still quite broad: 125–160°.[169]

TABLE 2.9 Average range of flexion at the knee joint with one standard deviation, and range of motion, for various age groups.

AGE GROUP	MAXIMUM KNEE FLEXION	RANGE OF MAXIMUM FLEXION
25–39	134° +/– 9°	130–160°
40–59	132° +/– 11°	125–155°
60–74	131° +/– 11°	125–150°

Sitting on your heels requires 160–170° of flexion. Sitting between your feet requires 170–180°.[170] From the above data we see that it is no surprise the average person cannot sit on their heels (Vajrasana or Thunderbolt Pose), let alone sit between their feet (Virasana or Hero's Pose), without working towards an expanded range of knee flexion. Some people will never be able to do these poses, due to compression of the tissues in the back of their knees, calves and thighs. Fortunately, for everyday life, full flexion ranges of up to 170° are not required: walking on level ground requires about 70° of flexion; climbing stairs and getting out of chairs requires about 106°; getting in or out of a bathtub needs around 152°; and squatting requires about 164°, regardless of whether the heels are lowered to the ground or raised.[171]

Extension

Moving the knee in the other direction is called extension. When the leg is completely straight, the knee is considered fully extended, but more movement beyond straight is available. This is called hyperextension, and it is normal and natural. By *normal* we mean that over 95% of people can and do hyperextend their knees. By *natural* we mean that this is a necessary movement for the knees and helps to reduce constant contraction and contracture of the quadriceps. The average person can hyperextend his or her knees 5–6°.[172] That is a good thing. Walking requires a small amount of hyperextension of the back leg—on the order of 2–7°. Descending stairs requires even more hyperextension—on the order of 3–15°.[173] Obviously, a bit of hyperextension is not evil.

Rotation

When the knee is flexed, the collateral ligaments become a little bit lax (see figure 2.115). Thanks to their orientation, they become more lax as the tibia externally (laterally) rotates but tighter in internal (medial) rotation. An often cited range of rotation suggests that normally, we only have about 10° of internal rotation available at the knee (i.e., with the foot pointing inward) but 30–40° of external rotation (the foot turning outward).[174] Remember that due to human variation, the reality will be quite a range, depending on the individual.

SOURCES OF TENSION

The answer to WSM? for movements at the knee is predominantly tension, with compression generally only occurring at the limits of flexion, where the back of the calves may contact the back of the thighs or the heels hit the buttocks. Tensile resistance can affect all ranges of motion possible at the knee, and this can come from the fascia surrounding the whole area as well as fascial restrictions far from the joint (the so-called anatomy trains), from the muscles that articulate and stabilize the joint, from the ligaments within and around the joint, as well as from the joint capsule. In general, we can summarize the sources of tension as follows:

- Resistance to flexion/extension: the fascia and muscles
- Resistance to twisting: the cruciate and collateral ligaments
- Resistance to valgus/varum: the collateral ligaments and joint capsule

Source of Tension from the Fascia

TENSILE RESISTANCE	COMPRESSION
Myofascial Meridians	

The myofascial meridians are continuous connections of fascia that envelop the muscles and joint capsules, forming trains of fabric that run around the whole body. The meridians that can impede movements at the knee include the superficial front line (which can inhibit flexion),[175] the superficial back line (which can inhibit extension),[176] the deep front line (which can also inhibit extension but mostly acts to stabilize the joint),[177] and the spiral line (which helps with proper tracking of the knee).[178] The lateral lines can work with or against the deep front line to either create side-to-side stability at the knee or cause valgum (knock knees) or varum (bow legs) problems.[179] See Volume 1, Appendix C on the myofascial meridians for more details about these lines.

Sources of Tension from the Muscles

TENSILE RESISTANCE	COMPRESSION
Muscles & Tendons	

The muscles acting at or around the knee help to both mobilize and stabilize it. No muscles at the knee can cause a sideways movement (valgus or varus).

There is one slight variation to the quadriceps that is important when we consider stabilizing stresses at the knee: the *vastus medialis obliquus* (VMO). The VMO consists of the lowest (distal) fibers of the vastus medialis, which run almost horizontally to the patella and assist in keeping the patella tracking in the intercondylar groove. Instead of pulling up on the patella, the VMO pulls medially, providing lateral stability. Strengthening of the VMO is often recommended for yoga students who have trouble aligning their knees in standing postures, perhaps because the vastus lateralis is too strong and thus pulls the knee to the side.

Although no muscles can *cause* varus or valgus movements of the knee, the vasti can help *prevent* them. While the side fibers of the vasti can help stabilize the kneecap and keep it tracking properly, the side fibers of the hamstrings serve a different function. When the knee is flexed, the hamstrings can either rotate the tibia or stabilize it and prevent too much rotation. The bicep femoris can laterally (externally) rotate the tibia or stabilize and prevent medial (internal) rotation and thereby prevent a valgus movement of the tibia. The semitendinosus, semimembranosus and sartorius can medially (internally) rotate the tibia or stabilize and prevent lateral (external) rotation and thereby prevent a varus movement of the tibia.

The popliteus supports the back of the knee and helps prevent too much hyperextension. The gastrocnemius crosses the posterior knee; thus, it can assist with flexing, but its primary function is to stabilize the back of the knee and prevent too much extension; loss of this function may lead to hyperextension.[180]

Sources of Tension from the Ligaments

TENSILE RESISTANCE	COMPRESSION
Ligaments & Joint Capsule	

THE CRUCIATE LIGAMENTS

The anterior and posterior cruciate ligaments are generally quite taut in all movements and throughout the knee's range of movement, but the anterior cruciate ligament (ACL) becomes especially taut as the knee approaches full extension, due to the tibia being pulled forward by the quadriceps. Co-contraction of the hamstrings with the quadriceps as you approach full extension can lessen the stress on the ACL. (To understand what we mean by "co-contraction," read It's Important: Co-contraction, on page 174.) The ACL, along with the posterior portion of the joint capsule and the collateral ligaments and hamstrings, prevents excessive hyperextension of the knee. Like the ACL, the posterior cruciate ligament (PCL) fibers are relatively taut throughout all knee positions and movements, but they become especially taut in full flexion, when the hamstrings try to pull the tibia backwards. Co-contracting the quadriceps with the hamstrings while the knee is in flexion decreases the stress on the PCL.

TABLE 2.10 Muscles causing or resisting knee movement

KNEE MOVEMENT	PRIME MOVERS	SYNERGISTS	MUSCLES THAT RESIST MOVEMENT
flexion	hamstrings	· sartorius · gracilis · popliteus · gastrocnemius	· quadriceps
extension	quadriceps	· tensor fascia latae · gluteus maximus	· hamstrings · gastrocnemius · popliteus
valgus	none	none	· semimembranosus · semitendinosus · sartorius · gracilis · medial gastrocnemius
varus	None	None	· biceps femoris · popliteus · lateral gastrocnemius
lateral (external) rotation of the tibia	bicep femoris	· tensor fascia latae · gluteus maximus	· semimembranosus[181] · semitendinosus[182] · popliteus · in full extension, all the muscles crossing the back of the knee[183]
medial (internal) rotation of the tibia	· semimembranosus semitendinosus · sartorius · gracilis · popliteus		· biceps femoris[184] · in full extension, all the muscles crossing the back of the knee[185]

The cruciate ligaments help prevent the femur from slipping off a stationary tibia—the ACL by inhibiting too much backwards movement and the PCL too much forward sliding. Alternatively, we can picture this with the femur fixed and stationary and the tibia moving. In this scenario, the ACL prevents too much anterior tibial movement under the femur and the PCL too much posterior tibial movement. When we do a deep squat—think of Chair Pose (Utkatasana) and sitting down into Squat (Malasana)—or jump and land with the knees flexed, there is a large shear in the knee from the femur trying to slide forward. The PCL resists this movement and is assisted by the joint capsule and the muscles surrounding the knee, and especially by the popliteus, which runs parallel to the PCL.[186]

The two cruciate ligaments stabilize the knee when twisting stresses occur at the joint. They cross and have slightly oblique orientations, so they press against each other and tighten up when the lower leg medially (internally) rotates, but they become a little lax when the leg laterally (externally) rotates (see figure 2.113).

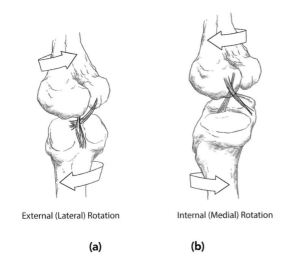

External (Lateral) Rotation   Internal (Medial) Rotation

(a)   **(b)**

FIGURE 2.113 The cruciate ligaments allow some external rotation of the lower leg (a) but tend to resist much internal rotation (b). The diagrams show a right knee.

THE COLLATERAL LIGAMENTS

The role of the collateral ligaments is to prevent too much side-to-side movement of the leg below the knee. The medial collateral ligament (MCL) prevents too much valgus movement (where the foot moves outwards and the knee inwards), and the lateral collateral ligament (LCL) prevents too much varus movement (where the foot moves inwards and the knee outwards). They are not alone; many of the soft tissues of the joint and the tone of the muscles also contribute to this sideways stability. Perhaps surprisingly, the collateral ligaments can also resist hyperextension of the knee, but again, many other tissues help in this function: the posterior joint capsule, the hamstrings, and mostly the ACL. Since the femur and tibia rotate a bit in opposite directions when locking the knee in full extension, the MCL experiences about 20% elongation at full extension compared to its length at full flexion.[187] This extra tautness makes the MCL more vulnerable to injury if the knee collapses inwardly while fully extended, such as can occur to football players who are clipped from the side when their foot is firmly planted and the knee fully extended.

We saw how both cruciate ligaments prevent too much rotation at the knee. The collateral ligaments also provide some stability here as well. Unlike the cruciates, however, which do allow more external (lateral) rotation of the tibia under the femur than internal (medial) rotation, the collateral ligaments become taut when the tibia externally rotates and slack in internal rotation (see figure 2.114). As

usual, some people can twist considerably, especially when the knee is flexed (as shown in figure 2.115), and this may be perfectly safe for them due to the laxness of the collateral ligaments.[188] Others can twist only minimally due to tautness in the cruciates and collateral ligaments, whether the knee is flexed or extended.

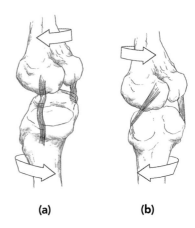

(a)   **(b)**

FIGURE 2.114 The collateral ligaments are lax with internal (medial) rotation of the leg (a) but more taut with external (lateral) rotation (b). The diagrams show a right knee.

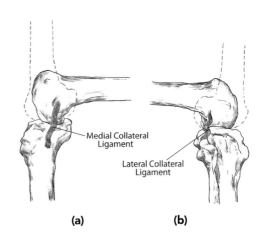

Medial Collateral Ligament

Lateral Collateral Ligament

(a)   **(b)**

FIGURE 2.115 The collateral ligaments are also lax when the knee is flexed: (a) the medial collateral ligament, (b) the lateral collateral ligament.

THE JOINT CAPSULE

The posterior fibers of the joint capsule reinforce the ligaments and fascia of a knee joint and help to resist hyperextension. The anterior portion can provide resistance to flexion. The medial and lateral aspects of the capsule can help to limit sideways (valgus or varus) movements.

TABLE 2.11 Sources of ligamentous tension restricting knee movements.

DIRECTION OF MOVEMENT	LIGAMENTS THAT RESIST MOVEMENT	JOINT CAPSULE FIBERS THAT RESIST MOVEMENT
flexion	· patellar ligament · patellar retinaculum · posterior cruciate ligament	anterior
extension	· anterior cruciate ligament · oblique popliteal ligament · arcuate popliteal ligament	posterior
valgus	· medial collateral ligament primarily[189] · cruciate ligaments · medial patellar retinaculum (when in full extension)[190]	medial
varus	· lateral collateral ligament primarily[191] · cruciate ligaments · lateral patellar retinaculum (when in full extension)[192] · iliotibial band	lateral
medial rotation of the tibia	· cruciate ligaments	
lateral rotation of the tibia	· arcuate popliteal ligament · lateral collateral ligament	posterior-lateral

IT'S IMPORTANT: Co-contraction

Knowing which muscle moves which limb when it contracts is valuable but is also an oversimplification of what really happens when we move. Very rarely is only one muscle involved in movement. To create stability around the joint and gain precision, we co-contract several muscles with each movement. One reason that our coordination is impaired and we become clumsy when we are tired or inebriated is that the co-contracting muscles lose their ability to guide our movements with the accuracy they provide when we are rested or sober.[193] Co-contraction of the agonist muscles (the prime movers and the ones that yoga teachers conducting anatomy training most often credit for movement) and the antagonist muscles (the opposing muscles that create stability and support in the articulating joint) occurs to ensure smooth, controlled movement.

> *To maintain and regain the health of a joint when it is bearing a load, stiffen the joint by co-contracting the muscles around it. To enhance mobility, move the joint through its full range of motion while there is no load.*

Stabilizing the joint while it moves prevents sudden stresses from exceeding its tolerance and stiffens the joint, making it better able to withstand the forces. Stabilization also provides a rigid frame upon which the muscles can act. In weightlifting, this is sometimes referred to as "locking it down." Another phrase is "make it stiff." Sprinters lock down and make their torso stiff to allow the greatest spring effect through the hips while running. To quote Stuart Mc-Gill, "a universal law of human movement is . . . 'proximal stiffness enhances distal mobility and athleticism.'"[194] In other words, have a firm, stiff core, then work to mobilize the extremities. In Anusara yoga, this same "hugging the muscles to the bone" is called "muscular energy."[195] We protect our wrist joints while moving from Down Dog (Adhomukhasvanasana) to Up Dog (Urdhvamukhasvanasana) by stiffening the fingers, palms and forearms, thus stabilizing the wrists. In Side Plank (Vasisthasana) we do the same to protect the shoulder: lock down and engage the shoulder muscles, making the joint stiff so that it is better able to withstand the stress of the posture. This "muscular energy" is another way of defining co-contraction of the muscles around the joint. We can also protect the knee joint while in standing postures such as Triangle (Trikonasana) and the Warriors (Virabhadrasanas) by co-contracting the hamstrings along with the quadriceps. This action will stiffen the knee and reduce stress on the knee ligaments.

Co-contraction has a minor cost that some yoga students may be reluctant to pay: it will reduce the range of motion around the joint. This is the standard trade-off between mobility and stability. If the goal of a yoga practice is to enhance range of motion at all costs, then there is the temptation to relax a joint too much when it is bearing a load. Unfortunately, this decision places the joint at risk. A better strategy, if the goal of a yoga practice is to build health, is to stabilize a joint, then work to mobilize it. This is especially important for the core joints of the spine, pelvis, shoulders and knees, but all joints will benefit from co-contraction of the surrounding muscles.

BALANCING TOO MUCH CO-CONTRACTION

If the muscles around a joint are constantly or chronically contracted, the fascia, ligaments and joint capsule can become remodeled and shortened to a reduced range of motion. While it is important to protect a load-bearing joint by co-contracting the muscles, too much protection is counter-productive and could make the joint fragile. Joints do need stress to remain healthy and open to their optimal range of motion. It is appropriate to stress a joint while it is not bearing a load and move it close to its end range of motion (the "edge"). This is the basis of yin yoga: a passive stress of the connective tissues around and through a joint.[196] To maintain or regain full health for a joint, use both co-contraction to strengthen it while it is bearing a load, and long-held, passive stress to increase its range of motion when it is not bearing a load.

SOURCES OF COMPRESSION

The knees support the full weight of the upper body, so there is a tremendous amount of compression of the femur onto the tibia, and of the patella onto the distal end of the femur. The stress at these compression sites can lead to pathology over years of doing too much or not enough. The joint needs stress to remain healthy and strong, but too much stress can wear out the cartilage and weaken the ligaments and joint capsule. However, these areas of compression generally do not limit range of motion.

Notice that not listed in the restrictions to movement shown in table 2.11 are any sources of compression. This is because, generally, there are none except in cases of pathology. However, there is one big exception: compression of the back of the calves against the back of the thighs can drastically limit flexion. People with big thighs and calves will find it difficult to sit on their heels, such as is required for Hero Pose (Virasana or Vajrasana—see figure 2.116). Compression here can also restrict range of movement in other postures, such as Squats (Malasana) or low lunges. With pathology, inflammation in the knee joint may also cause compression between tissues, but again, this generally affects flexion rather than extension and is felt in the back of the knees. Also, the presence of a fabella (the second knee-cap that many people have in the back of their knees) may restrict the range of flexion and thus a student's ability to sit with legs crossed.[197]

VARIATIONS IN RANGES OF MOTION

There are six possible movements at the knee: flexion, extension, lateral rotation, medial rotation, and the side movements of valgus and varus. These are all on display in a variety of yoga postures—even the side movements and rotations! Whether such movements *should* be allowed or should be corrected is highly dependent upon the student and her/his unique anatomical structure and history of stress on the knee. For many students, knee hyperextension or a large Q-angle may be harmless and does not need to be "corrected" via alignment cues. Such corrections may reduce the stress on the knees too much and could make them more fragile. For other students, however, these positions may be quite problematic, and great care must be taken to help stabilize the knees to prevent too much unwanted movement. Understanding this,

we can start to look at how these six kinds of movements arise in a yoga asana practice, and to learn what we should do—or need not do—to prevent injuries to the knee.

Flexion of the Knee

Flexion is the simplest movement of the knee to evaluate. Figure 2.116 shows the knees in full flexion as we sit between our heels in Hero Pose (Virasana). Many students, however, cannot do this posture because they can neither widen their feet enough to sit between them nor flex their knees sufficiently. The lack of flexion may be due to tension in the quadriceps (especially if the hips are extended) or compression in the back of the legs. These sensations are quite different: tension preventing flexion will be felt as a tightness or stretch on the front or top of the knees, whereas compression will be a softer, squishy feeling in the back of the knees, or between the calves and the thighs, or between the heels and the buttocks. Remember, tension can be worked on and reduced, but compression is the ultimate delimiter of movement in that direction. Over time, tension from the quadriceps can be reduced through lengthening the muscles or reducing their tone. If the tension is arising from fascial restrictions or adhesions, these too may be reducible in time and with practice.

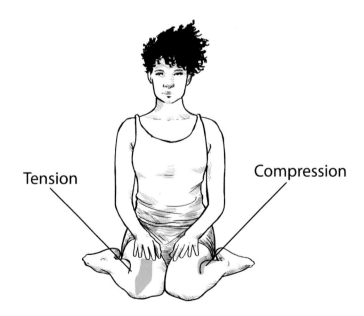

FIGURE 2.116 Sitting between the feet (Virasana) brings the knees close to their ultimate range of flexion.

The normal range of flexion for average people is somewhere around 0°–150°[198] What is the "normal" range of flexion for yoga students? The desire may be to get to the magical 180°, which allows the student to sit between the feet in reclining Hero Pose (Suptavirasana—see figure 2.88b), but there really is nothing magical about this position. It is not available to every body, but most bodies can approximate the position by sitting with a cushion or block between the feet so they can reach their maximum range of flexion while still in a variation of the pose.

Interestingly, one of the benefits of being able to sit on your heels is the *reduction* in stress in the knees. The amount of stress on the knees is less when we sit on the heels than when we kneel on both knees. Sitting on our heels distributes the body's weight from the thighs and gluteal muscles onto the calves and the heels. Kneeling on only one knee puts the greatest amount of stress on the knee, even more than squatting! Students with knee issues such as osteoarthritis in the medial tibia should avoid holding deep squats and doing prolonged kneeling on one knee.[199] This is important to understand for beginners or inflexible students who cannot move the leg far enough back in lunge postures; they often have their weight on the back knee instead of on the back foot or tibia. A better alignment for them may be to move the front foot forward so that the back knee is not flexed to a 90° angle (see figure 2.117). If that is not available, place support under the back shin and actively press it to the floor, to reduce stress on the back knee.

COMMON ALIGNMENT CUE FOR THE KNEE IN THE WARRIOR POSES (VIRABHADRASANAS)

Of more concern in yoga is the safest alignment of the front knee when it is close to 90° of flexion. This alignment issue arises quite often in the standing postures, such as the Warriors (Virabhadrasanas) and lunges (Anjaneyasana).

Figure 2.118 shows the most common alignment cue for the knee relative to the foot as given in the Warrior Postures (Virabhadrasanas): note how the bent knee does not extend beyond the ankle.[200] If the knee does wander in front of the ankle—as shown in figure 2.119, where the yogi is now in Side Angle Posture (Parsvakonasana, sometimes called Uttitaparsvakonasana)—the teacher will remind the student to draw the knee back or walk the foot further forward. Interestingly, the drawing in figure 2.119 represents Tirumalai Krishnamacharya,[201] the "man behind some of the most influential forms of international postural yoga today," according to Mark Singleton.[202] The previous figure, 2.118, represents Krishnamacharya's student and brother-in-law, B.K.S. Iyengar, the man often credited for creating the modern emphasis on alignment in yoga postures.

Why do we want the knee above the ankle in Warrior postures, lunges and other standing poses, such as Side Angle Pose? The frequent answer is that when the knee moves forward of the ankle, too much stress will be placed upon the knee—specifically the kneecap or perhaps the anterior cruciate ligament. This rationale ignores the observation we made in Volume 1: all tissues need stress to be healthy. If

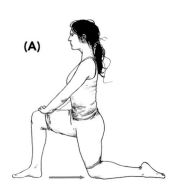
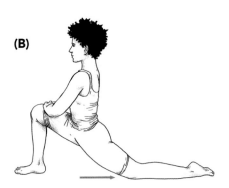

FIGURE 2.117 A low lunge (Anjaneyasana) with the back knee further back (b) may place less stress upon that knee than having the knee forward (a).

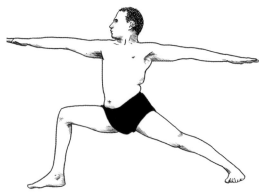

FIGURE 2.118 The standard alignment of Warrior Two (Virabhadrasana B). Notice the position of the knee over the ankle and the angle of the back foot.

we don't apply stress to the body, it becomes fragile. As one study has pointed out, if the patella is deprived of adequate stress because the knee is not deeply flexed, insufficient nourishment to the underlying cartilage can lead to degeneration and atrophy.[203]

Yes, some people may experience too much stress on the kneecap from having the knee in front of the foot in these postures; but is it a good idea to minimize the stress on everybody's patella? If that was really the intention of this alignment cue, why was Krishnamacharya risking injury to his knee? (If you are a yoga teacher, would you really go up to Krishnamacharya and try to correct his posture?) Indeed, is this a risky pose at all for him? Photos taken when he was 78 years old showed him in this position, and he lived to be 100. Clearly he was not damaging his knee by allowing it to come forward of the ankle. Clearly, also, he was unique—and so are you.

If you have been taught, and truly believe, that the knees must never come forward of the ankles, consider figure 2.120, which shows the position of the knees in Chair Pose (Utkatasana). These images depict the styles of yoga taught by B.K.S. Iyengar and Pattabhi Jois. Notice where their knees are in relation to their ankles: quite far forward, further than Krishnamacharya's knee in figure 2.119. Why is it okay for these yoga luminaries to have their knee forward of the ankles in Chair Pose but not in Warrior Pose?

The answer often comes down to aesthetics. Having the knee over the ankle in standing postures creates, in Iyengar's words, "a right angle between the right thigh and the right calf . . . keeping the right shin perpendicular to the floor."[204] It just looks right. But is it?

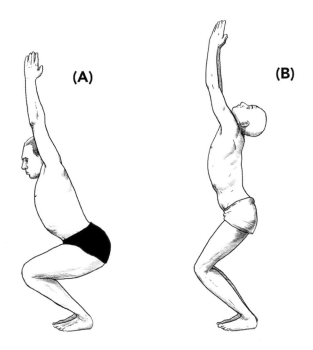

FIGURE 2.120 The Chair Pose (Utkatasana). Notice how the knees must come forward of the ankles to counterbalance the weight of the body going backwards. In (a), the version preferred in Iyengar yoga, the instruction is to make the thighs parallel to the floor. In (b), the version preferred in Ashtanga yoga, the style suggests aligning the hands, shoulders, hips, and heels. Students with flexion-intolerant back issues may be better off with option (b), while students with knee problems may do better with option (a).

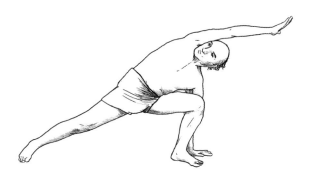

FIGURE 2.119 T. Krishnamacharya in Side Angle Pose (Parsvakonasana). Notice the position of the knee in front of the ankle, but also the alignment of both feet.

In everyday life we constantly allow—indeed, require—our knees to go in front of the ankles. Figure 2.121 shows what happens every time we climb stairs: the knee extends far in front of the ankle, and one leg bears the weight of the whole body as we climb. In other physical fitness modalities (e.g., weightlifting) and sports (e.g., fencing), the knee also comes forward of the ankle. Figure 2.122 shows an illustration of one of the greatest fencers in modern history, Aldo Nadi. Notice how in this lunging warrior posture, his front knee is well in front of the ankle; note, too, the position of the back foot and back hand, and the forward-leaning torso. If Aldo Nadi brought this posture to a modern yoga studio, he would be corrected, but he would be neither improved nor impressed.

Why is it okay for Aldo Nadi, Krishnamacharya and weightlifters to have their knees forward of the ankles, but not for modern yoga students? The answer is aesthetics. It is easy to see the alignment of the knee and the ankle and to modify students' postures to fit the image of a right-angle alignment, as Iyengar describes. However, if we take a *functional* approach to yoga, there may well be times when a student should, and indeed must, allow the knee to come forward. And there may well be times when a student should not allow the knee to go beyond the ankle. When we take a functional approach to our practice, decisions about alignment will be based upon the *appropriate* amount of stress we want to place on our tissues, not upon how the posture looks.

There is no question that having the knee forward of the ankle increases the pulling force of the quadriceps. One study examined how the degree of flexion changed the amount of pressure from the patella onto the femur. The researchers were looking at weightlifters performing deep squats with heavy loads.[205] To understand their findings, we need to understand the difference between *force* and *pressure*. Pressure (P) is the amount of force (F) *divided* by the surface area (A) over which the force is being applied: P = F/A. When we squat, we are creating a force in the quadriceps muscles, which causes the tendon surrounding the patella to press the patella onto the intercondylar groove of the femur.

As shown in figure 2.123, the surface area of the patella that contacts the femur changes as the knee flexes. When the leg is straight, the kneecap is high on the femur (see figure 2.141), and, due to the particular shape of the patella, there is little surface area contacting the femur and very little force being applied. Thus in full extension, the pressure is zero.[206] As the knee flexes, the patella begins to slide down the groove and can move 5–7 cm during this action.[207] Due to its shape, as it slides down the groove, more of the superior posterior (top underside) of the patella contacts the femur. The peak pressure in squatting comes between 80° and 90° of flexion. This is not the peak of the quadriceps' force! The force exerted by the quads continues to increase past 90°, but the surface area of the patella contacting the femur also increases past 90°, causing the pressure of the kneecap on the femur to lessen once we flex the knee past 90°.[208]

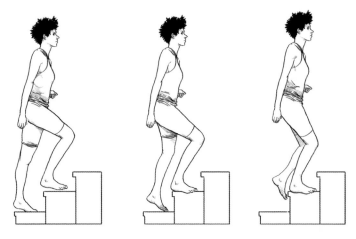

FIGURE 2.121 Climbing stairs. Notice that the knee must come forward of the ankle.

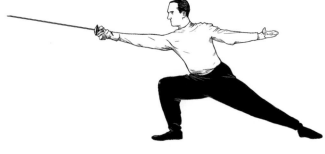

FIGURE 2.122 The fencing lunge of Aldo Nadi. Notice the position of the knee in front of the ankle. Also of interest is the position of the hands, the forward-leaning nature of his torso, and the turnout of the back foot. Note the similarities to figure 2.124b, below.

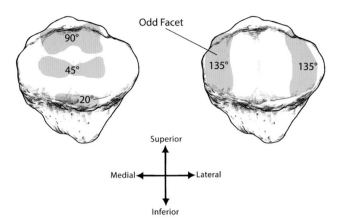

Odd Facet

90°

45°

135°   135°

20°

Superior

Medial ◀——▶ Lateral

Inferior

FIGURE 2.123 Contact between the posterior patella and the femur varies with the amount of knee flexion. At 20° of flexion, there is a small area of contact between the patella and femur, but at 135°, there is a large area of contact, which helps to reduce the pressure between the patella and the femur.

This is a very important point! If allowing the knees to go past 90° reduces kneecap pressure in squat, the same effect will occur in yoga lunges. As we increase our amount of flexion, we bring more patellar surface in contact with the femur and thus lessen the amount of pressure being applied. In other words, it is okay for most people to allow their knee to go forward of their ankle in lunges, just as Krishnamacharya and Nadi showed. Certainly this position is harder to maintain! The quadriceps have to be strong to stay here, but working the quads more is not necessarily a bad thing. It simply means that students with weaker quads will be challenged to stay here; they may need to back off due to a lack of strength, but not due to excess stress.

We are discovering that allowing the knee to come forward of the ankle in Warriors or lunges is not a problem for most students; it can work to strengthen the quadriceps and create more of a stretch in the back leg muscles, all while not increasing the pressure on the knee. However, what about the anterior cruciate ligament? Will letting the knee come forward place too much stress on the ACL? Studies have shown that stress on the ACL is greatest at 30° of flexion and decreases thereafter, so having the knee in front of the foot is not a problem for the ACL.[209] In any case, for most people, the amount of stress on the ACL in lunges is trivial compared to this ligament's tolerance levels. Even for students recovering from ACL injury, lunges and squats should not be a problem and may, indeed, be helpful.[210]

Of course, too much stress on the kneecap for *some* people could lead to degeneration, osteoarthritis or inflammation.[211] Squatting at knee angles (flexion) greater than 50° may be problematic for people with these knee issues. However, for people with healthy knees, this is not a concern.[212] Once again, we find that no one instruction will work for everybody. Hence, it is useful to offer students a range of options, perhaps creating three separate tracks they can choose to follow. [See the Sidebar *Note to Teachers: Customizing Classes.*] Students with degeneration in the knee (Track One) can be advised to ensure their thigh is at a 45° angle to the horizontal while in Warrior postures, as shown in figure 2.124a. This ensures that they do not worsen their situation by going past the 50° range. Students in Tracks Two and Three should be allowed to explore deeper variations. (Of note is figure 2.124b, which is an illustration of Pattabhi Jois's grandson, Sharat, doing Virabhadrasana II in the current Ashtanga style.[213] Observe how similar he looks to Aldo Nadi with the position of his front knee and back foot.)

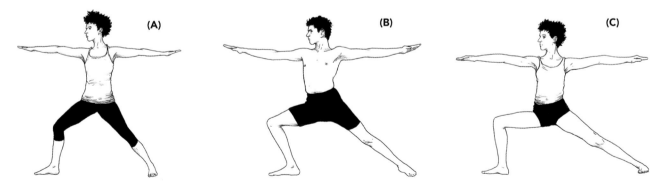

(A)   (B)   (C)

FIGURE 2.124 Three options for the knee in Warrior II Pose (Virabhadrasana B). For Track One students (a), the feet should be only wide enough to ensure the angle of the thigh to the horizontal is 45° or less. For Track Three students (b), the knee is perfectly okay coming forward of the ankle, but this may require the back foot being turned out and the torso leaning forward, which is more challenging but safe. For Track Two students (c), the knee may be aligned over the ankle, as is often described in standard yoga classes.

KNEE ALIGNMENT WITH THE FOOT: SUMMARY

Contrary to fitness folklore, and many yoga teacher training programs, for the vast majority of people there is no danger in allowing the knee to come forward of the ankle in lunges or standing postures. While the quadriceps will work harder to maintain this position, the stress in the knee is safe and may be required to keep the knees healthy. In any case, the stress on the knee is no greater than when doing Chair Pose (Utkatasana) or climbing stairs. However, for students who have pre-existing knee issues, it may be wiser to reduce to 45° the angle of the thigh to the horizontal by narrowing the distance between the feet.

FLEXION AND STRESS IN CHAIR POSE (UTKATASANA) AND SQUAT (MALASANA)

Studies of weightlifters in squats have shown that if the forward movement of the knees is deliberately restricted, the upper body leans more forward to compensate, and this reaction places extra stress on the spine's vertebrae and their ligaments. The recommendation is to not restrict how far forward the knees go when squatting.[214] This is instructive for yoga students when coming into the Chair Pose (Utkatasana). Sometimes, they are told to keep the knees back enough that the toes can be seen. At other times, they are told to squat down low enough that "the thighs are parallel to the floor."[215] Going low in these squats requires the hips to flex more deeply and move backwards. To maintain balance, the torso has to lean forward, which increases the hip flexion and causes increased flexion stress in the spine. In other traditions, however, the instruction is not to lower the hips so far but rather to attempt to align the hands above the shoulders, the shoulders above the hips and the hips above the feet. In figure 2.120 we see these two options. The first is the B.K.S. Iyengar version of Utkatasana,[216] while in (b) we have the Pattabhi Jois version.[217] Which one is correct? Both can be, depending upon your intention. With more hip flexion, more stress will occur in the hips and the spine; that may be good, but perhaps not if the student has trauma or weakness there. With less hip flexion and thus a straighter stance, more stress will occur in the knees;[218] again, that is not necessarily good or bad but depends upon the student. There is a trade-off, and which pose is right for you depends upon your biology, biography and intention.

Remember, the peak pressure in the kneecap occurs around 80–90° of knee flexion. Thanks to compression between the back of the thighs and the calves, the full Squat Pose (Malasana) puts far less pressure on the knees than the Chair Pose (Utkatasana).[219] Staying in the full Squat does not involve nearly as much stress on the knees as the Chair or the Warriors. In the upcoming section on the ankle—foot segment, we will look in more detail at the Squat Pose, including how far apart the feet can be and whether they should point straight ahead or outward.

Extension of the Knee

All tissues need stress to retain or regain their health. We know this, but often in our fear of doing too much we err on the side of doing too little. A case in point is hyperextension of the knee. It is common in the yoga community for teachers to suggest or demand that their students refrain from any hyperextension of the knee, especially in standing poses. The instructions are well intentioned; in *some* people, it is possible for a hyperextended knee to become injured. But out of the intention to do no harm, the teachers may be creating a situation where healthy knees, which are at no risk of damage in hyperextension, are prevented from receiving the stress that the knee needs to stay healthy. The fear of doing too much may be leading some teachers to offer too little. We risk fragilizing knees.

As noted earlier, hyperextension of the knees is normal and natural. The average person can hyperextend his or her knees 5–6° (see figure 2.125). Students interested in a more technical discussion of knee hyperextension can read the sidebar It's Complicated: Hyperextension of the knee, on page 186. Those less technically inclined needn't read the full sidebar but are advised to glance at figure 2.129.

NOTE TO TEACHERS: Customizing classes

Clothing manufacturers have long known that every body is different. So, they developed standardized ranges of offerings. From shoes to bras, from hats to pants, clothing comes in a variety of sizes. This variety has a cost: lots of inventory is needed to ensure that there is something for everyone—and even then, some people never seem to find the right sizes for their unique bodies. To save on inventory and cost, some manufacturers simply offer three sizes: small, medium and large.

If we adopt a functional approach to yoga that encourages us to seek an appropriate level of challenge and stress, rather than worrying about how we look aesthetically in the postures, we too can develop options for postures that fit students' abilities, just like clothing companies. A functional approach to teaching yoga requires that we have an intention for putting students into poses. We can consider several possible intentions for any posture: to build strength in the muscles, to stretch or lengthen tissues, to develop calmness in the midst of challenge, to prepare for more challenging postures to come, or any of many other possible goals. A generalized intention may be to build health, strength and resilience. Of course, our intention is also not to cause harm. Due to the reality of human variations, there are students who should take care with certain postures, there are students who are new to yoga and don't know the postures yet, and there are students who are naturally strong and flexible and require more challenge in various postures to benefit from them.

While it would be nice if we could custom tailor our classes to every individual student, unfortunately—except for private yoga instruction or very small classes—this is rarely practical. But, like the clothing manufacturers, we can group the students into one of three broad categories, offer different options, and allow the student to choose the most appropriate track to follow. For example:

- **Track One.** This track is aimed at students who are just beginning their yoga journey and do not yet know the postures, at students who have some pathology or inherent limitations to their ability to come into or remain in postures, or at students who simply want an easier challenge on the day. The teacher will offer options that make potentially challenging or dangerous postures more accessible and safer.
- **Track Two.** This track is for students who have been doing yoga long enough to know the nature of the postures being offered and of their own abilities. It is more challenging than Track One but not as advanced as Track Three. Teachers can offer options that take people deeper into the postures, but again not so deep that there is risk of injury.
- **Track Three.** This track is for experienced students who are healthy, strong and flexible, know their own limitations and can safely perform the more challenging versions of the postures. Teachers can now offer the more advanced variations but should continue to direct students to heed their bodies' signals to ensure they are not overdoing it.

The three tracks are not meant to be applied dogmatically. There are beginners to a yoga practice who are naturally strong and flexible and will be able to safely do the options offered in Tracks Two or Three. And there are students who after 10 years of a dedicated practice still cannot perform the options offered for Track Three. Ultimately, the student must decide which track is appropriate. However, the teacher can assist by reminding the student of her intention. Why is she doing yoga? Is it to build performance or to maximize health? Many students want to be Track Three but should keep to the Track One options. You may help students choose the appropriate track if you remind them: "Don't let your ego write checks that your body can't cash!"

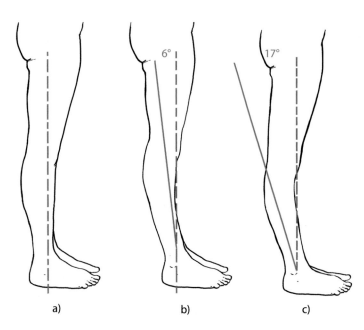

FIGURE 2.125 The ideal versus the reality of hyperextension. Anatomy books show the ideal alignment of the knees (a), but the average person hyperextends their knees ~6° (b). Some people, however, can hyperextend the knees to 17° or more (c).

IT'S COMPLICATED:
What is a newton?

A newton is a unit of force. Sir Isaac Newton's second law of motion states that force (F) is equal to the mass (M) of an object multiplied by its acceleration (A): F = MA. One newton (N) is defined as the force experienced by an object that has a mass of one kilogram and an acceleration of one meter per second squared (m/s²). The force of a person standing on the earth can also be calculated in newtons. For example, the acceleration (A) caused by gravity is 9.8 m/s². A man who has a mass (M) of 75 kilograms (165 pounds) exerts a force (F) on the ground of 735 newtons. (One N is equivalent to 0.225 pounds of force; one pound of force is equal to 4.45 N.) This same 75-kilogram man, when his knees are hyperextended passively, may experience a force on the ACL of about 120 N, which is about one-sixth of his body weight. The tolerance of his ACL to stress (assuming he is young) is around 2100 N, or almost three times his weight.

Opinion in the research community is divided on whether hyperextension leads to problems.[220] Most people do hyperextend, and most people do not have knee problems. In the case studies where hyperextension did lead to knee damage, the precipitating event was always dynamic: a blow to the knee in a contact sport, or a sudden stop, or a stop and turning (in sports parlance, "a cut and run"), or a hard landing after a jump. In none of the reported cases surveyed was *static* hyperextension cited as a cause of knee damage.

In the yoga environment, we rarely subject the knee to large, transient, dynamic stress. With the exception of Kundalini yoga and occasionally Ashtanga yoga, which may employ jumping into and out of postures, most yoga styles are slow. A hyperextended knee may experience static stresses while in the postures, but the levels of these stresses are far below the healthy knee's tolerance. Of most concern in hyperextension is the state of the ACL, as it provides 85% of the resistance to further extension.[221] (The posterior joint capsule and collateral ligaments provide additional but minimal support.) People between 22 and 35 years of age, with young, healthy ACLs, can tolerate over 2100 newtons (472 pounds) of force on the ACL before it becomes damaged. (What's a newton? See the It's Complicated sidebar on this page.) Even the ACLs of older students (over 60) can tolerate around 650 newtons[222] (146 pounds). The stress in a passively held hyperextended knee at 5° is around 120 newtons[223] (27 pounds), clearly well within the tolerance level of even old knees.

The amount of stress on the ACL in a hyperextended knee does depend upon the alignment of the leg with respect to the body and the ground, the degree of hyperextension, and the level of co-activation of the muscles surrounding the knee. People who have ACL damage, or who are recovering from surgery, or who are very lax in their ACL ligament and thus have a large degree of hyperextension may indeed be at risk of further damage to their knee if they allow static hyperextension to persist. For these individuals, it may be a good idea to back off and straighten a hyperextended leg. However, offering this advice to people with healthy knees may predispose them to a weakening of the ACL over time, because they are being prevented from applying a necessary stress to the joint. The challenge for teachers is how to instruct a class that may contain both kinds of students—those who can and should hyperextend, as well as students who should not.

Recall the philosophical approach to building health cited in Volume 1: To build muscular strength with little risk to the joints, load the tissues at low ranges of movement (this is a yang form of exercise); to build flexibility and connective tissue strength, stress the joints near their end range of motion when they are not bearing a load (which is a yin form of exercise). If we want to strengthen the knee joint and its associated connective tissue structures, we can do so in a yin way. Utilizing yin yoga postures such as Saddle Pose (Suptavirasana) will provide a nice amount of stress to the ACL and other knee ligaments, but it will do so in a very passive, non-weightbearing manner.[224] By incorporating yin stresses in our yoga practice, we do not need to stress the knee in our standing postures as well. In our yang practice, we are free to protect a hyperextending knee regardless of whether it needs protecting or not. We can combine yin and yang elements to maximize stress while minimizing risk.

It is worth noting that when the knees are hyperextended, some students compensate by tilting their pelvis anteriorly; this increases the normal lumbar curve (called hyperlordosis), which can have negative effects along the spine and higher up the body. Again, every body is different, and while hyperextension may be quite acceptable for the knees, for you it may cause lower back problems or other issues.

Let's summarize. It is okay for most people to hyperextend their knees in static yoga postures, but for some people it may be dangerous. To protect knees at risk, we can reduce hyperextension (see below), but this may prevent a stress needed to keep the knees healthy. One way to combine both intentions is to use a yin yoga practice to stress the joint safely and passively, and use our yang practice to stress the musculature of the body while refraining from hyperextension. In this way, we put no one at risk but are also not overly protective of those who need more stress.

REDUCING HYPEREXTENSION

If we do decide we need to reduce the level of stress on the ACL caused by hyperextension, the best technique is co-contraction of the quadriceps and the hamstrings. (See It's Important: Co-contraction on page 174.) To learn how to do this, sit in Staff Pose (Dandasana) with your legs stretched out in front of you (see figure 2.126). Relax, and feel the muscular tension around the knees: in the front of the thigh just above the knee, and at the back of the thigh. As shown in figure 2.126a, to deliberately hyperextend the knees, try engaging the

quadriceps. You may be able to do this by pulling up the kneecap, pushing your thighs into the floor and flexing your toes towards you. If you are prone to hyperextension, the heels will lift off the floor; feel how your quads are tighter. (Note that these cues won't work for some people, so they may have to do whatever it takes to lift the heel off the floor while pressing their thighs downward.) Hyperextension can be caused by overactivation of the quadriceps, or more weakly by the actions of the calf muscles, specifically the gastrocnemius. The common cue to lift the kneecap in standing postures, thus engaging the quads, does not stop hyperextension and may actually increase it. The quads pull the tibia forward, as shown in figure 2.127, creating more stress on the ACL. (The gastrocnemius pulls the femur backwards, again resulting in an increase in tension on the ACL.)

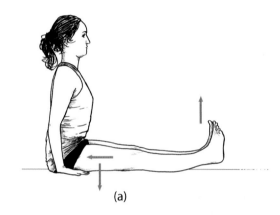

(a)

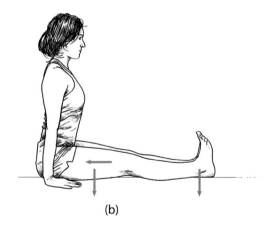

(b)

FIGURE 2.126 Hyperextending the knees in Staff Pose (Dandasana). (a) While sitting with the legs straight in front of you, tighten the thighs and notice whether your heels rise up; that signifies hyperextension. (b) Continue to push the thighs to the floor, but also push the heels down; this co-contraction engages the hamstrings and reduces hyperextension.

To reduce the stress on the ACL, we need to pull the tibia posteriorly, and we can do that by engaging the hamstrings. This co-contraction often happens unconsciously; people do it while they lift the kneecaps, without being aware of what they are doing. To do it consciously, try this. While sitting with legs outstretched, push your thighs *and* your heels to the floor, as shown in figure 2.126b. With your hands, feel the effects of this around the knee and the tension in the muscles. This action co-contracts the quadriceps and the hamstrings, firmly stabilizing the knee joint, reducing the amount of hyperextension and thus minimizing stress on the ACL.

Now that we know what co-contraction feels like, we can apply this technique to reducing hyperextension in all standing poses—for example, Triangle Pose (Trikonasana). Coming into the posture, we straighten the front leg so that it is not hyperextending, and we engage the quadriceps by lifting the kneecap or trying to stretch the mat with our feet. Now, we engage the hamstrings by simultaneously hugging the back of the thighs together or by simulating sliding the feet together. With your hands, you can feel the tension in the top and back of the thighs. This co-contraction should result in a stabilized and fully extended (but not hyperextended) leg.

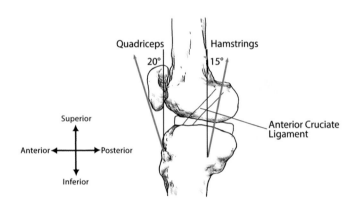

FIGURE 2.127 Co-contraction. Contraction of the quadriceps pulls the tibia anteriorly, creating stress on the ACL, but contracting the hamstrings pulls the tibia posteriorly, reducing ACL stress. Co-contracting both muscles at the same time helps to maintain extension but reduces ACL stress.[225]

Sideways Movement of the Knee: Valgus and Varus

What is the proper alignment for the front knee in Warrior Poses (Virabhadrasanas)? Figures 2.130 and 2.131 show an inward or outward orientation to the knees that can occur in a variety of postures, such as Warrior Poses, Wide-Legged Posture (Prasarita Padottanasana), sitting down into Chair Pose (Utkatasana) or Squat (Malasana), and the more challenging one-legged squat. The knees may fall inward towards each other (called valgum or abduction) or move away from each other (called varum or adduction.) Are these movements safe? As always, it depends!

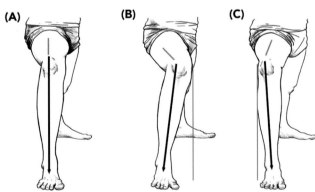

FIGURE 2.130 The alignment options of the knee in Warrior Poses (Virabhadrasanas. In (a), we see the knee aligned with the front foot and the hip socket. In (b), we see a valgus movement, where the knee collapses medially to the foot. In (c), we see a varus movement, where the knee is aligned laterally to the foot.

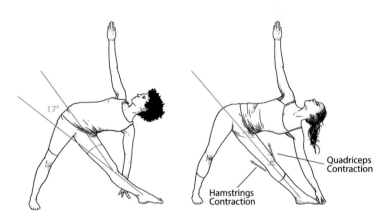

FIGURE 2.128 Co-contraction in the Triangle Pose (Trikonasana). We can engage the quadriceps by attempting to stretch the mat beneath us. We can engage the hamstrings by simultaneously hugging the thighs together or by simulating sliding the feet together. These two actions may reduce or eliminate hyperextension of the knee.

The medial collateral ligament provides 57% of the resistance to valgus movements when the knee is extended straight and 78% when it is flexed 25°.[250] In the yoga world, most teachers will suggest that the student align the knee so it points straight ahead, over the foot, as shown in figure 2.130a. The reason given is to reduce the stress on the medial side of the knee. This reasoning is not always valid for the Warriors. When the knee is flexed 90°, the collateral ligaments are at their shortest and thus most lax[251] (see figure 2.115), allowing both twisting of the knee and some lateral movement. There is very little stress on the medial ligaments of the knee in this position and very little danger of injury. Even if there were some stress, ligaments need stress to remain strong and thick.

In the other examples of valgum, shown in figure 2.131a, when the amount of knee flexion is reduced because the leg is straight or straighter, there is stress to the medial collateral ligament (MCL), and for some people, this is healthy. Avoiding stress on the MCL could lead to fragility. However, there are valid reasons why *some* students may wish to follow the alignment cue of "the knee pointing straight ahead"; there are also reasons why some students should not follow that cue. The "correct" position for the knee will depend upon each student's unique anatomical structure and the state of their ligaments, joint capsule and muscle tone.

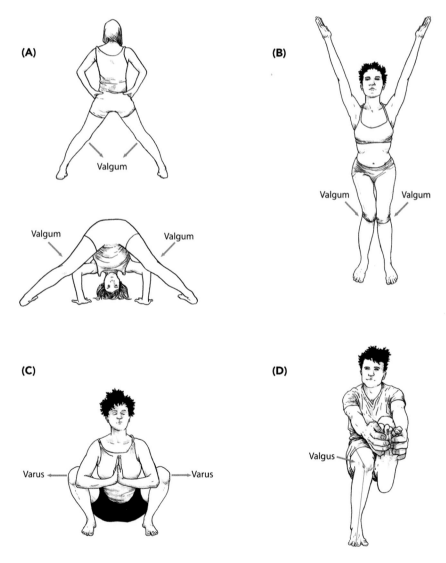

FIGURE 2.131 Knee valgum or varum may occur in many postures: (a) wide-legged postures (Prasarita Padottanasana), (b) Chair Pose (Utkatasana), (c) Squat (Malasana), (d) One-Legged Squat (Pistol Squat).

IT'S COMPLICATED: Hyperextension of the knee

Extending the knee straightens the leg. When in line with the thigh, the leg is considered fully extended. Figure 2.125a shows this "perfect" 180° alignment: the hip joint is above the knee joint, which is above the ankle joint. However, virtually everyone can go past the magical 180° line, a position called hyperextension of the knee. The average amount of hyperextension can vary greatly, but one study showed that 99% of women hyperextend, the average being 6.7° (with one standard deviation of 2.7° and a range from zero to 17°), while 95% of men hyperextend, their average being 5.5° (with one standard deviation of 2.5° and a range from zero to 17.5°).[226] Hyperextension greater than 5° is sometimes termed *genu recurvatum*[227] (Latin for "backwards-bending knee").[228] By this definition, most people have genu recurvatum.

Researchers are quite divided as to whether hyperextension of the knee predisposes us to injury.[229] Despite the inference in the literature and the yoga community that the 180° alignment of the knee is ideal, allowing the knee to be slightly hyperextended is necessary for human bipeds. By "locking the knees" and "hanging out" in the ligaments while we stand, we reduce muscular energy; the ligaments, rather than the quadriceps, are doing the work of supporting our posture. We evolved to do this. Walking chimpanzees expend far more energy than walking humans, because the chimps have to keep their knees constantly bent. Humans can completely extend the knee, and this saves on calories.[230] We use around 5° of hyperextension when we walk, which is, not surprisingly, the amount most people can do.[231] If we did not slightly hyperextend the knees while standing or walking, the quadriceps would be constantly working to hold our posture, which would be tiring and could lead to chronic shortening of the quadriceps.

On the other hand, we can do too much of anything. People who sit all day long, which allows their leg muscles to weaken, may tend to overdo hyperextension in the knees while standing. For these people, it may indeed be better to microbend the knees while in their yoga postures and work on strengthening their leg muscles.

All this is to point out that some hyperextension is very normal and useful. If we cannot hyperextend to our normal limit after a knee injury, the knee will feel constrained and stiff, and we may create unhealthy movement patterns to compensate for the loss of range of motion.[232] Restoring full range of motion, including hyperextension, prevents arthrofibrosis (abnormally thick scar tissue) and knee pain after surgery.[233] This 5–7° of hyperextension is important for full functional activity.

In figure 2.125, we see three variations on knee hyperextension. In the first drawing (a) is the common presentation found in many anatomy texts, illustrating the supposed ideal 180° alignment. The second drawing (b) shows the reality for the average person: a slight hyperextension of 6°. This is normal and healthy. The third picture shows a person with significant hyperextension of 17°.

There are two forms of hyperextension of the knee. The first is acute and the second chronic. In an acute hyperextension, the knee is forced backwards due to a sudden trauma or movement. The most frequently damaged ligament in knee injuries is the ACL, and a common cause of ACL injury is a sudden stress on the knee when it is hyperextended, such as a sports contact injury that forces the knee backwards. It more often occurs, however, when we make a sudden stop while running, especially when combined with a change of direction, or when we jump and land with the legs extended.[234] Landing from a jump and changing directions while running are the most common causes of ACL injuries.[235] Unfortunately, women are two to eight times more likely to damage their ACLs than men, and most often this happens from landing after a jump.[236] Women tend to activate their quadriceps initially upon landing, whereas men activate the hamstrings first.[237] However, this is due to geometry, not gender. (People with smaller bodies have shorter thighs and thus greater Q-angles and smaller tibial plateaus over which to distribute stress.) Excessive hyperextension of a knee bearing a load increases the risk of ACL damage. If the knee is twisted in addition to the hyperextension, the risk of damage increases.[238] Perhaps surprisingly, the incidence rate of ACL injuries is far lower in gymnastics than in skiing, handball, soccer, basketball or contact sports.[239]

Fortunately, in yoga asana practice, we do not subject the knee to sudden hyperextension stresses by changing directions of movement. The worry in yoga is related more to the second form of hyperextension: the chronically hyper-extended knee. In several standing postures, such as Triangle Pose (Trikonasana), King Dancer (Natarajasana), Tree Pose (Vriksasana) and Half-moon Pose (Ardhachandrasana), one leg is fully extended and supporting most or all of the body's weight. Figure 2.129 illustrates King Dancer and Half-moon. In photographs, B.K.S. Iyengar displayed the average amount of hyperextension in his supporting knee, 5–7°. Almost everyone can hyperextend their knee while standing, so it is to be expected that most yoga practitioners will do so in their postures. The question is: should they?

Static hyperextension of the knee can lead to increased tension on the ACL and the supporting structures at the back of the knee.[241] There is no bony stop at the back of the knee, like there is in the elbow. The ligaments, joint capsule and tendons have to restrict further posterior movement. About 85% of this stress is being absorbed by the ACL.[242] Recall that the ACL prevents the femur from sliding backward over the tibia, and the posterior cruciate ligament (PCL) prevents the tibia from sliding backwards under the femur (see figure 2.107). The greater the degree of hyperextension, the greater the degree of tension the cruciate ligaments will be under. A healthy ACL can withstand over 2,000 N (450 pounds) of force[243] and the PCL twice that.[244] The ACL experiences more tension than the PCL in hyperextension and thus is the main ligament we worry about in that situation. With 5° of passive hyperextension, the ACL experiences an average of only 118 N (26.5 pounds) of force, which is well within its tolerance levels.[245]

For most people, this amount of hyperextension is not a concern, but for some it may be. The causes of hyperextension beyond the normal range are many and varied: neurological differences, muscle weakness, ligament laxity or injury. While strong quadriceps engagement can cause hyperextension, quadriceps that are too weak to stabilize the knee may lead to compensation by movement into hyperextension, using the ligaments to provide stability that the muscles cannot.[246] For this reason, people with congenital muscle weakness, such as results from cerebral palsy or muscular dystrophy, or people who have suffered a stroke, often rely on hyperextension to support the knee, but over time this may create too much laxity in the joint.

Students who have damaged or compromised ligaments, people who hyperextend beyond the normal range (i.e., >10°),[247] older people who naturally have weaker ACLs,[248] or anyone recovering from knee surgery may well be advised to reduce the stress upon their ACLs encountered in hyperextension. However, while too much stress can be harmful, there is a danger in experiencing too little stress. "The absence of strain on ligaments, even those that have not been injured, has been shown to have harmful effects."[249] We need some stress on the ACL. The level of stress experienced by standing in hyperextension is quite moderate compared to the stress we experience while climbing stairs or running. For most yogis, hyperextension of the knee is not a problem. For some yogis, it may be. But correcting hyperextension in every body may not be a good idea, because, as just mentioned, we do need to stress the ACL to keep it healthy.

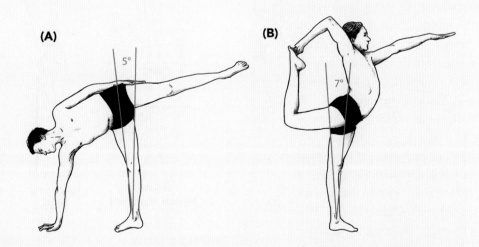

FIGURE 2.129 Hyperextension between 5° and 7° is normal. B.K.S. Iyengar hyperextended his knees in (a) Half-moon (Ardhachandrasana) and (b) King Dancer (Natarajasana).[240]

In valgus movement, as illustrated in figure 2.132c, the knee moves medially, lining up inside the foot. This does two things biomechanically to the knee when it is extended: (1) it stresses the MCL and ACL[252] and (2) it places more compressive stress on the lateral tibial condyle.[253] The opposite happens in varum, as shown in figure 2.132b, where the knee is lined up outside the foot: (1) it stresses the lateral collateral ligament and ACL and (2) it places more compressive stress on the medial tibial condyle.[254] Clinicians define the condition as valgum when the knee has a medial bend greater than 182°; if it has a lateral bend less than 178°, it is called varum.[255] Some researchers assert that the normal amount of angle is 5–7° of valgum. This means that on average, most people are slightly valgus, or knock-kneed.[256] Some individuals, however, are significantly different, and that may be normal for them, or it may be a sign of pathology. One survey found that 25% of people had varus alignment while 36% had valgus alignment, which means only 39% of those studied were neutrally aligned.[257] Another study found the reverse: 41% of people had varus alignment while 19% had valgus alignment, but still only 40% were neutrally aligned.[258] In which camp do you reside? To find out, read It's Important: Are you valgus or varus? on this page.

Again, our purpose is not to discover which number is "right" but to show how great human variability is. We do not know the typical amount of angle for the knees, nor what it should be. We do know that everyone is different. Thus, our quest is to find out what alignment works best for you.

THE CAUSE OF VALGUS OR VARUS KNEES

Unfortunately, the studies citing the frequency of varum or valgum did not correlate the causes as well. Knowing the cause is important. For some people, their varum or valgum is too much and can lead to pathology. For others, their valgum or varum is harmless, but trying to correct it may create harm. (See Appendix E: The Dangers and Benefits of Valgum or Varum Knee Orientation.)

IT'S IMPORTANT: Are you valgus or varus?

We are using the terms valgus and varus as adjectives to describe lateral movements in the knee (valgum and varum are the nouns). Valgus refers to inward movement of the knees, varus to outward movement. (To help you remember, you can associate the "g" in valgus with "g" for gluing your knees together and the "r" in varus for repelling the knees apart.)

Figure 2.136 shows examples of valgus and varus. When students stand and try to bring both their knees and their feet together, some cannot. If the knees are together but the ankles are 3 cm or more apart, this is termed *valgum*. If the ankles are together but the knees are 3 cm or more apart, this is called *varum*. Clinicians may use a different technique to measure the degree of varum or valgum, as shown in figure 2.132.

What is your situation? Measure yourself by coming into standing, bringing the knees and feet together and, if you tend to hyperextend, flexing your knees so that you are at 180° of extension and the legs are straight. (Hyperextension can mimic varum or valgum.)[263] Have a friend measure any gap between either the ankles or the knees. Are you valgum, varum or neutral? Keep your reality in mind as you read the rest of this section.

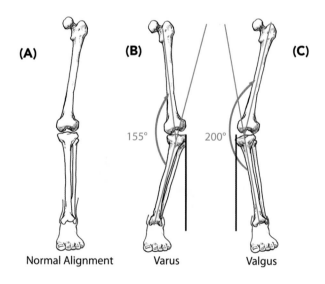

FIGURE 2.132 Valgus and varus alignment in the left knee. In (a), we see a knee aligned normally. In (b), we see a knee bowing outwardly or laterally, called varus. In (c), we see a knee falling inwardly or medially, called valgus.

Many anatomical and behavioral factors can lead to varum or valgum: pelvis width, acetabulum orientation, femoral torsion, tibial torsion, ankle and foot structure, ligament laxity, quadriceps weakness, proprioception deficiencies, pronation or supination of the feet, and other habitual movement patterns. (Relative to the feet, pronation means moving the soles down and outward, and supination means turning the soles inward and up.) The first few of these causes are beyond a student's control; the latter few are controllable. In figure 2.133 we see a range of tibial and femoral shapes that can create varum or valgum. These are not controllable or fixable. Fortunately, researchers have found that the *shape* of our joints is not the predominant factor in injuries attributable to varus or valgus alignment of the knees; instead, *how* we use our body is the important key to injury prevention.[259] The causes that are within our control include: weakness in the hip abductor and external rotator muscles (specifically the three gluteal muscles) and/or overactivity of the adductors; pronation of the foot, which can be caused by a restricted range of dorsiflexion; weakness in the quadriceps (specifically the vastus medialis obliquus); and weakness in the semimembranosus and semitendinosus hamstrings. These factors can be corrected, but if the relevant movements and use have become habitual, they are challenging to change. Attention and intention are required. Interestingly, a study of healthy tennis players found no correlation between valgus and varus orientation of the knee in lunges and muscular weakness or imbalance.[260] Just because something *could* be a problem does not mean that it *will* become a problem.

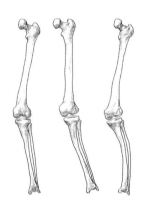 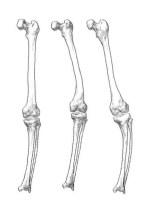

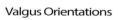

Valgus Orientations   **Varus Orientations**

FIGURE 2.133 Tibial and femoral shape may cause varum or valgum. On the left we have three examples of valgum caused by the shape of the tibia and femur. On the right we have three examples of varum. Yoga will not change the shape of these bones.

WHEN SHOULD WE CHANGE A VARUS OR VALGUS ORIENTATION?

First, let's restate what we have already discovered: not everyone needs to correct their valgus or varus orientation in yoga. For many people, their bones require their knee to line up inside or outside their foot in the Warrior Postures. It can be helpful to check whether the student's knees or feet can both come together when they stand in Mountain Pose (Tadasana). If only the knees are together (valgum), or if only the feet are together (varum), you should expect that the knee in the Warrior Postures is unlikely to be aligned straight ahead. Another way to determine whether this is a natural or unnatural position for a student is to look at the front foot in Warrior Pose. If the knee is valgus *and* the foot is pronated, then there is a good likelihood that the valgus can be corrected. However, if the knee is valgus and the foot is *not* pronated, then correcting the valgus position may result in the foot supinating unnecessarily. Be aware that the degree of pronation or supination may be subtle, on the order of only 10–20°, and thus hard to see. If the foot is neutral, regardless of what the knee is doing, there may be no need or point to correcting the varum or valgum. Figure 2.134 illustrates these situations.

NOTE TO TEACHERS: Do not offer a correction without knowing the cause!

If you do not know what is causing the alignment the student is presenting, "fixing" or correcting the alignment may put the student at risk. A good doctor does not prescribe medicine without first understanding what is causing the problem. Don't guess or assume—check it out. Ask the student what she is feeling. Notice her unique anatomy. If in doubt, leave it out. Don't adjust her, but do ask her to notice what sensations are arising.

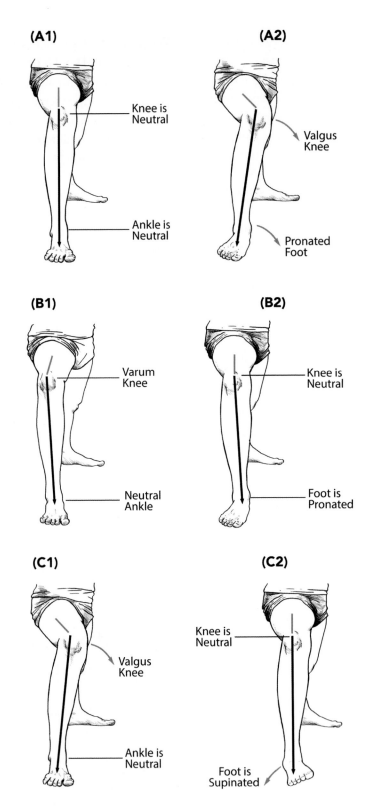

FIGURE 2.134 Fixing naturally occurring varum and valgus may cause pronation or supination of the foot. In (a1), we see a neutrally aligned knee and a neutral foot. In (a2), we see how pronation of the foot *creates* a valgus movement of a neutral knee, which could be corrected. In (b1), we see a natural varum knee with a neutral foot. In (b2), we see that "correcting" this knee pronates the foot. In (c1), we see a valgus knee with a neutral foot. In (c2), we see that "correcting" this knee supinates the foot.

In figure (a1), we see a neutrally aligned knee and a neutral foot. Beside it, in (a2), we see how pronation of the foot creates a valgus movement of a neutral knee. This is a correctable situation. We can do many things to realign the knee and the foot for this student, as will be discussed below. However, in (b1), we have a varum knee with a neutral foot. In (b2), we see that aligning this knee *creates* pronation of the foot. Pronating the foot to align the knee may create more problems than it cures. It would be better for this student to allow the knee to be slightly outside the foot in this pose. In (c1), we have a valgus knee with a neutral foot. In (c2), we see that aligning this knee creates supination of the foot, which again may not be desirable. It is easy, as yoga teachers, to see where a student's knee is pointing and make an aesthetic judgment, but just because a knee falls inside or outside the foot does not automatically mean we should change that orientation. We have to look more closely and check out what the ankle is doing, too.

HOW TO REDUCE VALGUS OR VARUS IF THE CAUSE IS CORRECTABLE

Sometimes the correction is very simple: stop pronating or supinating the feet. However, one reason for such foot motion may be a lack of strength higher up. Strengthening the hip muscles obviously will give greater control over what the legs are doing and their placement in static and dynamic positions. Strength training and re-education of the muscles around the knee and hip can improve knee tracking, where the knee is incorrectly tracking due to muscular imbalance or impaired motor control. Both strength and technique are needed so that the desired movements become habitual. Most yoga teachers know how to strengthen the muscles of the legs and hips, but particularly effective

in realigning valgus knees are postures that strengthen the abductors, external hip rotators and lateral hamstrings. One exercise taught to weightlifters and hockey goalies is the one-legged squat (but in this suggested version, as shown in figure 2.135a and b, ensure that the lifted leg is behind you or to the side, not in front).[261] To realign varus knees, strengthen the adductors and medial hamstrings. A very effective posture for both varum and valgum is Side Plank (Vasisthasana) and all its variations, as shown in figure 2.135c and d. Side Plank strengthens both the adductors and the abductors.

Lunges are not the only postures in which valgum and varum appear; they also show up in other standing postures with the legs apart. Figure 2.131 shows the Wide-Legged Posture (Prasarita Padottanasana) and Chair Pose (Utkatasana) with the knees tracking in a valgus alignment. Again, whether the valgus alignment is detrimental or normal and of no consequence depends upon the student's anatomical structure, the health and strength of the various tissues, and their proprioceptive abilities. If you know that your student is naturally valgus due to the shape of her bones (she can't bring her feet together in Mountain Pose—Tadasana), there may be no need to try to align her knees to neutral; indeed, doing so may lead to overly supinated feet. However, if you notice both the valgum and pronation of the feet, directions to move the knees apart may be warranted.

The Chair Pose can be held statically, or it can be a transitional position; as we move between squatting and standing, at some point we go through this chair-like position, and a momentary valgus movement may occur. This is common in weight-lifting with deep squats. Often, weightlifters, even Olympic athletes, will move through a small and brief valgus position as they rise out of a deep squat.

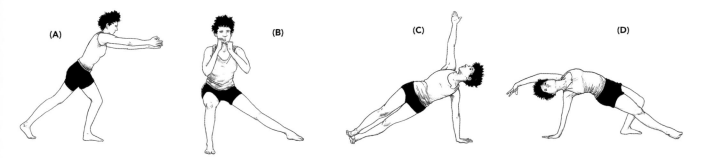

FIGURE 2.135 One-legged Squats and Side Planks (Vasisthasana) are particularly effective for strengthening the abductor and adductor muscles, which can help reduce valgus and varus tracking of the knee. (a) is the less stressful version of the one-legged squat. (b) offers another version, with the leg out to the side. (c) is the traditional Side Plank. (d) is an easier variation.

There is an ongoing debate in the literature as to whether this valgus movement is an "energy leak" or a necessary recruitment of other muscles, such as the bicep femoris and adductors, to help power through this sticky point.[262] We can see the same valgus movement occur when a student does a one-legged squat: coming up, the standing leg will often momentarily bow inward. This may be a natural and harmless movement. However, should the valgus continue throughout the whole movement or be larger than just a few degrees, there is consensus in the weightlifting community that better biomechanics are necessary.

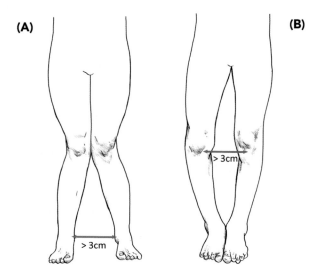

FIGURE 2.136 Valgus and varus can be determined by attempting to bring the knees and feet together. In (a), we see a student in valgus who can bring the knees together but not the ankles. In (b), we see a student in varus who can bring the ankles together, but the knees remain apart.

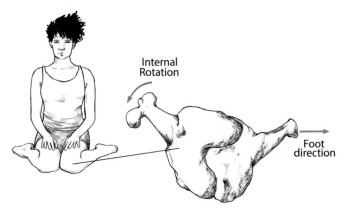

FIGURE 2.137 Internal rotation in Hero Pose (Virasana). The student allows her feet to point outward due to large internal rotation at the hip sockets. For her, there is no rotation occurring at the knee and thus, in this case, no risk to the knee.

Rotation at the Knee

Notice the woman sitting in Hero Pose (Virasana) in figure 2.137. Is the position of her feet safe for her knees, or is she risking death and destruction to her medial collateral ligaments, ACLs and menisci? As always, the answer is: it depends!

The collateral ligaments help to prevent twisting and side movements of the tibia under the femur when the leg is fully extended. The anterior cruciate ligament crosses to the lateral side of the posterior cruciate ligament; this arrangement causes the two cruciate ligaments to wrap around each other when the tibia is internally (medially) rotated under the femur (see figure 2.113). When the tibia externally (laterally) rotates under the femur, the two cruciate ligaments move away from each other, allowing more range of movement. An often given statistic suggests we only have about 10° of internal rotation available at the knee, but 30–40° of external rotation.[264] But is this the case for you?

It is useful to discover our own unique ability to internally and externally rotate the tibia. While clinicians use a more rigorous approach, we can approximate our range with the simple test shown in figure 2.138. Start by sitting with your legs extended. Hold the thigh steady just above the knee, to prevent any rotation arising from the hips. Without twisting your foot (keep the sole of the foot "flat," facing the wall), rotate your ankle/foot internally as much as you can. Again, make sure this is not coming from the hip; keep your kneecap pointing in the same direction throughout the movement. Notice how far you can internally rotate your ankle/foot. Now, do the same thing but with the knee flexed. As shown in (b), flex the leg about 90°, keep holding the thigh just above the knee, and try to internally rotate the ankle/foot as much as you can, again keeping the sole of the foot in the same plane (no twisting the foot). You will probably note an increased amount of rotation. The difference between what you can do now and what you did in (a) is the degree of your internal tibial rotation. While the average person may only achieve about 10°, what is *your* reality? The knee when passive can be rotated further than we can actively rotate it by ourselves. A clinician would do this measurement differently and would apply pressure on the foot to rotate the tibia while you relaxed your muscles. Thus, the clinician would get a slightly larger amount of rotation. What you have just observed is not your full limit, but it is indicative of what you can naturally achieve.

Now, try it with external rotation. Do the same as before, but rotate the foot outward. Notice the enhanced amount of external tibial rotation you achieve when the knee is flexed. Again, the average is 30–40°, but what is your reality?

The final part of this experiment is to note any sensations in the knee as you rotate the tibia. With the knee flexed, the collateral ligaments are slightly lax, so there should be no pain or stress on the sides of the knee, except possibly at the extreme limits to rotation. Restriction to further rotation may come from the cruciate ligaments. Do you feel any burning or pain deep inside the knee? If not, you have reached a healthy position for rotation. If there is pain, observe that and back off to where you do not feel the pain. That is your healthy limit to rotation, but it may not be your maximum limit. Only you can tell where this healthy limit is.

This experiment, as mentioned, did not test your full range of motion because you were actively trying to rotate the tibia. There is usually a little more range of motion available when we are passive, as we find in a few yoga poses, such as Hero (Virasana) and Lotus (Padmasana). Figure 2.137 is the version of Hero Pose we saw earlier, where the feet are pointing straight out to the side. Most yoga teachers will not allow this for fear of stressing the knee. However, there are three ways this can be achieved: (1) by internally

rotating your femur by 90°, (2) by relying upon your knees to provide external rotation of the tibia or (3) by both. The safest and easiest way to have the feet pointing to the side in Hero Pose is to do a deep 90° internal rotation of the femur at the hip socket. If you have this range of motion in your hips, no twisting occurs in the knee. Notice the position of the tibia relative to the femur in figure 2.137: the femur is internally rotated a full 90°. Since no external rotation is happening at the tibia, there is no danger to the knee in this posture for this person.

Most people, however, have nowhere near 90° internal rotation available from the hip. The average person has about 33° (with a standard deviations of 7°). Now, add to this the average range of tibial external rotation of 35° and we get to around 68° rotation—still not the 90° we need. But recall that the average person has a tibial torsion that twists the proximal end of the tibia externally by another 30°. All together, even a person average in all three ranges of motion can rotate the foot out to the side by 98°, which should be enough rotation to have little or no stress in the knees. This means that for most people, pointing the feet out to the side in Hero Pose is neither problematic nor dangerous.

However, you are not average! If you have limited internal rotation of the hip, if your external range of tibial rotation is considerably below 35°, if you have less tibial torsion, if you have particularly short cruciate ligaments, if you have had a

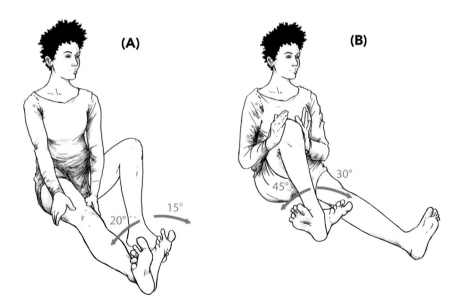

FIGURE 2.138 Determining your tibial rotation. (a) With one leg straight, and holding above the knee, rotate that ankle/foot inwardly and outwardly as far as it can go. Compare this to the range in (b) where, with the same leg now flexed, you rotate the ankle/foot as much as you can.

knee replaced, or if, due to any of many other variables, this posture feels painful for you, then don't point your feet out to the side. But if this pose is not available to you, please do not insist that no one else should ever do it.

Like every joint, our knees need stress to stay healthy. Twisting the knee while it is flexed can apply a healthy stress to the cruciate ligaments, cartilage and bones. Denying healthy levels of stress to these tissues will make them fragile. Putting too much stress on them also can destabilize them. Find out what is your appropriate Goldilocks' range of motion, where it is not too much but not too little either.

ROTATION AND VARUM (ADDUCTION) OF THE KNEE IN LOTUS POSE (PADMASANA)

Lotus Pose (Padmasana) is described in the Hatha Yoga Pradipika as the destroyer of all disease.[265] Ancient promises were often oversold. Lotus Pose is more often the destroyer of knees than of disease. The right foot should be drawn in first, then the left, and the soles of the feet supinated upwards.[266] For people who have a great deal of external rotation available in their hip socket, Lotus Pose is trivially easy. They were probably able to do the pose long before taking up a yoga practice. For most people, however, this pose is not and never will be available, and trying to make it available will damage the knees.

Lotus Pose requires around 100–110° of external rotation of the femur in the hip joint, or a combination of movement in the hip, knee and ankle/foot joints. To come into the posture, we first flex the right leg at the knee as much as

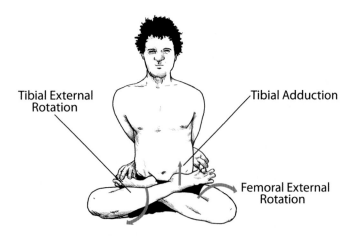

FIGURE 2.139 External rotations in Lotus Pose (Padmasana). Notice how the femur and tibia are both externally rotating and the ankle is forced upwards, created tibial adduction (varum) at the knee joint.

we can, then externally rotate the femur at the hip as much as possible, drawing the right foot onto the left thigh, and rotating the tibia so that the sole of the foot faces heaven—a natural direction for a sole to go. Then we do the same for the left leg. However, because the right foot is already in position, the left leg cannot flex as much (it is blocked a bit by the right leg) and must rotate even more to sit atop the right thigh; it has higher to go. Most people cannot flex the knee more than 150° without[267] training, and maybe 160–170° with training. Most people can externally rotate their femur 35–40°[268] before training. This is not sufficient for bringing the foot onto the opposite thigh; the missing ~70° of external rotation comes from the knee. Of course, when the knee is flexed and twisted, the collateral ligaments are lax and allow some sideways movement of the tibia (varum or adduction), but not 70°! So-called "hip openers" may increase the range of femoral external rotation in the hip socket that was restricted by muscular inhibitions, but ultimately, most people will be stopped well short of the magic amount by bone-on-bone compression in the hip socket.

The attempt to adduct and twist the tibia 70° will cause the medial femoral condyle to increasingly compress into the medial tibial condyle. Trapped between the two condyles is the medial meniscus. If a student persists in attempting to achieve a Lotus Pose at the expense of her knee, the medial meniscus will first complain, then tear. An early warning will come before the meniscus is torn: pain in the medial side (inside) of the knee. If the student experiences pain in the inner knees, she should cease the struggle immediately and back off. Other students may be graced with a warning pain in the outside of the knee; that is a signal from the lateral collateral ligament, which is complaining that the adduction being attempted is stressing it to the breaking point. Again, the attempt should be abandoned. Finally, when the student tries to turn the sole of the foot to heaven, the additional external rotation of the tibia required may be more than is available, and pain may arise in the cruciate ligaments. In all these cases, pain anywhere in the knee when attempting the Lotus Pose indicates that the knee either is not yet ready for the pose or never will be, due to insufficient external rotation in the hip and of the tibia at the knee.

Every student has to determine for herself whether the risk of the pose is worth the purported rewards. For students who have the bones to easily externally rotate the femur in the hip socket, there is probably little to no risk to their menisci. One study found that people who easily squatted or did Lotus all the time had no increase in their incidence of medial meniscal tears than the normal population.[269] However, another study showed that a lifetime of squatting and sitting in Lotus did increase the risk of osteoarthritis.[270] Again, everyone has to determine for themselves whether this posture is really worth the trouble.

The above warnings about Lotus Pose can be applied to any postures that require a great deal of external rotation of the femur in the hip socket, such as Pigeon Pose (Eka-padarajakapotasana) or Two-feet-behind-the-head Pose (Dwipadasirsana). If the femur cannot rotate, do not try to compensate by over-stressing the knee joint. Find a more moderate position where there is no pain. Stress in the knee is okay, but not to the point where there is pain while in the pose or after coming out of it.

LOCKING THE KNEE IN FULL EXTENSION (THE SCREW-HOME MECHANISM)

Rotation also occurs automatically as the knee approaches full extension. As the leg straightens, in the last 30° of knee extension, the tibia rotates about 10° externally (laterally) under the femur, which creates tension in the cruciate and collateral ligaments.[271] Alternatively, if the foot is fixed on the ground and the tibia cannot move, the femur will rotate internally (medially) over the tibia when the knee straightens. The rotation is caused by the different sizes of the condyles: the smaller lateral condyle has to roll further to match the larger medial condyle's motion, causing the tibia to rotate externally. The tautness of the ligaments gives the feeling that the knee has been locked into the final extension position. This is also known as the close-packed position of the knee, and it is important for minimizing the amount of effort and energy expended to keep the knees extended. This is often observable if we notice the orientation of the patella to the tibial tuberosity; just before we lock the knees, they line up almost vertically, but after locking, the patella will face slightly medially of the tibial tuberosity. To release the lock as flexion is initiated, the popliteus muscle pulls the femur into slight external rotation and/or the tibia into slight internal rotation, which then allows flexion to proceed.

Aligning the Knee with the Pelvis and Foot

So far, we have looked at the twisting torsion of the tibia, the Q-angle of the femur, and the fact that a flexed knee allows some degree of rotation of the tibia under the femur. We can now start to answer a question raised earlier: *What should be the alignment of the knee with respect to the pelvis when the knee is flexed, as found in standing poses like Warrior Two (Virabhadrasana II)?* We will see that the common cue of lining up the thigh to point straight ahead doesn't work well for everyone.

NOTE TO TEACHERS: Don't be afraid of locking the knees

Many yoga teachers suggest that students not lock the knees while in standing postures. They may disparagingly call this "hanging out in the joint." Their reason for suggesting that this is bad should be examined. The close-packed position of the knee is a natural place to be. It conserves energy and relies on the ligaments to stabilize the legs, which they were designed to do. If we never stress these ligaments, they will atrophy, becoming weaker and potentially causing instability in the knee. If we overstress these ligaments, they may also degenerate. Locking the knees is not bad per se—it is a natural position for most people to be in. But if a student already has knee issues and has been advised by her health-care consultants to avoid full extension of the knees and the close-packed position, it may be quite sensible to avoid locking the knees. Or perhaps the teacher wants the student to build strength in the quadriceps and thus suggests a slight micro-bend to the knees when in a standing posture. That may be a legitimate request, but why not give that direction to all students, even those who are not in hyperextension? Why shouldn't all students strengthen their quads, if that is the intention?

Figure 2.140 shows a few variations that are possible when we look at how the femur is oriented with respect to the knee and the foot in standing postures and lunges. In (a), we have the commonly sought alignment of the knee over the ankle, the foot pointing straight ahead and the femur perfectly in line with the foot. Some teachers suggest using a yardstick to guide the correct alignment, aligning the hip joint, knee and foot with the stick. The reason given for this cue is that it reduces stress on the knee by minimizing the twist of the cruciate ligaments. While some twist in the knee is fine when it is flexed, it is very important that there be no twist in the knee before we straighten the leg—for example, as we transition from Warrior (Virabhadrasana) to Triangle (Trikonasana). Unfortunately, the alignment shown in (a) does twist the cruciate ligaments for some people, and transitioning from this position to a straight-legged posture may overstress these ligaments.

Most teachers seeing someone with the thigh pointing inside the foot, as shown in figure 2.140b, will ask the student to point the knee over the foot or will perhaps give a more precise instruction: "Point your knee over your second toe." Some teachers ask for the knee to point over the little toe. In any case, they will not tolerate a knee pointing inwardly. If this alignment is accompanied by a pronated foot, aligning the knee with the foot may indeed be a wise thing to do, but as we have seen, if the foot is solid and neutral, adjusting the knee may end up supinating the foot, and this is not always a great alignment. Some students do need to keep their knee inside the line of the foot.

Figure 2.140c shows a different case. Here, the knee is above the ankle, but the line of the thigh points inside the foot. The thigh and the foot are not pointing in the same direction. Should they be? Remember that the Q-angle (see figure 2.111 again) is the angle between the pull of the quadriceps (basically, indicating the line of the femur) and a vertical line passing through the tibia. While clinicians no longer bother much with the Q-angle because it has very little relevance to knee pathology or problems, it is a reflection of anatomical structure. Some people have larger or smaller Q-angles. An average Q-angle is somewhere between 14° and 17°. For someone with a large Q-angle, the femur naturally is going to point inward of the foot in a lunge. This is

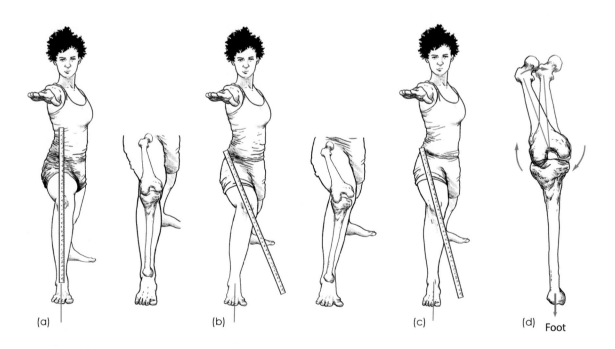

(a)　　　　(b)　　　　(c)　　　　(d) Foot

FIGURE 2.140 Alignment options of thigh to foot: (a) the standard requested alignment—thigh, knee, ankle and foot all pointing along the same line; (b) the thigh is not aligned with the foot, and the knee is inside the foot; (c) the knee is not aligned with the hip but is over the ankle; (d) shows the twisting in the knee joint that will occur when the hip in (c) is forced to align with the knee as shown in (a).

not a problem, but if a well-meaning teacher tries to fix the line of the thigh, she may end up creating the very twist in the knee that she was hoping to avoid.

Certainly, some students, especially beginners, may be adopting this posture due to tightness in the myofascia of the inner legs. Their adductors may be too tight to allow the degree of abduction at the hip sockets shown in figure 2.140a. In this case, trying to open the inner thighs by moving the knee outwards may be helpful. However, if the restriction to that movement is not tension but rather compression in the hip socket, then if the student has opened as much as she can, trying to come into the "proper" aesthetic alignment may not be in her best interest. Figure 2.140d shows what may happen. Moving the hip so that the thigh is in line with the knee and the foot means the femur has to externally (laterally) rotate over the tibia. This is equivalent to internally (medially) rotating the tibia. With this movement, the cruciate ligaments come into contact. Recall that most people can only internally rotate the tibia about 10° before the cruciates cross. The crossing of the cruciate ligaments is the natural barrier to deeper internal rotation.

Remember also that the tibia has torsion. For most people, the tibia rotates about 30° from top to bottom, causing the foot to point outward in its neutral position. The cue to point the foot straight ahead requires internal rotation of either the femur at the hip socket or the tibia at the knee. When the knee is bent, as it is in lunges and Warrior Poses, the internal rotation mostly comes from the knee. Aligning the foot straight ahead in a lunge, for most people, already twists the tibia internally, taking up whatever laxity the cruciate ligaments had to offer. Adding more twist in the knee by aligning the pelvis, knee and foot creates even more stress in the cruciate ligaments. Without meaning to, the teacher who encourages the student to keep the hip and the knee in line with the foot, and to keep the foot pointing straight ahead, may create a twist in the knee that will remain as the leg straightens when the student moves into Triangle Pose from Warrior Pose.

It is easy to see when the knee is not aligned with the foot, but that aesthetic observation alone should not be used to "correct" a student. A deeper inquiry is needed before trying to change whatever alignment the student is presenting. Is there pain? Is the foot pronating? Does the student have a history of arthritis or other knee pathologies? Does she have a large Q-angle, observable when she is standing? Is she varum or valgum? If so, is this due to muscular weakness or anatomical structure? Correcting someone without understanding why they are presenting a particular alignment may lead to more problems than the student currently has, if any. It is okay for many students to have their knees pointing inside the foot in Warrior Two.

Tracking of the Patella

Recall that the patella never comes in contact with the tibia and only slides up and down on the distal end of the femur. It glides through the patellar groove (also called the *intercondylar groove* or the *trochlea*). How far it moves is variable and depends upon the size of the groove, the length of the femur and the tension in the patellar tendon, but on average, the patella can move 5 cm from full flexion to full extension. Of course, everyone is different: for some people the patella can move up to 14 cm—almost 6 inches.[272]

Figure 2.141 shows the position of the patella at various stages of knee flexion and extension. In (a), we see that the patella is lifted upwards on the femur in hyperextension. (The common cue to avoid hyperextension by lifting the kneecaps actually serves to deepen the extension—the quadriceps, while lifting the kneecap, pull the tibia forward when engaged.) In (b), we see that in full extension, but not hyperextension, the patellar ligament is lax and the patella sits a bit lower than its highest point. Once we start flexing the knee, the quadriceps again engage to guard against too much flexion too quickly, and this action once more causes the patella to rise up slightly. By about 20° of flexion (c), the patella comes in to the top of the patellar groove and starts to make initial contact with the insides of the condyles. At this stage in its travels, the shape of the condyles does little to prevent the patella from sliding laterally, the direction in which it would tend to move due to the stress of the quadriceps, which are aligned laterally and superiorly to the knee. The primary restraint here preventing the patella from a lateral excursion is the stability of the medial patellofemoral ligament.[273] With greater flexion, the patella begins to track down the groove. At 90° of flexion (d), the superior portion of the patella is in contact with the groove. From here, the patella now starts to slide down deeply into the groove. At 135° of flexion (e), it is sitting well embedded, and the side facet (called the *odd facet*) is now touching the inner medial condyle.

If the patella is prevented from gliding up the femur (superiorly) to its normal limit, extension may be limited: if it cannot glide down the femur (inferiorly), flexion may be limited.[274] A common problem that arises with the patella is dislocation, where it slides out of the valley of the condyles. In figure 2.110, we saw the shape of the patella and the shape of the groove in which it slides. If the lateral side of the groove is too shallow or the shape of the patella too flat, the patella is more likely to be pulled laterally out of the groove by the quadriceps. It can also be pulled out of the groove to the medial side, but dislocation to the lateral side is much more common. As the knee straightens (extends), the Q-angle, which represents the line of pull by the quadriceps, increases.[275] As the knee flexes, because the patella is more distal from the pelvis, the Q-angle decreases, and the quadriceps exerts less of a lateral pull. It is quite unlikely that you will dislocate your kneecap when the knee is fully flexed. It is more likely to happen as the knee approaches full extension. This would imply that we have to take greater care to avoid dislocation of the patella when the knee is straight or approaching straight than when the knee is flexed 90° or more.

As mentioned earlier, there is no consensus that the Q-angle has a bearing on patellar problems. We do not really know whether the Q-angle is a factor or not. This confusion may be due to human variation. People with a low profile for the lateral condyle or a flatter patella may be far more likely to suffer knee problems if they also have a high Q-angle, whereas someone with a higher lateral condyle or more triangular patella may have no problem at all with a high Q-angle. In the absence of clear findings from the research community, what do we do? Apparently, it does not cause additional problems to ensure that the quadriceps' lateral pull is balanced with an offsetting pull from the medial muscles of the quads—the vastus medialis, or more specifically the lowest portion, called the vastus medialis obliquus (VMO). Our challenge is, how can we specifically strengthen the VMO? Many researchers do not believe it is possible to isolate just those muscle fibers.[276] Instead, we need to strengthen the whole quadriceps group of muscles, but that may also make the vastus lateralis stronger, which may have caused the problem in the first place. Indeed, several researchers have proposed that too much quad strength can cause or worsen osteoarthritis in the knees.[277] Perhaps the safest approach is to utilize co-contraction of all the thigh muscles, specifically the hamstrings and the quads, to stabilize the patella and ensure it tracks smoothly.

If you or your students have kneecap tracking issues, it is a good idea to employ co-contraction of the quadriceps and the hamstrings. Even if you have no kneecap problems, it is not a bad idea to keep stabilizing co-contraction around the knees, especially in standing postures where the knees are flexed less than 90°. Remember, stiffness is stabilizing.

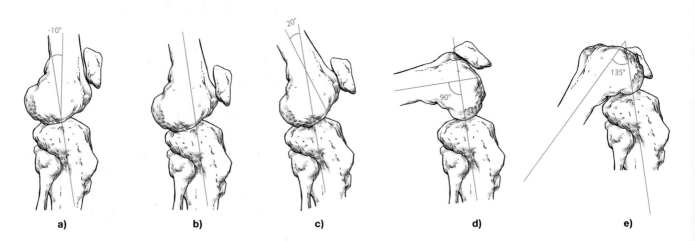

a)   b)   c)   d)   e)

FIGURE 2.141 Tracking of the patella. (a) In hyperextension of −10°, the patella is pulled up high on the distal femur. (b) In full extension, it sits slightly above the femoral condyles but not as high as in hyperextension. (c) With 20° of flexion, the patella is now contacting the femoral condyles. (d) At 90° of flexion, the superior portion of the patella is in contact with the condylar groove. (e) At 135° of flexion, the patella is sitting well embedded in the groove.

Knee-Joint Summary

We can employ the WSM? spectrum to summarize which tissues can be counted on, or employed, to stabilize the knee in all its possible directions of movement. Table 2.12 answers WSM? question as it pertains to the knee.

Warning: This table does not indicate *why* the tension may have arisen. As we saw in Volume 1, tension is caused by many things, not always short muscles. Other causes include emotions, nervous system interactions, hydration and pathologies. Scar tissue, arthritis or inflammation can cause or increase tension. The limitations suggested in the table are not static facts but indicators of possibilities. The table is for general guidance, not for specific evaluation. Everyone has to answer for themselves, "What is stopping me?"

TABLE 2.12 WSM? spectrum for the knee joint

MOVEMENT OF THE KNEE	TENSILE RESISTANCE				COMPRESSION
	MYOFASCIAL MERIDIANS*	MUSCLES	LIGAMENTS	JOINT CAPSULE	SOURCE
flexion	• superficial front line	• quadriceps	• patellar ligament • patellar retinaculum • posterior cruciate ligament	anterior	• back of thighs against calves • buttocks against heels
extension	• superficial back line • deep front line	• hamstrings • gastrocnemius • popliteus	• anterior cruciate ligament • oblique popliteal ligament • arcuate popliteal ligament	posterior	
valgus**	• deep front line • lateral lines	• semimembranosus • semitendinosus • sartorius • gracilis • medial gastrocnemius	• medial collateral ligament (primarily) • cruciate ligaments • medial patellar retinaculum (when in full extension)[278]	medial	
varus**	• deep front line • lateral lines	• biceps femoris • popliteus • lateral gastrocnemius	• lateral collateral ligament (primarily) • cruciate ligaments • lateral patellar retinaculum (when in full extension) • iliotibial band	lateral	
medial rotation of the tibia***		• biceps femoris[279] • in full extension, all the muscles crossing the back of the knee[280]	• cruciate ligaments		
lateral rotation of the tibia***		• semimembranosus[281] • semitendinosus[282] • popliteus • in full extension, all the muscles crossing the back of the knee[283]	• arcuate popliteal ligament • lateral collateral ligament		

* See Volume 1, especially pages 71–74, for a description of the myofascial meridians.
** Flexion, valgus and varus are also resisted in part by the pressure of the femoral condyles against the tibial plateau.[284]
*** The tibial eminence can make a small contribution to limiting rotation.[285]

CHAPTER 4
The Joint Segments of the Lower Body:
The Ankle–Foot Segment

We have journeyed down from the pelvis and through the knee, and now we reach the most distal joint segment: the ankle and foot, which we are calling the ankle–foot segment. As we saw with the knee, the lower we go, the more important stability becomes. The whole weight of our body is supported on two small pylons called our ankles, and our ability to walk is governed by the stability our feet provide. But this does not mean that mobility is unimportant; our ankles and feet are designed to absorb energy and redirect it while we walk, making walking an energy-efficient process. It is the ability of the foot to move in response to the changing stresses of standing, balancing, walking or running over varied terrain that allows us to be bipeds. This combination of mobility and stability is important in our yoga practice as well.

The usual terminology in discussions about the feet and ankle is strange and often confusing. Unfortunately, anatomists have not helped this situation, for they often disagree on the meaning of certain terms and apply the same terms in varying ways. We will try to be consistent in our usage and, where practical, will choose the simpler terms.

Our first simplification will be in describing the movements of the ankle and foot. The ankle moves in two directions, like a hinge—it dorsiflexes (the top of the foot comes closer to the shin bone) and plantarflexes (the bottom of the foot moves away from the shin). The foot is much more complicated, but we will still restrict our evaluations to two main movements: supination and pronation. In supination, the sole moves closer to the inner (medial) ankle, and in pronation, it moves away from the inner ankle and closer to the outer (lateral) ankle. Even with our simplifications, understanding the effect of moving our feet is not easy, because we can choose to move the foot when it is not bearing any weight (this is referred to as an "open chain"), or we can fix the foot on the floor and move our leg while the foot is bearing weight, such as when we are standing (this is called a "closed chain"). In other words, we can move the foot or we can move the leg, and what appears to be supination in one situation may appear to be something different in the other. With some patience, however, all will become clear.

Sometimes, the foot will be referred to in segments: the hindfoot refers to the heel and ankle (the talus and calcaneus); the forefoot refers to the front of the foot, consisting of the metatarsals and phalanges; the midfoot is what's left—the other tarsal bones in front of the heel and ankle.

Form

There are 31–33 joints in the foot and ankle (depending upon the person and how you define the joints).[286] That allows for a lot of different movements. Although the foot is a very complicated structure, for our purposes we need to understand just four movements: dorsiflexion and plantarflexion of the ankle (see figure 2.200) and supination and pronation of the foot (see figures 2.201 and 2.202). These are the four movements yogis need to understand to answer our WSM? question when it comes to the foot.

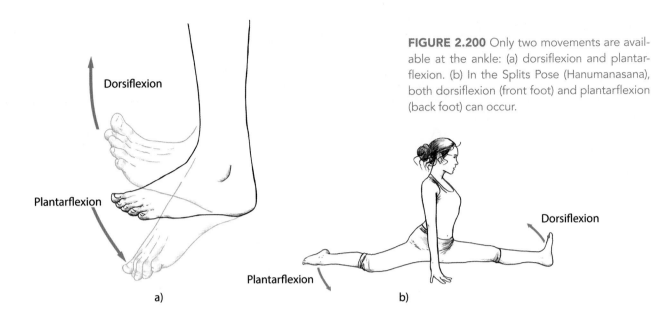

FIGURE 2.200 Only two movements are available at the ankle: (a) dorsiflexion and plantarflexion. (b) In the Splits Pose (Hanumanasana), both dorsiflexion (front foot) and plantarflexion (back foot) can occur.

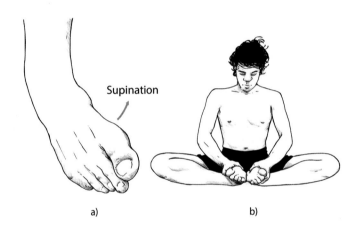

FIGURE 2.201 Supination opens the sole of the foot towards the midline of the body in (a). This can be done passively to the feet, as shown in (b) Butterfly Pose (Baddhakonasana).

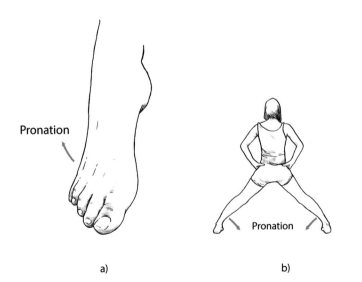

FIGURE 2.202 Pronation opens the sole of the foot away from the midline of the body (a). This often occurs in standing postures when the feet are far apart, as in (b), Prasaritapadottanasana. In this case, the foot doesn't move but the leg does, creating pronation at the ankle.

THE ARCHITECTURE OF THE ANKLE–FOOT SEGMENT

We are calling the ankle and foot a joint segment because it involves many joints. An average person has 28 bones in the foot, and these articulate with each other in complicated ways. Some of them do not touch; these are the floating sesamoid bones under the balls of our feet, which provide stiffness to the fascia in these locations. One bone (the *talus*) has no connecting muscles or tendons and moves only by the stress of its neighboring bones. To get a clear picture of what is happening when we move our feet, and appreciate the limits to movement, we need to look at the structure of the bones and ligaments, then add the effect of the muscular attachments and tendons. As always, we will look at the extent of human variation in the size and shape of our bones and see how this may affect some people's available range of movement.

Landmarks

THE ANKLE JOINT

Technically called the *talocrural* joint (*crural* means "leg," and the *talus* is the bone the leg rides upon), the ankle is the joining of three bones: the fibula, tibia and talus. As shown in Figure 2.203, the fibula and tibia form a "mortise," an "n" shape. The talus fits inside the mortise like a "tenon." For thousands of years, woodworkers have used mortises and tenons to fit one piece of wood into another with simplicity and great stability.

Figure 2.204 shows a mortise and tenon structure. You can see how similar our ankle is to this arrangement. Unlike a carpenter's joint, however, the arrangement of the tibia, fibula and talus allows the talus to move; like a hinge, it can flex and extend (called dorsiflexion and plantarflexion), but that is all. The medial (inner) and proximal (top) part of the mortise of the ankle joint is formed by the tibia. The lateral (outer) part of the mortise is the fibula. The sides of the mortise prevent the talus from abducting, adducting or twisting. Notice, though, how one side of the mortise is longer than the other: the fibula extends lower than the tibia, providing greater resistance to lateral movement of the foot at the ankle. Of course, the ankle joint is not made of wood and glue, so there is some wiggle room, but not very much. (We say that the only movements here are plantarflexion and dorsiflexion, but that is a very convenient approximation of reality; there is some wiggle room, and if the ankle is damaged, there unfortunately may be more room.) The stability of the joint is enhanced by a series of ligaments, which also bind the bones together.

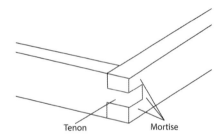

FIGURE 2.204 Mortises and tenons have been used by carpenters for millennia to form a stable joint.

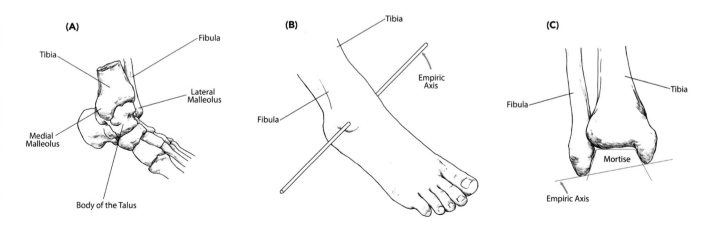

FIGURE 2.203 (a) The ankle is the joining of the fibula, tibia and talus. (b) The empirical axis runs from the distal fibula (lateral malleolus) to the distal tibia (medial malleolus). (c) The top and inner side of the tibia, along with the inner side of the fibula, form a mortise.

At the distal end of the tibia is your inner ankle prominence, a bulge or bump called the medial *malleolus* (Latin for "hammer"). The outer bulge, your lateral malleolus, is the distal end of the fibula. Notice in figure 2.203 how the lateral malleolus is a bit lower and more backwards than the medial, inner ankle. The average amount of backward rotation from tibia to fibula is 20–30°, while the downward inclination is about 10°.[287] (This is also shown in figures 2.307 and 2.223.) This alignment means that a line through the ankle, from lateral to medial malleolus, is not in just one of the three key planes of the body. In turn, this means that dorsiflexion and plantarflexion of the ankle are not simple planar movements in the sagittal (side) plane. Another reason this is so is tibial torsion, which we discussed in Chapter 3.

To be complete, we must also consider the joining of the tibia and fibula separately from their relationship with the talus. The fibula joins with the tibia at the top, at their proximal ends, just below the knee; they then join together again at the distal ends, just above the talus. This lower joining is a *syndesmosis* joint, which means the two bones are held together by connective tissue. There is no joint capsule here; the joint is held together only by the syndesmosis ligaments. Damage to this joint is often referred to as a "high ankle sprain," which means the sprain is above the joining of the talus to the mortise of the fibula and tibia. High ankle sprains are relatively uncommon, occurring in about 15% of ankle injuries.[288] This injury usually only occurs during a sporting accident where the foot is dorsiflexed and then receives a sudden externally rotating force—highly unlikely to happen during a yoga class.

At the proximal ends, just below the knee, the fibula and tibia join within a synovial joint. There is some slight movement available here. When we dorsiflex the ankle or pronate the foot, the fibula slides forward (anteriorly) and upward (superiorly) against the tibia. When we plantarflex the ankle or supinate the foot, the opposite happens: the fibula slides backwards (posteriorly) and downwards (inferiorly).[289] Sometimes, the proximal end of the fibula can get stuck against the tibia or jammed against the tibia's lateral condyle by too much upward traction from the bicep femoris or too much pronation of the foot and dorsiflexion of the ankle.[290]

Along the middle lengths of the tibia and fibula is the interosseous membrane (shown in figure 2.100), which vertically joins the two bones, stabilizing them and separating the muscles on the front of the leg from those on the back.

THE FOOT

Figure 2.205 shows the 26 bones of the foot, skipping the sesamoids. As shown, the talus (also called the "anklebone") is considered part of both the ankle and the foot, reflecting its important position between them. (*Talus* is Latin for "ankle" or "slope.") The full weight of the body rests on the talus bones of each foot. Directly below the talus is the heel bone, called the *calcaneus* (Latin for "heel"), the largest bone in the foot. The talus and calcaneus are two of the foot's seven *tarsal* bones. In front of the talus and calcaneus are the *navicular* (so named because to some eyes it looks like the hull of a navy ship), the *cuboid* (which to other eyes looks like a cube) and three *cuneiform*, or wedged-shaped, bones. In front of

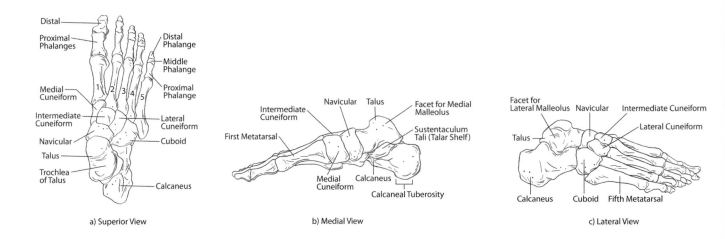

FIGURE 2.205 The bones of the foot. (a) superior view; (b) medial view; (c) lateral view.

the tarsal bones are the five metatarsals; *meta* means beyond, hence, these extend beyond the tarsals. Even more distal than the metatarsals are the rows of *phalanges* (from the Greek *phalanx*, meaning "log"), starting with the proximal phalanges, the intermediate ones, and finally the most distal ones—the tips of your toes. Notice that your big toe, extending off proximal phalanx #1, does not have a middle phalanx; your big toe has only two bones, whereas all the other toes have three. The lines of metatarsals and phalanges form *rays* radiating out from the tarsals. Each ray is numbered, with the first ray including the big toe and the fifth leading to the little toe.

Twenty-six bones sounds like a lot to remember, but it is actually quite easy, as you only have to remember seven bones and two other names—the rest is a matter of numbers. The ankle bone (talus) and heel bone (calcaneus) are pretty easy to remember. The other five are the navicular (navy bone) on the big-toe side (medial), the cuboid (cube-shaped bone) on the little-toe side (lateral), and the three cuneiform (wedge bones): lateral, intermediate and medial. Then remember the "beyond the tarsals"—the metatarsals: #1 is on the big-toe side, and #5 is on the little-toe side. Finally come the three rows of phalanges: proximal (closest), middle and distal (furthest). The only trick is to remember that the big toe has no middle phalange and all the rays follow the numbering schema from 1 to 5.

THE THREE ARCHES

Our feet are springs! That's one of the features helping us to run and jump, but even walking requires these springs. They reduce the amount of energy we need to expend. Springs are simple concepts, and so are arches, but our feet are far from simple. The way the arches become loaded, converting the kinetic energy of walking into potential energy and releasing this stored energy back into movement, is complex. The bones of the feet form three main arches (see figure 2.206): two longitudinal ones (the higher one medially and the lower one laterally) and a transverse arch running from the outside of the foot to the inside.

The medial longitudinal arch, formed by the calcaneus, talus, navicular, medial cuneiform and first metatarsal, is very important for propulsion. The lateral longitudinal arch, which is much lower than the medial, is formed by the calcaneus, cuboid and fifth metatarsal and is very important for weight bearing; it is hidden by the muscles of the sole and is therefore a bit mysterious. Unlike the medial, this arch contacts the ground. The transverse arch is formed by the three cuneiform bones and the cuboid but continues to be seen in the metatarsals and, to a lesser degree, the phalanges.

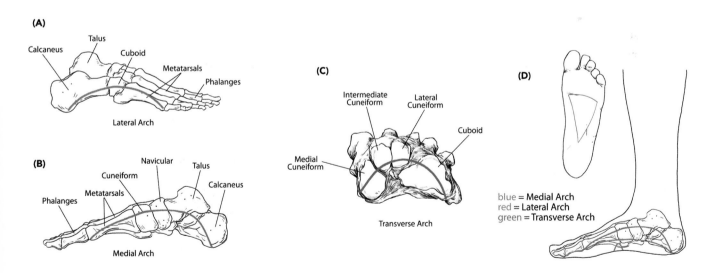

FIGURE 2.206 The arches of the foot: (a) lateral, (b) medial, (c) transverse (posterior view, looking forward from the ankle) and (d) all three.

Together these three arches form a curved triangle (see figure 2.206d), with one vertex at the heel, a second at the distal, medial metatarsal (#1) and a third at the distal lateral metatarsal (#5). Often, in standing yoga postures, the teacher will encourage the student to feel three points of contact between the foot and the earth and become grounded at each point. The teacher is referring to these three vertices. When we stand, the weight of our body is distributed among these three points, but the heel receives most of the weight, which is why it is thicker and more padded than the other vertices.

While the bones form the arches, they are like the wood of a bow: the bow string gives the bow its springiness, and the ligaments keep the arches springy. If the ligaments become lax or the bones lose their alignment, the arch collapses; this is termed a fallen arch, or *pes planus* (Latin for "flat foot"). There are two distinct kinds of pes planus: a flexible version, where the foot remains flexible even though the arch has fallen, and an inflexible version, where the bones of the hindfoot have fused or were never separated in the first place. The person with a flexible flat foot may be fully functional and need no intervention, whereas someone with a rigid flat foot may require surgical intervention to recover full utility of the foot. Popular estimates show that 20% of the population has fallen arches[291]! Children often have flat feet, but they grow out of this condition in time.

In the other direction, some people have very high arches, a condition called *pes cavus* (Latin for "hollow foot") or claw foot. One study estimates that 10% of people have pes cavus,[292] but another claims it occurs in 20% to 25% of the adult population.[293] The cause of this condition is most often neuromuscular; for example, a disease called Charcot Marie Tooth causes muscle weakness, creating pronounced persistent flexion of the first metatarsal and phalangeal ray that leads to a permanently raised arch.[294]

NOTE TO TEACHERS: Getting grounded

In our standing postures, we are often advised to broaden the base of our feet and get grounded. There is a technique that can help with this. When we pronate the foot while it is bearing weight, the bones of the forefoot are loosened a bit, which allows us to spread our toes, creating a wide base of support. This wider base is great but may also now be too flexible—it is not stiff or solid. If we next supinate the foot, the bones of the forefoot come closer together and wedge themselves into a very stiff structure. Now we are solid. (To understand why, see Appendix F: The Movements of the Foot and Ankle.) We can combine pronation with spreading the toes, and then supination, which stiffens the forefoot. This creates a broad, grounded base. You can experiment with this yourself and then share this with your students. Come into a standing position with your feet slightly apart. Now, roll the ankle of one foot slightly inwards towards the floor so that you can lift the lateral (outer) edge of your foot off the floor (that is pronation), and notice how easy it is to spread your toes. Do that: spread your toes. Now, keep the spread, firmly plant the outer edge of your foot back on the floor, and move your inner ankle away from the floor (supinate). Notice how your foot stiffens. You are solid, grounded, but with a nice wide base. Next, do it with the other foot. You can practice this every time you are in a standing pose.

This is a natural process that we do every time we walk. When our foot first comes into contact with the ground, the ankle plantarflexes and the foot pronates; the bones in the midtarsal region separate slightly, and the forefoot becomes flexible. This pronation creates a flexible structure and spreads out our base as wide as possible by spreading the toes. Pronation also allows us to accommodate varied terrain beneath our feet. Plus, the greater the area of contact the foot has with the ground, the more rebound we can create. When we push off with that foot, the ankle again plantarflexes, and we now supinate the foot, creating a stiffer structure; the midtarsal bones press into each other, which allows a more elastic recoil to propel us forward.[296] This is a very efficient process, which again involves pronation to broaden our base, then supination to become stable—what we try to emulate in standing yoga postures.

Many factors affect arch function: the foot's overall shape, the shape of the individual bones, the stability of the ligaments, muscle fatigue, ethnic background, gender, age and type of footwear.[295] So, who shall we say is normal? If 20% of the population has fallen arches and 20–25% have overly high arches, that does not leave many people who are in the supposedly "right" range. There is also little correlation between left and right feet; sometimes, people have fallen or raised arches in just one foot. Clearly, whether your arches have fallen or are very high, the range of motion in your ankles and feet will be quite different from other people's.

THE BONES OF THE ANKLE AND FOOT

Who has normal feet? You do, of course. Your feet look the way feet are supposed to look. But everybody else has strange feet—they just don't look right, do they? Their shoe size is likely different from yours; they have toes that are too long or too stubby, arches that are too high or low, heels that seem wrong. This known variability in everyone's feet is for some reason often ignored in yoga classrooms. Shape determines function, and if everyone is different, what they can or can't

do will also be different. The shape of our feet is due to the shape and size of the 28 foot bones and their ligaments, and it is no surprise that these bones vary greatly from person to person.

The Talus

The talus—our ankle bone—connects the foot to the leg. Above, it fits into the mortise formed by the tibia and fibula. Below, it rests upon the heel bone (calcaneus). To the front, it articulates with the navicular bone. This means that the talus has a lot of articulating surfaces and a lot of cartilage; indeed, no other bone in our body has as much articular cartilage in relation to its total size. All this bone-on-bone contact leaves no room for any muscles or tendons to attach to the talus, so it moves only due to the pressure and movement of its neighboring bones and their ligaments. This lack of muscular attachment affects the blood supply to the talus, which is tenuous at best.[297]

Figure 2.207 shows several views of the talus. Like a little, yellow, rubber duck, it has three main parts: the body, the head and the neck, which joins the body to the head. The body is the superior surface of the talus, connecting with the mortise of the leg formed by the tibia and fibula. The head is the anterior portion, connecting the talus to the navicular bone. The neck is relatively thin.

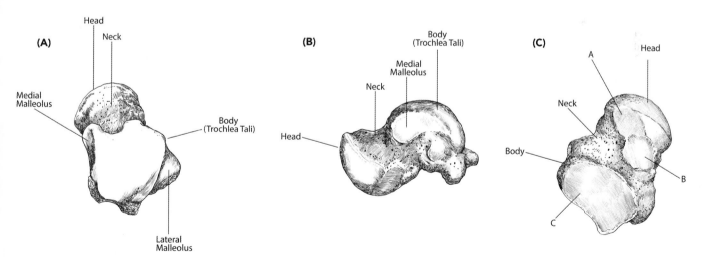

FIGURE 2.207 Three views of a right talus: (a) superior, (b) medial and (c) inferior, showing three facets for articulation with the calcaneus (A, B, C).

The top of the talus, an area called its *trochlea*, articulates with the mortise of the tibia and fibula.[298] The trochlea is rounded in several directions to allow easy movement, and its particular shape contributes greatly to the ankle's stability.[299] From front to back the trochlea is convex, but from side to side it is slightly concave. On the sides of the trochlea are smooth surfaces for articulating with the distal ends of the tibia and fibula.

The Calcaneus

The inferior (underside) of the talus articulates with the heel bone. This is called the *talocalcaneal* joint and is where the ankle bone meets the heel bone. Often it is referred to as the *subtalar* joint because it is "below" the talus. This is the term we will use. The calcaneus is the largest bone in the foot. It is angled posteriorly (backward) and inferiorly (downward) from the ankle and acts like a short lever for the various tendons that pass around it or attach to it, like the *Achilles* tendon, sometimes called the *calcaneal* tendon (see figure 2.208). The plantar (bottom) surface of the calcaneus is the site of attachment for many of the foot's intrinsic muscles and the plantar fascia. The extreme posterior, inferior part of the calcaneus has a tuberosity (bump) that contacts the ground. There is a lot of softer, cushiony material under this tuberosity, and these fibers become part of the plantar fascia, which continues forward and divides into five slips of fascia that attach to the toes. At the distal end (the front) of the calcaneus is a smooth surface that articulates with the cuboid bone.

The Navicular, Cuboid and Cuneiform Bones

Distal to the talus and calcaneus are the remaining five tarsal bones, also called the *anterior tarsals*. The hull-shaped navicular joins with the head of the talus, forming the *talonavicular* joint, while the cuboid joins with the calcaneus, creating the *calcaneocuboid* joint. When the foot is planted on the ground, in the closed-chain position, and when the talus tries to pronate, it drops down and medially, but the navicular moves upward and laterally, effectively flattening the arch. This movement makes the foot more flexible and pliable, better able to conform to a varied ground terrain. It is easier to spread your toes when the talus pronates. When the talus tries to supinate, the opposite happens: the navicular moves downward and medially, increasing the arch.[300] Supination of the talus stiffens the forefoot, making it more stable, which helps the foot spring off the ground as we walk. It is very difficult to spread your toes when the foot is supinating.

The cuboid has six surfaces (like a cube) and several interfaces: proximally it joins with the calcaneus and helps to form the foot's lateral longitudinal arch; distally it joins with the fourth and fifth metatarsals (you can palpate this latter joint on the lateral side of your foot—it is the major bump you will feel about halfway between the heel and the ball of the little toe); and medially it articulates with both the navicular and the lateral cuneiform.

The three cuneiforms articulate with the navicular proximally and with the first three metatarsals distally. The cuneiform and cuboid form the transverse arch of the foot (see figure 2.206c). All are gliding joints and do not have

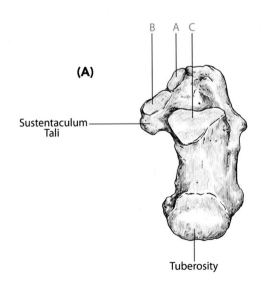

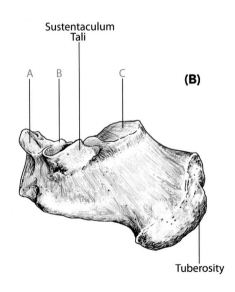

FIGURE 2.208 The calcaneus: (a) superior view and (b) medial view of a right heel bone.

extreme ranges of motion. They are restricted primarily by their close proximity to each other and by stabilizing ligaments.

Most of the movement in the foot occurs around the bones we have already mentioned: the tarsals. Usually, the tarsals move as one structure around the talus. There are two functional parts of the subtalar joint: the talocalcaneal articulation and the talocalcaneonavicular movement.[301] More distally in the foot, movement is limited, but there is some.[302]

The Other Bones: Metatarsals and Phalanges

At the ends of the cuneiforms and cuboid sprout the five metatarsals. These miniature long bones (similar to the tibia and femur but much shorter) are triangular in cross-section and taper distally. Proximally their base is cube-shaped, but distally their ends are spherical. The first metatarsal, which leads to the big toe, is the shortest but thickest of the five. The second is usually the longest and the stiffest in its connection to the tarsals. The first and second metatarsals are the strongest because the medial side of the foot resists the greatest forces when the foot pushes off in walking or running. Each metatarsal has a slight longitudinal curve on the plantar side, which helps with the foot's ability to bear loads. Not only do the metatarsals articulate with the distal ends of the tarsals and the proximal ends of the phalanges, but they also articulate slightly with each other. However, some people are lacking the facet on the first metatarsal that would allow some articulation with the second.[303]

Distal to the metatarsals are 14 little logs: the *phalanges*. Also numbered from 1 to 5, from medial to lateral, the phalanges have three rows, except for the big toe. The big toe is also called the *hallux*; it has only two phalanges, but they are big. Unlike its counterpart in the hand (the thumb), the big toe is not so mobile, nor is it opposable to the other toes. Unlike the fingers, the toes are designed to extend (dorsiflex) considerably but flex (plantarflex) minimally; this is an important design requirement for a walking biped.

When we look at the foot as whole, we find on the lateral (outer) side that the calcaneus, cuboid, fourth and fifth metatarsals, and fourth and fifth phalanges form the lateral arch. The medial (inner) side of the foot has the calcaneus, talus, navicular, cuneiform and first to third metatarsals and phalanges, which form the medial arch (see figure 2.206).

IT'S COMPLICATED: The trochlea of the talus

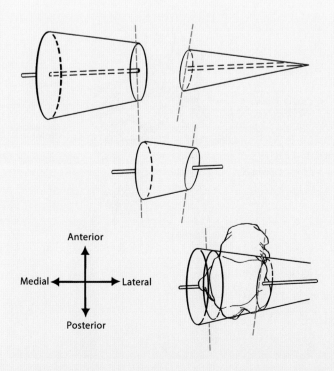

Anterior

Medial ◄──────► Lateral

Posterior

We could look at the trochlea of the talus as rounded, much like the surface of a cylinder, but the medial edge of the trochlea is bigger than its lateral edge, which means that the surface of the trochlea is actually more like a cone, as shown in figure 2.209.[304] The cone shape of the trochlea means that as the talus rotates under the leg, the medial (larger) edge will move further and faster than the outer (lateral) edge. This differential can cause some medial or lateral movement to the foot as the ankle flexes, or some internal or external rotation of the leg if the foot is fixed.

FIGURE 2.209 The surface of the trochlea tali is cone-shaped. The lateral edge is smaller than the medial edge, so the later edge of the cone is smaller and more oval due to the obliqueness of the fibular facet.

THE LIGAMENTS

While most of the joints in the foot are gliding joints, they are still surrounded by joint capsules. However, these fibrous joint capsules are thin and reinforced by ligaments. Often, the synovia of one joint is continuous with that of a neighboring joint. The ankle (talocrural joint) has both medial and lateral collateral ligaments, providing stability to the joint and preventing too much movement. The medial ligament of the ankle is called the *deltoid collateral* or sometimes simply the *deltoid* ligament, and it fans out in a triangular (delta) shape with fibers running from the medial (inner) malleolus anteriorly to the navicular and talus, inferiorly to the calcaneus, and posteriorly to the back of the talus. These ligaments, as shown in figure 2.210, are respectively called the anterior tibiotalar ligament, the tibionavicular ligament, the tibiocalcaneal ligament and the posterior tibiotalar ligament. Together these ligaments provide medial stability to the ankle. Chronic instability in these medial ligaments is rare.[305] Due to the length of the fibula on the lateral side of the ankle, extreme pronation of the foot causes bone-on-bone opposition; the distal end of the fibula contacts the lateral talus, and this provides medial stability.

On the outer (lateral) ankle we find three lateral ligaments, which radiate out from the fibula's malleolus. The calcaneofibular ligament, as shown in figure 2.211, runs almost vertically downward from the distal end of the fibula to the lateral side of the calcaneus. The posterior talofibular ligament runs from the posterior distal end of the fibula to the posterior side of the talus, and the anterior talofibular ligament runs from the anterior distal fibula to the talus. In addition, there are two ligaments that bind the mortise: the posterior tibiofibular ligament reinforces the back side of the mortise, and the anterior tibiofibular ligament reinforces the front side. The lateral ligaments play an important role in preventing too much supination or inversion of the foot and are the ones most likely to be sprained when we "roll our ankle." (The posterior talofibular ligament is usually spared when this happens.)[306] Unlike the medial ligaments, the lateral ligaments are more easily injured because supination is not prevented by the distal tibia in the same way that too much pronation is resisted by the longer, lower distal fibula.

The talus and calcaneus are also strongly bound together by their ligaments (as shown in figure 2.210), specifically the medial and posterior talocalcaneal ligaments and (as shown in figure 2.211) the lateral talocalcaneal and interosseous talocalcaneal ligaments. Figure 2.212 shows several of the ligaments already mentioned, from a posterior view. Figure 2.213 shows a plantar view, wherein we can see ligaments binding the calcaneus to the cuboid and the navicular—the plantar calcanealcuboid ligament and

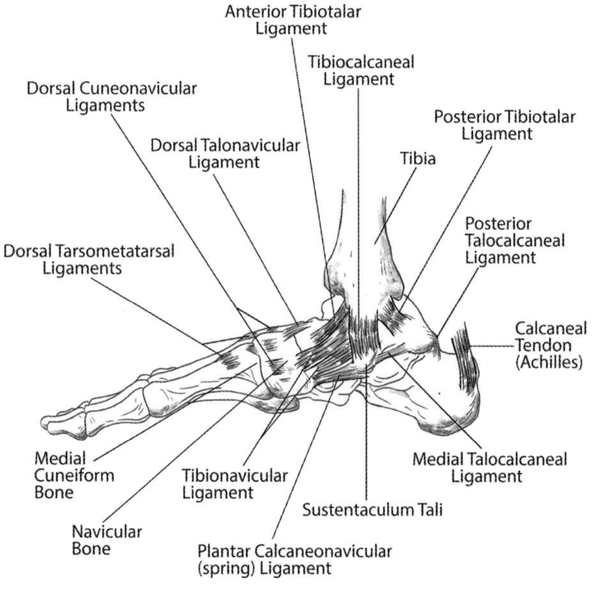

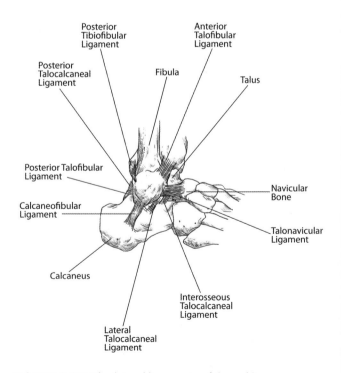

FIGURE 2.210 The medial ligaments of the ankle and hindfoot (right foot).

FIGURE 2.211 The lateral ligaments of the ankle.

plantar calcaneonavicular ligament (also called the spring ligament)—and the plantar cuboideonavicular ligament, binding the navicular bone to the cuboid. Stability between the talus and calcaneus is mostly due to the conformation of the bony surfaces, although these ligamentous connections also play an important role. However, which ligaments play the most important role is still a mystery.[307] We also see in figure 2.213 the long plantar ligament, which runs from the heel to the metatarsals. The spring ligament (plantar calcaneonavicular) has a very important role in stabilizing the medial arch of the foot, as it is a very thick, broad band of fibers upon which the head of the talus "rests." Not shown are the myriad of other ligaments joining the anterior tarsals, metatarsals and phalanges. While the stability of the tarsal joints is mostly due to the tight interfaces between the bones and the tough, fibrous ligaments, the tarsometatarsal and phalangeal joints are stabilized mostly by their ligaments.

The Retinacula of the Foot

Surrounding all these ligaments around the ankle and the top (instep) of the foot are various retinacula. The purpose of a retinaculum is to help keep tendons in their proper alignment and to act as pulleys, changing the direction of the applied forces. These structures don't actually exist as separate entities; they are carved and created by anatomists out of the ubiquitous fascia.[308] In some places, this fascia becomes thicker, forming strong bands that serve the function attributed to the retinacula, but these are not separate slips of fascia—they are part of the whole. The foot's several retinacula guide specific tendons to their homes and form the pulleys needed to redirect the force created by the distant muscles.

The retinacula of the foot prevent the peroneal tendons (the flexor and extensor tendons) from "bowstringing"— that is, from straightening and losing their effectiveness (bowstrings are straight, but these tendons stay curved). The peroneal and extensor retinacula have superior and inferior aspects, as shown in figure 2.214. The superior peroneal retinaculum, which is a continuation of the deep transverse fascia of the leg, runs from the posterior (back) of the lateral (outer) malleolus down to the calcaneus; the inferior peroneal retinaculum is distal to this and is continuous with the flexor retinaculum. The flexor retinaculum runs from the anterior (front) of the medial (inner) malleolus down the inside of the ankle and connects with the dorsum (top) of the foot and the plantar (bottom) aponeurosis. There is again

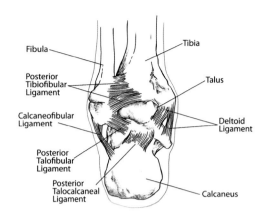

FIGURE 2.212 Posterior view of the ankle's ligaments.

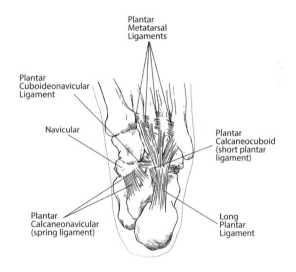

FIGURE 2.213 Plantar view of the calcaneal ligaments.

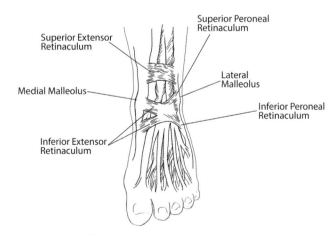

FIGURE 2.214 The retinacula of the foot.

no clear delineation between where the lower leg's deep fascia ends and the flexor retinaculum begins.[309] There are two extensor retinacula. The superior extensor retinaculum is a band that runs from the front of the fibula to the front of the tibia; its proximal border is continuous with the leg's crural fascia. The inferior extensor retinacula is Y-shaped. One upper end of the Y begins just distal to the lateral (outer) malleolus, then runs across the top of the foot to the medial (inner) malleolus; the other upper end runs to the navicular.

Each retinaculum constrains a group of tendons to their proper positions, as indicated in table 2.13.

Fascia of the Foot

An *aponeurosis* (from the Greek for "becoming a tendon") is a broad, flat sheet of fibrous collagen. We find them in various locations around the body. The most famous one in the foot is called the *plantar fascia*. This is a thick band of fascia stretching from the tuberosity of the heel to the balls of the foot (the metatarsal heads). It has three main strips: lateral and medial, and a wider, tougher, central band (see figure 2.215). This central band is often referred to as the plantar fascia proper, and it plays the most important structural and functional role. All three bands get thinner as they flow forward. At the midtarsal area, the central fascia divides into five individual bands that fan out to the heads of the metatarsals, under the balls of the foot.

Due to its position on the foot's lateral and medial sides, the plantar fascia contributes to the stability and height of the longitudinal arches, and to resisting movement; it helps to bind the bones together, like a bowstring binds the ends of a bow. (It is not alone in this function, as the long plantar ligament and the spring ligament also contribute.) One study found that without our plantar fascia, our arches would be 25% weaker.[310] However, despite the contributions of the fascia, tendons and ligaments to maintaining the arches, the bones' shape and structure are responsible for 65% of the arches' rigidity.[311] As with the curved stones of an ancient Roman arch, the geometry of the bones and their compression against each other are the primary factors.

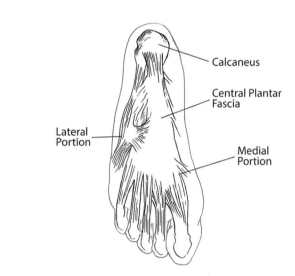

FIGURE 2.215 The plantar fascia.

TABLE 2.13 The retinacula of the feet and the long tendons they guide in the lower leg.

EXTENSOR RETINACULA	PERONEAL RETINACULA	FLEXOR RETINACULUM
Tibialis anterior	Peroneus longus	Tibialis posterior
Extensor hallucis longus	Peroneus brevis	Flexor hallucis longus
Extensor digitorum longus		Flexor digitorum longus
Peroneus tertius		

The amount of stress that we can load onto the plantar fascia without damage is similar to the amount of stress that our ACL can withstand: the plantar fascia has a strength–safety factor of about 2.5, which is comparable to the ACL's factor of 2.4. (By comparison, bone has a factor of six, most tendons have a factor of eight, but the tendons that we require to be springy have factors between two and four. This shows that our plantar fascia is also meant to serve us like a spring.)[312]

Occasionally, the plantar fascia is the site of great pain; 10–20% of injured athletes complain of pain here, but athletes are not the only ones to suffer *plantar fasciitis*—it occurs more often in sedentary middle-aged people.[313] To learn about what causes plantar fasciitis and what we can do about it, read It's Complicated: What causes plantar fasciitis? below.

As we have seen, fascia is ubiquitous and has no clear boundaries. The plantar fascia is continuous with the Achilles tendon, at least while we are young. (In elderly feet, no connection is apparent.)[314] The plantar fascia throws off deep septa that flow between and around the foot's muscles and tendons. A continuation can be traced from the fascia at the bottom of the foot to the retinacula on the top of the instep, and this in turn can be followed upwards to the crural fascia, in the lower leg.[315] The movements, contractions and tensions created by the muscles of the foot and lower leg can affect the foot's deep fascia and either enhance or restrict the range of motion. In the other direction, limitations and tightness in the plantar fascia can show up as tight hamstrings, increased lumbar lordosis and even neck problems. In these situations, a lot of massage of the plantar fascia with knuckles, tennis balls or, for the hardier, golf balls may be required to release the tension.[316]

IT'S COMPLICATED: What causes plantar fasciitis?

Plantar fasciitis manifests as sharp, stabbing pain in the heel that is worse first thing in the morning and gets better as the fascia stretches out and begins to move, but it can be aggravated by long periods of standing. Any condition that ends in "itis" is usually an inflammation condition, so plantar fasciitis would be an inflammation of the plantar fascia; however, rarely are any inflammation factors found with this condition.[317] Plantar fasciitis is a misnamed problem! We really don't know what causes it. Until recently, we believed it was caused by overuse of the foot, leading to a thickening of the fascia near the heel, eventual degeneration of the collagen fibers, and the development of chronic inflammation.

Intrinsic and extrinsic factors were also believed to lead to plantar fasciitis. Intrinsic risk factors included age, weight, and the nature of the foot—its arches, heel pad thickness, and ankle range of motion. Extrinsic factors included prolonged standing, walking on hard surfaces, footwear style, and sudden bouts of unfamiliar exercise. All of these factors were thought to result in degeneration of the fascia around the heel. The problem with this lovely theory is that such degeneration seems to occur quite often in a lot of people, but they do not suffer the pain of plantar fasciitis! These factors can arise without any symptoms, so they are,

by themselves, unlikely to be the cause of plantar fasciitis. Indeed, the normal bio-markers of chronic inflammation do not appear to be present in sufferers of plantar fasciitis—it does not seem to be an inflammation issue at all.

This painful problem is closer to *tendinosis* (degeneration of the collagen) than tendinitis (inflammation). Indeed, some therapists are recommending we change the name of the condition to *plantar fasciosis*.[318] We are not sure—it may be that inflammation begins the degeneration, then the inflammation disappears, leaving only the degeneration. Researchers today believe that the factors we once thought caused plantar fasciitis are exacerbators, not initiators, of the condition. Repetitive stressing of the fascia is not by itself a problem, and indeed, such stress is essential to keeping the fascia healthy.

New research is looking at other possible causes of plantar fasciitis, including inherent fascial deficits (some pre-existing mechanical fault in the fascia) and neuromuscular deficits, which make the fascia less able to withstand normal cyclical loading or may cause it to experience an abnormal level of stress. While a minority of sufferers do opt for surgery (5–10%), most cases of plantar fasciitis resolve on their own within six to 18 months of conservative therapy.[319]

THE MUSCLES AND TENDONS

The foot is moved by both extrinsic and intrinsic muscles. The extrinsic muscles run from the leg to the foot, originating on either the femur, the tibia or the fibula and narrowing into long tendons that attach to the foot. The intrinsic muscles are much shorter and are found entirely within the foot, mostly in the plantar side—the bottom, fleshy part.

Extrinsic Muscles: Posterior Leg

To aid in remembering the extrinsic muscles that run from the leg to the foot, it is useful to consider them as groups of three muscles in four distinct locations—posterior, lateral, anterior and deep—with each group having a distinct function. On the posterior (back) side of the leg, we find the three muscles that plantarflex the ankle. These are the *gastrocnemius*, *soleus* and *plantaris*, shown in figure 2.216. (*Gastroc* is from the Greek for stomach, and *kneme* means leg, so the gastrocnemius is the belly of the leg. *Soleus* is Latin for sole, as in a type of fish—flat and round.) The gastrocnemius and soleus come together in one tendon and attach to the calcaneus; this is the *calcaneal tendon*, or as it is more commonly known, the Achilles tendon. The "gastrocs," as it is sometimes called, is the most famous calf muscle due to its prominent bulge at the back of the calves. However, it is not the bulk of the calf muscles. That honor goes to the soleus; the gastrocnemius is quite thin by comparison.

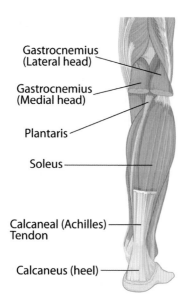

FIGURE 2.216 The posterior plantarflexors.

Together the gastrocnemius and soleus are often referred to as the *triceps surae*, due to their having three "heads" or origins. The gastrocs has two heads on the posterior (back) of the femur, proximal (above) the condyles. This attachment means the gastrocs can either plantarflex the ankle or flex the knee or do a bit of both; or it can resist extension of the knee or dorsiflexion of the ankle or a bit of both. (However, if the foot is fixed on the ground, in a closed-chain position, the gastrocnemius working concurrently with the hamstrings can actually act to extend and straighten the knee! So, are the hamstrings and gastrocs flexors of the knee or extensors? It all depends! They can be either, depending upon the situation.) If the knee is bent, the gastrocnemius is not stretched very much when the ankle dorsiflexes; that sense of stretch you may feel in a low lunge at the back of the calf of the forward leg when the knee goes well past the foot, or in a deep squat, is probably due to the soleus' resistance tensing the Achilles tendon. However, when the knee is extended, as it is in Down Dog (Adhomukhasvanasana), the stretch in the calf may well be due to the gastrocs, because now it is being stretched across both the ankle joint (which is dorsiflexing) and the knee joint (which is extending).

The soleus arises from the proximal, posterior (upper, backside) tibia. It lies underneath the gastrocs, so it is a bit hidden by its more famous brother, but you can feel it: when you dorsiflex the ankle, the soleus flattens out to the side of the calves and goes a bit lower than the gastrocnemius. Sometimes the soleus goes by the alias "second heart" because its contraction as we walk helps pump blood from the lower body to the heart.[320]

The third member of this "back of the leg" group is the plantaris, but about 12% of people don't have one![321] Some anatomists consider the plantaris a vestigial muscle, once important to our reptilian ancestors but not needed much today.[322] It has a very small belly, arising from the medial side of the lateral, posterior femoral condyle, and its tendon runs to the medial side of the calcaneus. Like the gastrocs, it can assist in flexing the knee or plantarflexing the ankle, but its contribution is minimal in both cases.

Figure labels:
- Gastrocnemius (Lateral head)
- Gastrocnemius (Medial head)
- Plantaris
- Soleus
- Calcaneal (Achilles) Tendon
- Calcaneus (heel)

LATERAL LEG MUSCLES

The term *peroneus* comes from the Greek for the pin of a brooch or buckle, which the peroneal muscles sort of resemble. A synonym would be *fibularis*, which is fitting because the peroneals run alongside the fibula. There are two peroneal (or fibularis) muscles: one longer and one shorter, as shown in figure 2.217. The *peroneus longus* arises from the proximal head of the fibula and has a long, slender tendon that goes under the lateral (outer) malleolus, under the tuberosity of the fifth metatarsal, along the bottom arch of the foot to the first metatarsal head. Its shorter brother, the *peroneus brevis*, arises about halfway down the fibula, also runs under the lateral malleolus and attaches to the fifth metatarsal tuberosity. Both of the muscles serve to evert the foot (turn the sole outward) and assist in plantarflexion of the ankle. In most people there is a third peroneal muscle called the *peroneus tertius* (also called the *fibularis tertius*). It attaches distally to the dorsal (back or top) of the fifth metatarsal (the base of the little toe.) Most studies say it is present in about 90% of the population, but some studies have found it occurring only about 50% of the time, depending on ethnicity. It seems to be a bit more frequent in men than women.[323] Although a rudimentary muscle, it assists in eversion like the other peroneals, but unlike them, it also aids in dorsiflexion of the ankle, like the anterior leg muscles.

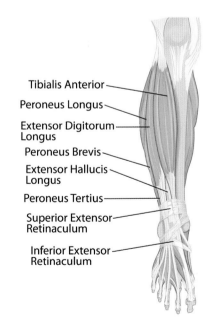

Tibialis Anterior
Peroneus Longus
Extensor Digitorum Longus
Peroneus Brevis
Extensor Hallucis Longus
Peroneus Tertius
Superior Extensor Retinaculum
Inferior Extensor Retinaculum

FIGURE 2.217 The lateral plantarflexors and anterior extensors.

ANTERIOR LEG MUSCLES

Sandwiched between the peroneal muscles and the tibia are the extensors of the ankle and toes. Again we find three: the *tibialis anterior, extensor digitorum longus* and *extensor hallucis longus*, as shown in figure 2.217. The tibialis anterior is the muscle you feel when you run your hand along the outside of your shin bone. You can easily detect it when you dorsiflex your foot, because it shortens and bulges. It arises from the anterior, lateral tibial condyle and runs to the medial cuneiform and first metatarsal. The extensor digitorum longus is not easily palpated. It is just lateral to the tibialis anterior, so as you run your hand down the leg and onto the bony surface of the foot, you may easily feel its four tendons, especially when you dorsiflex (extend) your toes; each tendon runs to one of the toes, the distal phalanges (but not the big toe). The big toe is moved by the third in this group, the extensor hallucis longus, which runs under the extensor retinaculum.

The names of these muscles tell us what we need to know: *extensor* tells that these muscles *extend* (or dorsiflex) the *digits* (the toes) or the *hallux* (the big toe). And they are *longus*, which means their bellies are long. The extensors not only extend the toes but also help dorsiflex the ankle. The extensor digitorum longus can also assist with everting the foot, while the extensor hallucis longus can help invert it.

DEEP LEG MUSCLES

The last group of three are the deep flexors of the ankle and toes: the *tibialis posterior, flexor digitorum longus* and *flexor hallucis longus*. The names are very similar to the extensors we just looked at, but these muscles are deeper, almost impossible to palpate, and of course move the toes and foot in the opposite direction—they flex (or plantarflex). As shown in figure 2.218, the three are found behind the shinbone, deep in relation to the gastrocs and soleus. Their tendons follow a medial path that mirrors the lateral muscle tendons: they pass under the medial malleolus and under the flexor retinaculum. The tibialis posterior runs to the bottom of the five anterior tarsal bones and to the second to fourth metatarsals. The flexor digitorum longus runs to the second to fifth digits (toes) and their distal phalanges, while the flexor hallucis longus runs to the big toe's distal phalange. Both of these muscles also help to invert the foot and provide a little bit of ankle plantarflexion service as well.

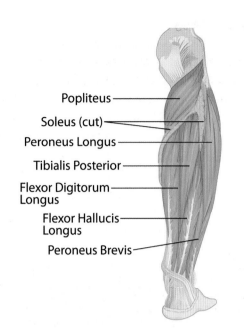

- Popliteus
- Soleus (cut)
- Peroneus Longus
- Tibialis Posterior
- Flexor Digitorum Longus
- Flexor Hallucis Longus
- Peroneus Brevis

FIGURE 2.218 The deep flexors are the tibialis posterior, flexor digitorum longus and flexor hallucis longus.

Muscles can contract to initiate movement, assist with movement, or resist and help control movement. Remember that no muscle works in isolation, and this is so in the foot as well. For example, the peroneus longus and the tibialis posterior often engage together, forming a strap or sling under the midsole of the foot (as shown in figure 2.222), assisting with maintaining the arch of the foot, especially when we stand on our toes; these co-contractions provide stability, which is very important when we attempt to maintain our balance in this position.

Intrinsic Foot Muscles

So far, we have described the muscles that are found outside the foot, which send tendons to its various bones. There are also many smaller and shorter muscles inside, called the intrinsic muscles. These can be described as dorsal (on the top of the foot) and plantar (in the sole).

Right on the top of the foot, as shown in figure 2.219a, is the extensor digitorum brevis; it runs from the front, top, lateral side (anterosuperolateral) of the calcaneus and joins with tendons two to four of the extensor digitorum longus, except for one slip that runs independently to the big toe. Sometimes, this slip is given the name extensor hallucis longus.[324] The extensor digitorum brevis assists with dorsiflexion of toes one to four.

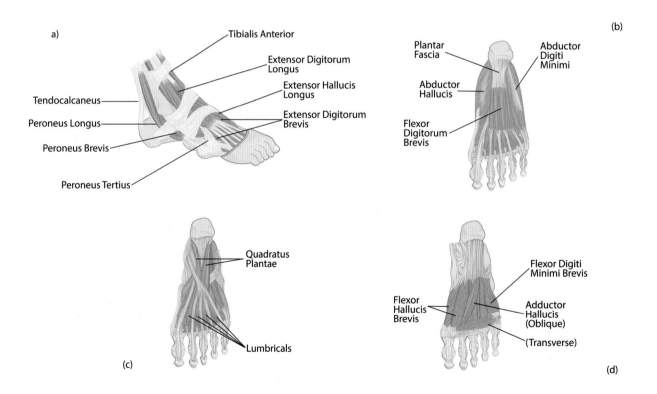

a)
- Tibialis Anterior
- Extensor Digitorum Longus
- Extensor Hallucis Longus
- Extensor Digitorum Brevis
- Tendocalcaneus
- Peroneus Longus
- Peroneus Brevis
- Peroneus Tertius

(b)
- Plantar Fascia
- Abductor Digiti Minimi
- Abductor Hallucis
- Flexor Digitorum Brevis

(c)
- Quadratus Plantae
- Lumbricals

(d)
- Flexor Digiti Minimi Brevis
- Flexor Hallucis Brevis
- Adductor Hallucis (Oblique)
- (Transverse)

FIGURE 2.219 The intrinsic foot muscles. The muscles along the dorsal side (a) generally extend the toes, while the muscles of the plantar side (b, c, d) generally flex them.

THE SOLE

Many books on the anatomy of the feet describe the intrinsic muscles in the sole as forming four plantar layers and one dorsal layer, reflecting the order in which these muscles are exposed during dissection. While this does not necessarily provide a functional approach to understanding these muscles, it is a useful convention. It is even more helpful to look at the muscles in positional groupings: lateral (pertaining to the toes or "digits"), medial (pertaining to the big toe or "hallux") and central. Using this approach, we can work through the sole's layers, investigating 10 muscles.[325] (This number is not fixed, as some people are missing some of these muscles while others may have a few extra. Also, different texts on anatomy will have different naming conventions, which can increase or decrease the number.)

FIRST LAYER

This is the most superficial layer of the sole and contains the *abductor hallucis, abductor digiti minimi* and *flexor digitorum brevis*, as shown in figure 2.219b. The abductor hallucis, as its name implies, abducts the big toe. It arises from the medial side of the calcaneus and plantar fascia and ends on the medial side of the proximal phalange of the big toe. The abductor digiti minimi, as the name indicates, abducts the little toe. It arises on the lateral side of the calcaneus and plantar fascia and ends on the lateral side of the proximal phalange of the little toe. The function of our abductors is weakened or lost entirely when we wear shoes. But in yoga classes, we can regain this lost ability by learning to spread our toes in all our standing postures.

Note that when we talk about abduction or adduction of the toes, we are not using the medial plane of the body as the reference plane, as we normally do; rather, just for the feet, we use the plane of the second toe. Abduction is movement of the big toe away from the second toe, and adduction is movement towards it. Similarly with toes 3, 4 and 5 (the little toe), when they move away from the second toe, they are said to be abducting, and when they move towards it, they are adducting. Naturally, then, the second toe cannot abduct or adduct, because it can't move away from itself.

The flexor digitorum brevis (the short version of the flexor digitorum longus) flexes all but the big toe. It runs from the calcaneus to the middle phalanges of toes two to five.

SECOND LAYER

Deeper than this first layer is our second group of intrinsic muscles, consisting of the flexor digitorum accessories and the four lumbricals. These accessories help the flexor digitorum longus and the flexor hallucis longus flex the toes. They are also known as the *quadratus plantae*. As shown in figure 2.219c, the quadratus plantae has two heads coming off the calcaneus, and it ends on the flexor digitorum longus—it actually becomes the flexor digitorum longus (which is why it is an accessory to it). This allows the quadratus plantae to redirect the pull of the flexor digitorum longus to be more in line with the axis of each of the four toes (but not the big toe). Curiously, this muscle is missing in about two percent of the population, while up to 20% of people might be missing one of the two heads, which can affect the way their feet work.[326]

The lumbricals also assist the flexor digitorum longus and therefore can be considered accessories, too. (Their funny name is due to their worm-like appearance: *lumbric* is Latin for earthworm.) The lumbricals arise from the tendons of the flexor digitorum longus and end on the dorsal side of the tendons of the extensor digitorum longus. They go from tendon to tendon! They also insert onto the base of the proximal phalanges, so they can flex proximal phalanges two to five at the metatarsophalangeal joints, even though they can extend the second to fifth toes at the interphalangeal joints. They assist in plantarflexing the interphalangeal joints when we push off from the ground.

THIRD LAYER

This layer, shown in figure 2.219d, includes the short muscles assisting the big toe and the little toe: the flexor hallucis brevis, adductor hallucis (transverse and oblique heads) and flexor digiti minimi brevis. The flexor hallucis brevis is short, as its name implies, running from the cuboid and lateral cuneiform to either side of the proximal phalange of the big toe. It has two insertions onto the big toe phalange, and the sesamoid bones form within these two tendons. These sesamoid bones provide a fulcrum that increases the muscles' leverage and pulling power, helps absorb and distribute pressure, and can reduce friction when the tendons slide over the bones.

The adductor hallucis has two heads: one arising at the bases of the second to fourth metatarsals, the other arising from the plantar ligaments across the third to fifth metatarsophalangeal joints. It runs to the lateral side of the proximal phalange of the big toe. Although it adducts the big toe, it can also assist with maintaining the foot's transverse arch and may minimally assist in flexing the big toe. If this muscle is not working well—for example, if it is too tight—the result can be a condition called *hallux valgus*, in which the big toe overlaps the second toe and the first metatarsal is significantly abducted medially.

Flexor digiti minimi brevis plantarflexes the little toe. It arises on the base of the fifth metatarsal and runs to the base of the fifth proximal phalange.

THE DORSAL LAYER

On the dorsal (top) of the foot, we cannot feel many muscles, but here we find the interossei and the extensor digitorum brevis. There are two layers of interossei: four on the dorsal side of the metatarsals (2–5) and proximal phalanges, and three on the plantar side of phalanges 3–5. They help to plantarflex the proximal phalanges, which is again important for the push-off phase of walking. Since they attach to the distal metatarsals, as shown in figure 2.220, they help keep them together and support the transverse arch. The dorsal interossei can help to spread (abduct) toes 3 and 4 apart, while the plantar interossei can adduct toes 3–5.[327]

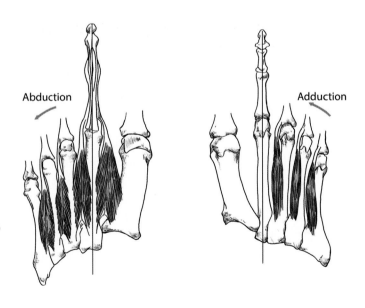

FIGURE 2.220 The interossei of the left foot: (a) dorsal interossei seen from above; (b) plantar interossei seen from below.

THE TYPES AND RANGES OF VARIATIONS

Variations in the Tibia

The distal end of the tibia articulates with the talus. This end, shown in figure 2.221, is called the *tibial plafond*; "plafond" is the French word for ceiling, and this is the ceiling of the ankle joint. We could also call it the tibial portion of the ankle's mortise.

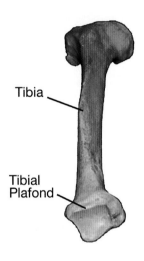

FIGURE 2.221 The tibial plafond is the distal end of the tibia, which sits atop the talus.

The width of the anterior side of the plafond varies by gender and within gender. A study of Italian and French populations using radiology found the average width in men to be 34.5 mm, with one standard deviation (SD) of 2.3 mm. The average width for women was 30.8 mm, with one SD of 3.0 mm.[331] However, another study of dry bones from a museum in Nairobi, Kenya, found significantly narrower widths as well as significant variation by gender.[332] Again, the point is not to determine what is the true average width of the tibial plafond but to point out that this width is quite variable. For the French and Italian studies, the width in men varied from ~30 to ~39 mm for 95% of the population examined. For women, the two SD range was 25–37 mm. This variation is significant because smaller widths are generally associated with smaller ranges of dorsiflexion.[333]

Another significant variation in the leg is the alignment of the distal ends of the tibia and fibula, which forms the *empirical axis*. The axis is angled both inferiorly and *(continued on page 221)*

TABLE 2.14 Summary of extrinsic and intrinsic muscles (M = main movers; A = accessory movers).

EXTRINSIC MUSCLES	DORSI-FLEXOR	PLANTAR-FLEXOR	PRONATOR (EVERTOR)	SUPINATOR (INVERTOR)	TOE EXTENDER	TOE FLEXOR
Gastrocnemius		M				
Plantaris		A				
Soleus		M				
Peroneus brevis		M	M			
Peroneus longus		M	M			
Peroneus tertius	A		M			
Tibialis anterior	M			M		
Extensor digitorum longus	M		M		M	
Extensor hallucis longus	M			A	M	
Tibialis posterior		M		M		
Flexor digitorum longus		M		A		M
Flexor hallucis longus		M		A		M

INTRINSIC MUSCLES	TOE EXTENDERS	TOE FLEXORS	TOE ABDUCTORS	TOE ADDUCTORS
Abductor hallucis		M	M	
Abductor digiti minimi		M	M	
Flexor digitorum brevis		M		
Flexor digitorum accessories		M		
Lumbricals	M	M		
Quadratus plantae		M		
Flexor hallucis brevis		M		
Flexor digiti minimi brevis		M		
Adductor hallucis		M		M
Extensor digitorum brevis	M			
Interossei (dorsal)	M		A	
Interossei (plantar)		M		A

IT'S COMPLICATED: Arch support

While the shapes of the bones determine the curve of the arches, and their congruence with each other contributes 65% of the arches' stability,[328] ligaments and muscle tendons are also important contributors to that stability. The flexor hallucis longus is the main bowstring tendon for the medial arch, running under the posterior groove of the talus and the sustentaculum tali of the calcaneus—effectively lifting it up and thus supporting the medial arch. The peroneus longus, tibialis posterior and abductor hallucis also support the medial arch. Two muscles are mainly involved in supporting the lateral arch: the peroneus brevis and peroneus longus. Their actions are very important in maintaining our lateral balance when we are standing on our toes. The transverse arch's muscular support comes from the adductor hallucis, peroneus longus, tibialis posterior and interossei.

Two muscles in particular really help to support all three arches: the tibialis posterior and peroneus longus.[329] As shown in figure 2.222, each tendon comes from the opposite side of the foot and thus they form a "sling." These two muscles pull up and help to maintain the arches, but only in certain circumstances. In an open-chain position, with no weight on the foot, when the tibialis posterior is engaged, it will supinate (invert, plantarflex and adduct) the forefoot. However, in a closed-chain, weightbearing position, the foot will not easily move. Now, engaging the tibialis posterior will cause the arch to rise higher, as long as the foot remains solidly planted on the ground, with the ball of the big toe and the inner heel pressing firmly into the earth. We can build this supination habit by rolling the inner ankle away from the floor, rooting down through the big-toe mound, thus strengthening the tibialis posterior and its arch-preserving ability. We can do this whenever we feel our feet are overly pronating, such as often happens in wide-legged forward folds (Prasaritapadottanasana—see figure 2.235b).

The other major arch supporter is the peroneus longus. Whereas the tibialis posterior wraps around the medial side of the foot, the peroneus longus approaches the arch from the lateral side. In an open-chain, non-weightbearing position, it will evert, plantarflex and abduct the forefoot, but in a closed-chained position, with the foot firmly planted, it will lift the lateral and transverse arches. Together, these two muscles act like a stirrup, pulling up the arches and thus stabilizing the foot. Yoga practices that strengthen these muscular actions may assist with maintaining healthy arches.

Research in 2014[330] discovered that three intrinsic foot muscles also play a significant, active role in supporting the arches under weightbearing conditions: the abductor hallucis, flexor digitorum brevis and quadratus plantae. Not only do they react to a flattening of the longitudinal arch, but they are strong enough to resist the deformation and contribute to its rebounding. Indeed, the greater the load on the arch, the more active these intrinsic muscles become. It seems, in fact, that these muscles are activated only when the plantar fascia is approaching the limit of what it can withstand on its own.

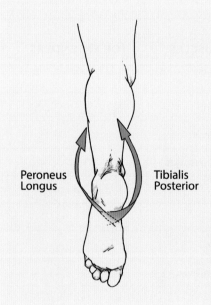

FIGURE 2.222 The sling of the foot.

posteriorly from medial to lateral. Figure 2.223 illustrates the angle of the empirical axis in the frontal (coronal) plane, which averages 10° below the horizontal plane. However, one SD is 4°, so the range of values for the degree of variation from the horizontal for the empirical axis for 95% of the population is 2–18°.[334] Due to tibial rotation, the empirical axis is laterally rotated in the horizontal (transverse) plane anywhere from 14° to 45°, the average being 30°.

Variations in the Talus

The alignment of the talus is not in line with one of the three cardinal planes of the body; instead, it points along the first ray of the foot or to the inside (medial or big-toe side). The talus dips below horizontal, as shown in figure 2.224a, its longitudinal axis angled downward at about 30° to a horizontal plane. The average angle between the neck of the talus and the ray of the second toe is 30° (see figure 2.224b). This angle is much larger in children, closer to 40–50°, often making children's feet appear more inverted.[335] (The orientation of the neck of the talus is not to be confused with the orientation of the subtalar joint—the joint between the talus and the calcaneus—which is also quite variable and can have an effect on the foot's range of pronation and supination.[336] This aspect of the subtalar joint involves the calcaneus as well as the talus, so we will discuss it when we look at variations in the calcaneus.)

Of great interest for yoga students and teachers is the trapezoid shape of the trochlea—the top of the talus—because it is wider at the front than at the back. This means that as the ankle dorsiflexes, the talus eventually becomes wedged into the mortise of the tibia and fibula; so, our

ultimate limit to dorsiflexion is dictated by the shape of our talus trochlea! This is the ankle's "close-packed" or rigid position. (Trying to force the talus into the mortise too deep, too quickly can sprain or rupture the ligaments joining the tibia and fibula.) In the other direction, when we plantarflex the ankle, the narrower part of the trochlea (its posterior part) has less contact with the mortise. The ankle is therefore less stable in plantarflexion. This lack of stability is one reason that most ankle sprains occur when the ankle is plantarflexed, and why wearing high heels is riskier than wearing no heels, because in high heels, the foot is constantly plantarflexed, making the ankle is less stable.

Unsurprisingly, the particular shape of the talus' trochlear trapezoid is highly variable. Some people have a wider distal end of the trapezoid, and they are more likely to be limited in their range of dorsiflexion. The width of the mortise also plays a role in limiting dorsiflexion, and it too is variable. Of course, the range of motion is also affected by the shape of the distal end of the tibia, as just discussed. Hence, the unique shapes of the talus and tibia affect our ankle's range of motion.

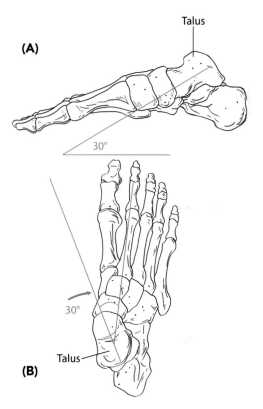

FIGURE 2.224 The axis of the talus is (a) below horizontal and (b) runs medially.

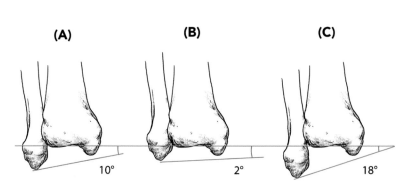

FIGURE 2.223 The tilt of the ankle. The empirical line of the ankle forms an angle of 10° to the horizontal plane, as shown in (a); however, that is just an average. The range of variation below the horizontal for this angle for 95% of the population is from 2° (b) to 18° (c).

Figure 2.225 shows the key parameters of the trochlea: length, posterior width, anterior width and angle of the trapezoid.[337] The anterior width varies from 28 mm in women (1 SD = 1.7 mm) to 32 mm in men (1 SD = 2.4 mm). The posterior width varies from 23 mm in women (1 SD = 1.6 mm) to 26 mm in men (1 SD = 2.1 mm). Thus, the trochlea of an average woman is 5 mm wider at the front than at the back, compared with 6 mm wider for men. This, of course, is only an average. The angle of the trapezoids ranges from 7° to 18°.[338] Someone with a greater angle is more likely to reach dorsiflexion compression earlier than someone with a smaller angle, all other conditions being equal. These other conditions would include the width of the mortise, the laxity of the ligaments, the length of the plantarflexing tendons and the tightness of the plantarflexor muscles, which again are all variable. Women tend to have narrower trochlea than men, but the angles of their trapezoids are virtually the same. The smaller values for women may be because shorter people tend to have narrower anterior trochlea, and women, on average, are shorter than men.

When we described the femur in the discussion on the hip (see page 110), we discovered that the femur neck in some people has a very different shape, thicker than normal. This cam-shaped variation may also show up in the talus. As shown in figure 2.207, the neck normally curves away from the body of the talus, creating a saddle-shaped depression. However, about 2.5% of the population has a less dramatic curve, giving the neck a cam appearance (shown in red in figure 2.226), which flattens the neck. We will look later at how this variation can affect the range of dorsiflexion available, but researchers have noticed that people with post-traumatic ankle pain tend to have this talus cam much more frequently than the normal population.[339] It may be that having a cam predisposes you to injury in the front of the ankle. Having a significant cam shape to your talus is also correlated to pes cavus—a high arch in the midfoot.[340]

Looking at the posterior (back) of the talus, we find other variations that can also lead to pain and pathology. A 1931 study found that 43% of people have a growth of bone there, called a *Stieda process*, named after the German anatomist Ludwig Stieda, who first described this variation[341] (figure 2.227a). Many people also have an extra bone situated just behind the posterior talus, called the *os trigonum* (figure 2.227b). From 2.5% to 14% of the population has this bone,[342] although one estimate was as high as 50%![343] Lots of people have an os trigonum or a Stieda process, so clearly not everyone who has one or the other will suffer pain due to its presence. However, footballers, gymnasts and ballet dancers do seem to have a disproportionate occurrence of a painful condition called *posterior ankle impingement syndrome* (PAIS),[344] which may be caused by either the Stieda process or the os trigonum. Either situation can affect the range of plantar flexion available. While elite athletes used to be the ones most often diagnosed with PAIS, today it is recognized that impingement syndrome is a common cause of persistent ankle pain in the general population.[345]

In some people, the neck of the talus develops distinct facets from physical contact with the tibia and fibula, caused by frequent squatting. These are called *squatting facets*. The incidence of these squatting facets is much higher in Indian

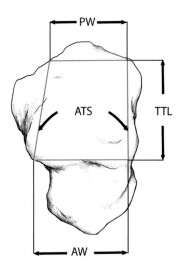

FIGURE 2.225 The trapezoid of the trochlea tali (shown in red): PW = posterior width, AW = anterior width, TTL = trochlea tali length, ATS = angles of the trapezoid shape.

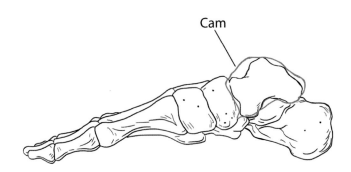

FIGURE 2.226 The talus cam (outlined in red). Notice how the neck is not curved downwards, as in the normal talus.

populations than in European populations, probably because of the greater frequency of squatting in India than in Europe, although there is some indication that the difference may be due to genetic inheritance.[346] (Interestingly, Europeans of the 13th century had similar squatting facets as modern Indians: undoubtedly, the rise in popularity of the chair in the West had something to do with Europeans squatting less.[347])

By and large, the right and left tali are quite similar and symmetric; the average amount of variation between them is less than 7.5%.[348] Some people do have a significant difference between their left and right ankles, though. You might be one of them.

Variations in the Calcaneus

Usually, there are three articulating sites forming sliding joint surfaces between the calcaneus and the talus, labeled in figure 2.207 as A, B and C. However, some people only have one large articulating surface connecting all three spots. Other people have only two facets, with points A and B merged into one. Normally, facet C, between the inferior side of the talus body and the superior surface of the calcaneus, is the biggest interface and is ovoid. There is not much variation in its area. The head of the talus has both a middle and an anterior interface with the calcaneus as well. These facets show considerable variation by ethnicity.

These variations are speculated to be related to the incidence of arthritis as well as to a lack of stability in the subtalar joint.[349] (Some researchers believe that if there are two facets at the head of the talus, there is greater subtalar stability and a lower likelihood of arthritis. These two facets, along with the facet at the body of the talus, form a nice, stable tripod that helps to prevent excessive movement in the subtalar joint. The pattern of two separate facets in the head of the talus is more common in people of European descent than in people of Indian descent.[350])

The axis of the subtalar joint is quite oblique, as shown in figure 2.228. The angle of this axis is tilted about 42° from the horizontal (transverse) plane and 16° from the side (sagittal) plane. Note that this is not the same as the orientation of the talus, which averages 30° to the ray of the second toe. Also, recall that we are restricting ourselves to using just two directions of movements for the foot (pronation and supination) and two for the ankle (dorsiflexion and plantarflexion). With the oblique axis of the subtalar joint, it is easy to see how pronation and supination occur: they are rotations of the foot around the red line shown in figure 2.28a. So basically, the majority of the movements we will concern ourselves with are happening at either the talocrural joint (the ankle) or the subtalar joint.[351] The subtalar axis is not fixed; as we dorsiflex or plantarflex the ankle, this axis traces a cone, as shown in figure 2.228c.

Stieda
Process
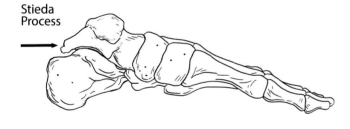

Os
Trigonum
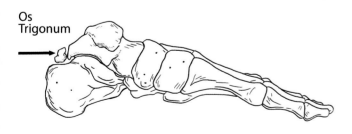

FIGURE 2.227 Stieda process (top) and the os trigonum (bottom).

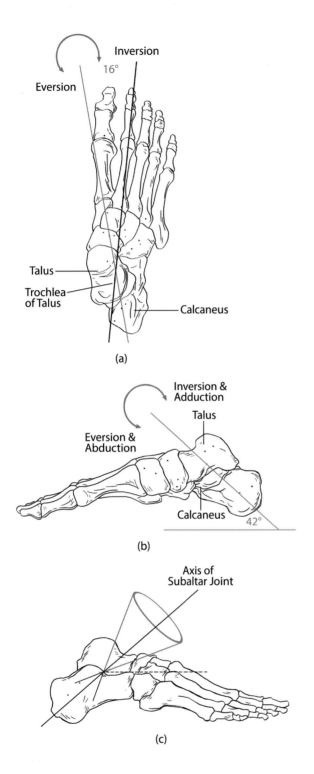

(a)

Inversion
16°
Eversion
Talus
Trochlea of Talus
Calcaneus

Inversion & Adduction
Talus
Eversion & Abduction
Calcaneus
42°

(b)

Axis of Subaltar Joint

(c)

FIGURE 2.228 The oblique axis of the subtalar (talocalcaneal) joint, shown in the superior view (a) and the medial view (b). Rotation around the more horizontal axis (a) creates inversion and eversion. Rotation around the more vertical axis (b) yields both inversion/eversion and adduction/abduction. Together these create the movements of supination and pronation. When plantarflexion and supination are combined with dorsiflexion and pronation, movement around this axis describes a cone (c).

The subtalar orientation angles of 42° and 16° are, again, averages.[352] Several sources cite the side plane variation as ranging from 16° to 23°.[353] These differences are significant. A larger angle leads to less supination of the heel when we stand or walk but greater pronation of the forefoot. Reducing the angle leads to greater supination of the heel but less pronation of the forefoot.[354] One researcher noted: "Since the relative position of the subtalar joint axis in the foot is not constant among individuals, it is reasonable to assume that variations in the location of the subtalar joint axis have a significant effect on the torques and the motions about the subtalar joint during standing and during walking."[355] We might add "and during standing yoga postures." A foot that seems overly supinated or pronated while in Warrior 2 Pose (Virabhadrasana II) may be due to the orientation of that student's subtalar joint.

The angle that the calcaneus alone forms to the horizontal is also variable: for people with high arches, the angle is higher than for people with fallen arches. As the arch of the foot falls, the foot grows longer. (One thing to look forward to as you grow older is that your shoe size may increase! Your foot gets longer as the arch gets shorter.) Another effect of arch height is the relative positioning of the heel behind the ankle. If the ankle is more over the heel, as shown in figure 2.229b, the body's center of gravity is precariously far back; this requires the body to lean forward, placing the pelvis and/or knees slightly in front of the ankles, which could lead to tightness in the superficial back line meridian of the

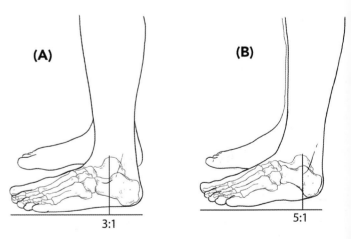

(A)   (B)

3:1   5:1

FIGURE 2.229 Positioning of the ankle with respect to the heel. In (a) we see an average alignment of the ankle to the heel, where the ratio of the length of foot in front of the lateral malleolus to behind is 3:1. In (b) there is more foot forward of the lateral malleolus: the ratio is now 5:1.

fascia and joint problems in the knees and pelvis. Thomas Myers believes that a ratio of 1:3 between the hindfoot and the forefoot provides the most effective support.[356] A ratio of 1:5, however, may result in minimal support. Whether this variation is due to genetics or faulty biomechanics is debated; it could be due to both or either. When it is due to faulty biomechanics, it can be fixed through repatterning movements or physiotherapy. If the shape and length of the calcaneus are the cause, however, it will not change without some sort of surgical intervention.

Of course, another reason for the back of the heel being closer to the ankle could simply be that the calcaneus is shorter; it may have nothing to do with the angle of the heel bone. Some people do have shorter heels than others. Several studies have shown that calcaneus lengths in humans are quite variable, ranging around a mean for adults of 5.4 cm (with 1 SD of 0.36 cm). This means 95% of people are within the 4.7–6.1 cm range.[357] Despite the apparent disadvantage of having a shorter heel, this could be a big advantage in a race![358] Surprisingly, the fastest sprinters are found to have the shortest heels.[359] This seems counterintuitive at first, but the shorter the heel, the greater the stress in the triceps surae (calf muscles) and the Achilles tendon, which means runners with shorter heels get a greater energetic rebound from their Achilles tendons. Also, those with longer heels require their plantarflexing calf muscles to contract further to move the lever of the foot, and that means they have to contract faster. (See figure 2.303 to review the way levers work.) Quicker muscular contraction is weaker muscular contraction. People with shorter heels, thus shorter levers, don't have to contract their plantarflexors as fast, which enables the muscle to generate more force.[360]

Not only is a shorter heel an advantage for sprinting (it has no advantage at walking speeds), longer toes are also advantageous for running, especially in sprinting; the longer the toes, the more time the foot can stay in contact with the ground and thus the more time there is for pushing off when we run.[361] This works well for the first few paces of a race when it is necessary to get up to maximum speed as quickly as possible. Evolutionary biologists believe shorter calcanei and longer toes may have been one of the adaptations that homo sapiens evolved to help with persistence hunting—our ability to run down faster animals over long distances and times.[362] Our shorter heels may have helped us supplant the Neanderthals, but even today there are many people with short toes and long heels, or long toes and short heels.

Other Variations of the Foot

Most anatomy texts will claim that the foot has 26 bones, those discussed earlier. Some will claim 28, as they include the two sesamoid bones found just below the big toe. Remember that these are averages. You may have more than 26 or 28—some people have extra sesamoid bones at the base of their other toes.[363] Normally, sesamoid bones are embedded in the tendons. There is no consensus on their exact role; they may prevent injury by reducing friction on the tendons,[364] or perhaps they are shock absorbers, or maybe they serve as pulleys, increasing the effective force of the muscle or changing the direction of the force. The fact that they exist probably means that they are doing something valuable.

Many people have other floating bones called *supernumerary* bones (or *ossicles*, which means "small bones"), such as the *os peroneum* within the peroneus longus tendon near the cuboid, or the *os trigonum*, which is a small bone just behind (posterolateral) the talus; the os trigonum should have become the talus, but it never joined with the talus and remained a separate bone.[365] Approximately 3–15% of people have an os trigonum,[366] and about 26% have an os peroneum.[367] While often these supernumeraries are the remnants of bones that should have fused together, sometimes, they can grow inside fascia when stress becomes chronic; the body reacts to constant stress by thickening the fascia, and the area may ossify (become bone). We saw a case of this in the knee, where around 20% of the population grows a second kneecap, called the fabella, behind the knee, in the fascia of the gastrocnemius. The same thing can happen in the foot. How many bones do you have in your feet? Only an imaging radiologist can tell you for sure. Having these sesamoid and supernumerary bones is rarely a problem, but in a few cases, they can cause pathology and become problematic.

Less than one percent of people have a condition called a *tarsal coalition*, which often arises in their second decade of life.[368] Like two or more political parties joining together in a coalition, two or more tarsal bones may forgo their normal articulating joint and become fibrously connected, thus eliminating independent movement. People with tarsal coalitions have much less flexibility in their feet and often have fallen arches as a result.[369] This inhibition to movement is not caused by tight, short muscles but by the binding together of the otherwise sliding surfaces of the bones.

Function: Application in Yoga Postures

We have seen how the architecture and form of the ankle–foot segment allow the movements of dorsiflexion/plantarflexion at the ankle and pronation/supination in the foot. We will now look at the ranges of possible motions for an average person, and for all those yoga students who are not average. In answering our WSM? question, we will also look at the sources of tension and compression and how compression may arise in different places due to natural variations in the bones and joints.

NORMAL RANGES OF MOTION

As we have already noted, the foot is a very complicated structure, but fortunately, for our purposes we can whittle down the number of movements we need to understand to just four: dorsiflexion and plantarflexion of the ankle; and supination and pronation of the foot. Of course, many more movements are possible, and those who want a deeper understanding of the movements called eversion, inversion, abduction and adduction should read Appendix F: The Movements of the Foot and Ankle. The four movements we will look at here can seem complicated, but yogis need to understand them to be able to answer the WSM? question.

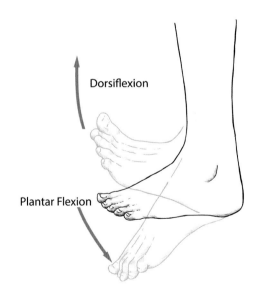

FIGURE 2.230 The ankle can only dorsiflex or plantarflex.

Dorsiflexion and Plantarflexion

There are only two movements available at the ankle: dorsiflexion and plantarflexion. That's easy to remember. For now, don't worry about the fact that our toes can also dorsiflex and plantarflex; let's keep it simple.

Dorsiflexion

The *dorsum* is the top of the foot, analogous to the back of your hand. (The word *dorsum*, from Latin, generally means "back"—the back of our body is the dorsal side. However, it seems strange to say the "back of the foot," so we say the "top of the foot," although we do mean "back," just as we refer to the back of our hand.)

Dorsiflexion results in the top of the foot coming closer to the shin or, if the foot is fixed, the front of the shin coming towards the top of the foot. We do this latter movement in many yoga postures: Chair Pose (Utkatasana), Squat (Malasana), Down Dog (Adhomukhasvanasana), and the back leg in Warrior Postures (Virabhadrasana) and Egyptian or Pyramid Pose (Parsvottanasana) (see figure 2.231). Any time the knee is over the toes or in front of the foot, we are dorsiflexing at the ankle. Often, the movement is passive (which is good, because our dorsiflexing muscles are far weaker than our plantarflexors). For example, in Chair Pose, as the knee comes forward, the ankle naturally and passively dorsiflexes. But occasionally, we have to actively dorsiflex the foot, which we may do with the front foot in Pigeon Pose (Kapotasana) to stabilize the knee. The amount of dorsiflexion we can achieve may dramatically affect how deeply we can go into many of these poses; if we can't dorsiflex the ankle enough, we may have to let our heels come off the floor (a common occurrence in Down Dog) or rotate the foot and leg more externally (which many people do for the back foot in Warrior 1 Pose or for both feet in Squats).

Our ability to dorsiflex may decline somewhat as we age, and there seems to be a slight gender difference, as table 2.15 shows. This table presents the results of a study of 600 healthy individuals. The ranges shown in brackets are at the two standard deviation (SD) limit, which means 95% of the people surveyed fall within that range.

TABLE 2.15 The average amount of dorsiflexion by gender and age. The ranges indicate where 95% of people will fall.[370]

AGE	WOMEN	MEN
2–8	24.8° (22.5–27.1°)	22.8° (21.3–24.3°)
9–19	17.3° (15.6–19.0°)	16.3° (14.9–17.7°)
20–44	13.8° (12.9–14.7°)	12.7° (11.6–13.8°)
45–69	11.6° (10.6–12.6°)	11.9° (10.9–12.9°)

Studies vary! Another found that most people can dorsiflex 25°.[371] Daily functional activities require a wide range of dorsiflexion ability:[372]

- Walking on level ground: 1–22°
- Climbing stairs: 7–30°
- Descending stairs: 14–38°
- Rising from a chair: 23–38°
- Kneeling (toes tucked under/ankles dorsiflexed): 26–45°
- Sitting cross-legged: 26–39°
- Squatting with heels on the floor: 33–45°[373]

One study found that everyday walking on level ground requires about 9° of dorsiflexion.[374] Why do these studies vary so much? One reason is the way the researchers take the measurements.[375] Another is the reality of human variation. Is the average amount of dorsiflexion available really in the 10–25° range shown in table 2.15, because if it is, then most people will have difficulty rising from a chair, kneeling or sitting cross-legged. Squatting with the heels on the floor is not going to happen for 95% of the population, give the results of that study.

However, another study found that the average amount of dorsiflexion available is 39°, with one SD of 7°; thus, 67% of people studied fell within the 32–46° range, and 95% were within the 25°–53° range.[376] Again, we should not focus on the exact number but instead realize that everyone is different. What is important is *your* range of motion and whether it is healthy for you. Is it enough, not enough or too much? For some people, dorsiflexion beyond 45° could result in damage to the ligaments in front of the ankle or damage to the bones themselves. Fortunately, such extreme dorsiflexion is not required in everyday living or even in most yoga postures.[377]

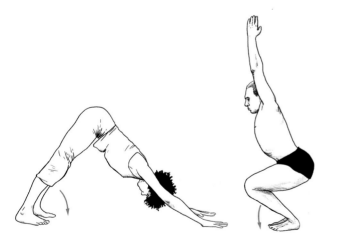
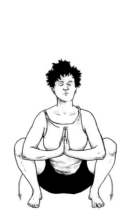
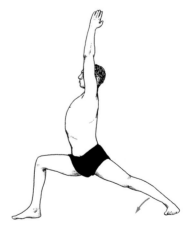

FIGURE 2.231 Yoga postures that require dorsiflexion: Down Dog (Adhomukhasvanasana), Chair (Utkatasana), Squat (Malasana) and Warrior 1 (Virabhadrasana 1). In all these cases, the foot is fixed and the shin moves towards the floor.

Plantarflexion

The plantar side of the foot is the bottom, homologous to the palm of the hand. Plantarflexion of the ankle occurs when we move the foot away from our shin or if our foot is fixed when we move our shin away from our toes. When we balance on tiptoes, we are plantarflexing, and again, this is occurring at the ankle, as shown in figure 2.232a.

Our ability to plantarflex may decline slightly as we age, and there seems to be a gender difference, as table 2.16 shows.[378]

TABLE 2.16 The average amount of plantarflexion by gender and age. The ranges indicate where 95% of people will fall.[379]

AGE	WOMEN	MEN
2–8	67.1° (64.8–69.4°)	55.8° (54.4–57.2°)
9–19	57.3° (54.8–59.8°)	52.8° (50.8–54.8°)
20–44	62.1° (60.6–63.6°)	54.6° (53.2–56.0°)
45–69	56.5° (55.0–58.0°)	49.4° (47.7–51.1°)

Everyday walking on level ground requires about 24° of plantarflexion. However, the range goes from as little as 7° to as much as 36°,[380] so it is hard to say what is normal. Other functional activities show similarly wide ranges of plantarflexion:[381]

- Climbing stairs: 18–40°
- Descending stairs: 20–46°
- Kneeling (sitting on heels/ankles plantarflexed): 8–40°
- Sitting cross-legged: 15–37°

Given that the average person, even at 69 years of age, has at least 48° of plantarflexion available, performing these everyday tasks is not a problem for most of us.

Supination and Pronation of the Foot

The ankle can only move in two directions, but the rest of the foot has lots of other possibilities. Again, to simplify the situation we will mostly look at the two major ones: supination and pronation. These can occur in the hindfoot or in the midfoot and forefoot. In the hindfoot, it happens at the tarsal joints below the ankle.

Figure 2.233 shows the foot supinating and pronating in an open-chain (non-weightbearing) mode. The axis of rotation through the subtalar joint is oblique, as was shown in figure 2.228. The transverse tarsal joint (see figure 2.310) also plays a strong role in controlling both pronation and supination, as does, to a much more limited degree, the talocrural (ankle) joint. Consequently, supination is a combination of movements across several joints and consists of inversion, adduction and plantarflexion; pronation is a

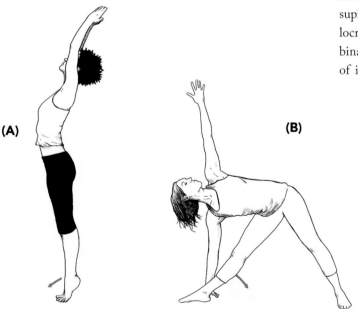

(A)

(B)

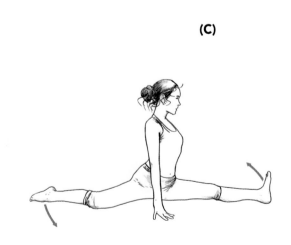

(C)

FIGURE 2.232 Plantarflexion occurs when we move the foot away from the shin: (a) when we stand on our tip toes or (b) when we move the shin away from the foot for Triangle Pose (Trikonasana). In (c), the Splits Pose (Hanumanasana), both dorsiflexion (front foot) and plantarflexion (back foot) can occur.

TABLE 2.17 The average active range of motion for the talocrural and subtalar joint complex.[384]
The ranges indicate where 95% of people will fall.

	INVERSION	EVERSION	ABDUCTION	ADDUCTION
Average	22.6°	12.5°	38.3°	33.6°
Range	16.1–30.2°	10.1–16.1°	29.8–48.3°	25.8–45°

combination of eversion, abduction and dorsiflexion. It is not simple to quantify the ranges of motion for supination or pronation, because these movements occur in multiple planes. However, the ranges for eversion, inversion, adduction and abduction in the ankle-joint complex, which consists of the subtalar joint and the talocrural joint, have been compiled (table 2.17).[382] In general, our peak flexibility occurs around the age of 15, so the older we get, the less range of motion we have in all directions. Females between nine and 20 average a greater range of motion than men, but women as they age also tend to lose range of motion more quickly than men.[383]

As always, do not take these figures as exact representations of humanity. Other studies have found much larger ranges of motion.[385] The point is always: we are different, and there is no one right range of motion for healthy people.

Supination

If we consider the sole of the foot (the plantar side) to be similar to the palm of our hand, supination is when we turn the palm up or the sole inward. Figure 2.234 shows the foot supinating as the sole moves towards the mid-plane of the body; the sole moves closer to the medial (inner) ankle. We do this in Butterfly Pose (Baddhakonasana) when we open the soles towards the sky, or in Lotus Pose (Padmasana) when we open the sole as we draw the foot onto the opposite thigh. These are open-chain movements: the foot is free to move. However, in a closed-chain movement, when the foot is fixed on the ground, moving the medial ankle towards the sole is, counterintuitively, pronation of the hindfoot, because the heel everts and moves outward as the talus moves inward. In the closed-chain situation, moving the inner ankle up and away from the floor is supination of the hindfoot. (Again, this is challenging to understand, so see Appendix F: The Movements of the Foot and Ankle, for more information.)

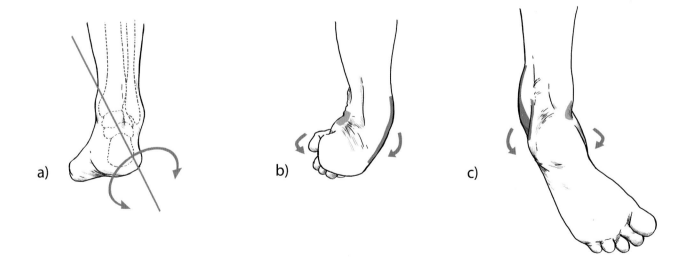

a)   b)   c)

FIGURE 2.233 Supination and pronation of the foot: (a) the neutral foot, showing the axis of rotation through the subtalar joint; (b) supination with inversion and adduction; (c) pronation with eversion and abduction. The red shading indicates areas where compression could arise, while the blue shading indicates areas where tension may limit movement.

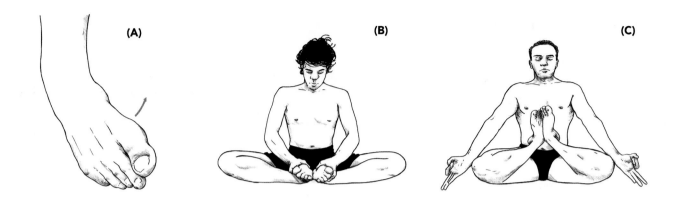

FIGURE 2.234 Supination opens the sole (a) towards the midline of the body. This can be done passively, as shown in (b) Butterfly Pose (Baddhakonasana), or (c) more extremely in Kandasana.

Pronation

Pronation, as shown in figure 2.235a, is movement in the other direction from supination; as with our hands when we turn our palms down, when we roll the sole away from the mid-plane of the body, towards the lateral or outside, we are pronating. That is in the open-chain case, but remember, for the closed-chain situation, where the foot is fixed (figure 2.235b) and we move the medial (inner) ankle toward the mid-plane, we are pronating the hindfoot. (If it seems confusing that the foot is pronating in this closed-chain situation, please read Appendix F: The Movements of the Foot and Ankle. While it looks like the talus is coming closer to the heel, which would be supination, in reality, the calcaneus everts away from the talus, while the talus adducts and plantarflexes. This is pronation.)

We are often advised to supinate the foot in our standing yoga postures to correct the tendency to over-pronate. In the example of Wide-legged Standing Forward Fold (Prasaritapadottanasana), it is natural to pronate the foot (see Figure 2.235b); we must to get the foot fully grounded when our legs are apart, but once the foot is grounded, supination will stiffen it and make it more stable. For this reason, most yoga teachers will encourage supination and discourage pronation. While the feet mostly pronate in our standing postures, the fear is that they will pronate too much, so supination is encouraged to stabilize the foot.

To be more complete, supination is actually a combination of three movements: plantarflexion, inversion and adduction. Pronation is a combination of dorsiflexion, eversion and abduction. These movements occur not just

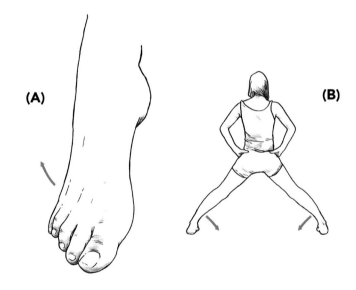

FIGURE 2.235 Pronation opens the sole (a) laterally away from the midline of the body. This often occurs in standing postures when the feet are far apart, as in (b) Prasaritapadottanasana. In this case, the foot doesn't move but the leg does, creating pronation at the ankle.

at the subtalar joint (the hindfoot) but also at the hard to pronounce *talocalcaneonavicular* joint and the *calcaneocuboid* joint (the midfoot). While we could use these other terms of eversion, inversion, etc., for our purposes we can stick with supination and pronation. However we will occasionally use these other terms for greater clarity.

The Four Movements of the Toes

Just as we have simplified the movements of the ankle and foot to four, we can also simplify the toes' movements to just four: dorsiflexion (which we can also call extension), plantarflexion (which is often simply called flexion), abduction (the toes spread apart) and adduction (the toes come together). Normally all five toes move together, but the big toe can move independently of the others. Some yoga teachers suggest doing exactly this, as shown in figure 2.250: we can flex the big toe while extending all the others, then reverse this and extend the big toe and flex all the others.[386] This can be done while in seated forward-folding postures, like Head-to-Knee Pose (Janusirsasana), and it can help to realign the toes and strengthen the arches of the foot.

The range of movement in the toes is much greater when we passively move the joint than is available when we use the foot's own muscles to try to articulate the joints. For example, we can use our hands to dorsiflex (extend) our big toe almost 90° or more, but we can't do it by just extending the toe on its own. Try it yourself. Firmly plant your foot on the floor, pressing the big-toe mound into the ground, and use one hand to pull up the big toe; you can probably get close to 90° or even beyond. But then release the toe, ground down into the big-toe mound again, and try to raise (extend) the toe by itself. You won't have as much range of movement. The same applies in flexion and abduction—the passive range of motion is greater than the active range. Normally, walking without shoes requires about 65° of extension of the big toe at the metatarsophalangeal joint.[387] Walking with shoes allows less movement because the shoe is doing the work.[388] Because toe flexion is assisted by the heel rising, not purely by active flexion of the big toe, the toe is flexed both passively and actively while walking. Most people's range of motion is adequate for walking. However, in yoga classes, dance and other athletic endeavors, 90° is often required.

When we dorsiflex our toes, as shown in figure 2.236, we increase the stress in the plantar fascia, so the arch become higher. This also happens when we supinate our foot and externally rotate our lower limbs; the plantar fascia and the arches become stiffer. This is necessary for increasing the springiness of our step as we push off from the ground when we walk or run.

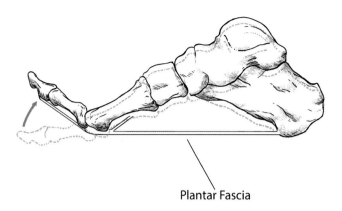

Plantar Fascia

FIGURE 2.236 Dorsiflexing the big toe increases the height of the arch.

SOURCES OF TENSION

The answer to WSM? for movements at the ankle and foot is either tension or compression. The sources of tensile resistance can affect all ranges of motion possible there. In general, we will look at the sources of tension affecting the movements of dorsiflexion/plantarflexion at the ankle and pronation/supination in the foot.

Source of Tension from the Fascia

TENSILE RESISTANCE	COMPRESSION
Myofascial Meridians	

As mentioned earlier, the myofascial meridians are continuous connections of fascia that envelop the muscles and joint capsules, forming trains of fabric that run around the whole body. The meridians that can impede movement in the ankle and foot include the superficial front line (SFL), the superficial back line (SBL), the deep front line (DFL) and the lateral lines (LL).[389] (See the detailed description of myofascial meridians in Appendix C of Volume 1.)

The SFL fascial meridian may restrict both plantarflexion and dorsiflexion if it becomes stuck in the area of the retinacula that passes over the tendons of the dorsiflexors. Fascial restrictions may be found along the dorsum (top) of the foot up onto the anterior (front) portion of the lower leg.[390] Manual therapy may be helpful in releasing any adhesions or stuckness along this line.

The SBL myofascial meridian runs from the soles of the feet, up the back side of the body (which includes the calves and hamstrings, the spine and the back of the neck), to the eyebrows. While it creates extension of the body and plantarflexion of the foot, it limits dorsiflexion. Part of the SBL is the fascia of the sole, the plantar fascia, which resists dorsiflexion and, in so doing, causes the longitudinal arches of the feet to deepen. If we also dorsiflex (extend) the toes, especially the big toe, this puts even more tension in the plantar fascia, making dorsiflexion at the ankle more difficult. Flexible yoga students who don't feel much of a stretch at the back of the calves while in Down Dog, even though their legs are extended completely straight and their heels are on the ground, may be advised to try lifting their toes (but not their heels!). This instruction puts more tension in the plantar fascia, which, thanks to its fascial continuity with the Achilles tendon, stresses the calf muscles. With toes extended, even flexible students may feel a stretch in their calves in Down Dog.

The DFL and LL can limit the foot's range of movement. If the DFL is unusually short, the tightened tibialis muscles tend to supinate the foot and resist pronation. When the LL are overly tight, the shortened peroneals tend to pronate the foot and resist supination. Working together, the DFL and LL help to stabilize the mortise of the tibia and fibula on top of the talus while maintaining the medial arch of the foot.[391]

Sources of Tension from the Muscles

TENSILE RESISTANCE			COMPRESSION	
		Muscles & Tendons		

RESTRICTIONS TO DORSIFLEXION

To a clinician, a lack of dorsiflexion has many names, including *equinus*, *gastrocnemius contracture* and *limited ankle dorsiflexion*.[392] These terms are used when the maximum dorsiflexion achieved is less than 5° while the knee is extended, or less than 10° when the knee is flexed.[393] The muscles that resist dorsiflexion are the same ones that cause movement in the opposite direction: the plantarflexors. The biggest cause of limited ankle dorsiflexion is tightness in the gastrocs.[394] It can become tight for a number or reasons, including sitting at a desk for long hours with the foot plantarflexed and the knee flexed, or sleeping with the foot in plantarflexion, or simply overtraining the gastrocnemius, making them stronger but shorter and tighter.[395] Having limitations to your range of dorsiflexion may

bring dire consequences; your midfoot may pronate in order to compensate for lack of dorsiflexion, meaning your leg will become functionally shorter and internally rotated, which can cause problems in your knee, hip and lower back, not to mention severe foot problems.[396] Limited ankle dorsiflexion can cause a host of problems: low back pain, hallux rigidus, hyperextension of the knees, bone spurs on the heel, chronic plantar pain and plantar fasciitis, callus on the forefoot and other foot problems.[397] Dorsiflexion limitations may be a reason for patellofemoral pain (pain under the kneecap).[398]

For yoga students, probably the most frustrating part of having limited ankle dorsiflexion is the inability to get their heels to the floor in Down Dog or Squat; they want to look like the teacher, and their inability to achieve the same aesthetic appearance makes them feel inadequate. Fortunately, several studies have shown that being unable to lower your heels to the floor in Down Dog will not prevent you from entering heaven![399]

The strongest plantarflexors of the ankle are the calf muscles of the gastrocnemius and soleus. If the gastrocs is not the primary cause of limited ankle dorsiflexion, the soleus may be. How to tell? Notice what you are feeling and where. As shown in figure 2.239, gastrocs tension may tend to be noticed as a stress a bit higher up the calf, in its belly or above, while tension due to the soleus may be more in the mid to lower calf. Or, their tendon, the Achilles tendon (*calcaneal tendon*), may be where you experience the tension; this can be felt as a stress lower down the calf or around the back of the ankle. There are other plantarflexors as well: the tibialis posterior, the peroneus longus and brevis, and the flexor digitorum longus and flexor hallucis longus. Tightness or shortness in these muscles can interfere with the range of dorsiflexion available. The solution then is to stretch out those muscles. But as already noted, these are rarely the main contributors to limited ankle dorsiflexion.

RESTRICTIONS TO PLANTARFLEXION

There are not as many sources of muscular tension restricting plantarflexion as there are for dorsiflexion. Tension resisting plantarflexion will be felt on the top of the foot, in front of the ankle, or even in the front of the shins, (as shown in figure 2.242c). The dorsiflexor muscles are not nearly as strong as the plantarflexors, but even so, the three dorsiflexors—the tibialis anterior, extensor hallucis longus and extensor digitorum longus—can limit some people's amount of plantar flexion. If these muscles are contracted, short and tight, they will be a limitation. Fortunately, they can be stretched out over time, and the range of plantarflexion can thereby be increased.

RESTRICTIONS TO PRONATION

As shown in table 2.17, the ranges of abduction and adduction are similar, but the range for inversion is almost twice that for eversion; it is easier to turn the sole of your foot inward than outward. Tightness or tension in the invertors of the foot, the tibialis anterior and tibialis posterior, can restrict eversion and thus pronation.

RESTRICTIONS TO SUPINATION

Moving the foot in the opposite direction, supination, may be resisted by tension in the evertor/pronator muscles: the peroneus longus, brevis and tertius.

Sources of Tension from the Ligaments

TENSILE RESISTANCE			COMPRESSION
	Ligaments & Joint Capsule		

RESTRICTIONS TO DORSIFLEXION

A source of limitation to ankle dorsiflexion is capsular adhesion; the joint capsule may have lost some flexibility or become contracted.[400] This can often happen when someone has had to immobilize their ankle, perhaps to recover from a broken foot or bad ankle sprain. When the ankle is immobilized, the joint capsule undergoes contracture, which can significantly reduce range of motion in all directions.

Resistance to dorsiflexion may also arise in the ligaments that bind the tibia, fibula, talus and calcaneus. On the medial (inner) side of the ankle, the deltoid ligament's tibiotalar fibers and the tibiocalcaneal ligament may resist further dorsiflexion. On the lateral (outer) side, the ligament that joins the heel to the fibula (the calcaneofibular

TABLE 2.18 Muscles causing or resisting ankle and foot movements.

MOVEMENT	PRIME MOVERS	SYNERGISTS	MUSCLES THAT RESIST MOVEMENT
Ankle dorsiflexion	Tibialis anterior, extensor hallucis longus, extensor digitorum longus	Peroneus tertius	Gastrocnemius, soleus, peroneus brevis, peroneus longus, posterior tibialis, flexor digitorum longus, flexor hallucis longus
Ankle plantarflexion	Gastrocnemius, soleus, peroneus brevis, peroneus longus, posterior tibialis, flexor digitorum longus, flexor hallucis longus	Plantaris	Tibialis anterior, extensor hallucis longus, extensor digitorum longus
Foot pronation	Peroneus brevis, peroneus longus, peroneus tertius, extensor digitorum longus		Tibialis anterior, tibialis posterior
Foot supination	Tibialis anterior, tibialis posterior	Extensor hallucis longus, flexor digitorum longus, flexor hallucis longus	Peroneus brevis, peroneus longus, peroneus tertius

ligament) and the ligament that joins the talus to the fibula (the posterior talofibular ligament) may resist further dorsiflexion. Finally, the back side of the talocrural joint, the posterior joint capsule, may resist as well. All these ligaments become taut when the ankle dorsiflexes.[401]

If someone sprains their ankle, these ligaments can become lax and thus be unable to prevent further dorsiflexion. It can take a long time for lax ligaments to shrink back to their original lengths, so if this happens, either the person has to strengthen the musculature around the ankle to prevent hypermobility, or the ankle continues to dorsiflex until it reaches the ultimate delimiter of movement: compression. However, for many people, compression can be reached even without the ligaments being lax and even with the muscles strong and tight. It may depend upon the shape of their bones.

RESTRICTIONS TO PLANTARFLEXION

Tension that resists plantarflexion can arise in the medial aspect of the joint capsule, and in the deltoid collateral ligament found on the medial (inner) side of the ankle that binds the tibia to the talus, navicular and calcaneus (see figure 2.210). The anterior talofibular ligament—the band across the front of the mortise—and the tibionavicular fibers of the deltoid ligament will also constrain too much plantarflexion.

RESTRICTIONS TO PRONATION

Tension preventing pronation can arise in the medial aspect of the joint capsule and in the deltoid collateral ligament found on the medial (inner) side of the ankle, binding the tibia to the talus. These ligaments, as shown in figure 2.210, are respectively called the anterior tibiotalar ligament, tibionavicular ligament, tibiocalcaneal ligament and posterior tibiotalar ligament.

RESTRICTIONS TO SUPINATION

Tension preventing supination may arise in the lateral ligaments binding the ankle joint: the calcaneofibular ligament, posterior talofibular ligament and anterior talofibular ligament, as shown in figure 2.211. As well, tension in the lateral side of the talocrural joint capsule assists in preventing too much supination.

TABLE 2.19 Sources of ligamentous tension restricting ankle and foot movements.

MOVEMENT	RESISTING LIGAMENTS
Ankle dorsiflexion	Tibiotalar ligament Tibiocalcaneal ligament Calcaneofibular ligament Posterior talofibular ligament Posterior joint capsule
Ankle plantarflexion	Deltoid collateral ligament Tibionavicular ligament Anterior talofibular ligament
Foot pronation	Deltoid collateral ligament Medial aspect of the joint capsule
Foot supination	Calcaneofibular ligament Posterior talofibular ligament Anterior talofibular ligament Lateral aspect of the joint capsule

SOURCES OF COMPRESSION

Once the tensile resistance of the tissues described above has been reduced sufficiently, the next answer to WSM? becomes compression. In general, we will look at the sources of compression affecting the movements of dorsiflexion/plantarflexion at the ankle and pronation/supination of the foot.

Restrictions to Dorsiflexion

TENSILE RESISTANCE	COMPRESSION
	MEDIUM: bone on flesh

Ultimately, the talus may come into contact with the tibia or the fibula, or some tissues may become pinched in between these bones; that is compression. You will know that you have reached compression when you feel sensations in the front of the ankle while you dorsiflex. You may still have some residual tension in the muscles, tendons or fascia along the back of the foot, ankle or calf when you reach compression, but it will now be compression that is stopping you. There are two qualities you may observe with compression at the ankle: (i) a hard edge that you feel you can't go past—this will be the case when the anterior, superior body of the talus is wedged into the mortise; or (ii) a medium feeling of being stuck but a sensation that you could push a bit deeper—this is caused by tendons being trapped between the talus and the tibia.

This medium quality may arise when we actively try to dorsiflex the foot or extend the toes. The tendons of the extensor digitorum longus, extensor hallucis longus and tibialis anterior all run in front of the ankle and under the extensor retinaculum (see figures 2.214 and 2.217), and when engaged, they tend to rise up, pressing against the retinaculum. They are in a prime position to be caught between the dorsiflexing talus and the mortise of the tibia. You can check this out for yourself. Come into an easy lunge position with the front knee slightly in front of the foot. This places the front ankle in a passively dorsiflexed position. With your hand, feel the front of your ankle; it should feel soft. Keep feeling the front of the ankle as you extend (lift) the toes and try to lift the forefoot off the floor. Notice how these tendons are now bulging outward, limiting how much dorsiflexion you can do.

This medium feeling of compression can also arise when the ankle is inflamed. If you have some pathology in the foot or ankle whereby the tissues are inflamed and swollen, compression may easily be reached. This often occurs for people with diabetes.[402] In these cases, the chronic swelling of the tissues restricts the range of dorsiflexion available.

Finally, the anterior inferior tibiofibular ligament can get pinched in between the talus and tibia, creating compression.[403] This generally arises only after a severe ankle sprain.

TENSILE RESISTANCE	COMPRESSION
	HARD: bone on bone

The hard feeling of compression occurs when the talus hits the tibia or fibula—when bone hits bone. There are several reasons why this may occur. It may be due to the size of the body of the talus (as discussed when we looked at the talus bone in detail—see figure 2.225 on page 222), the width of the anterior border of the talus or the width of the mortise. Or, as shown in figure 2.226, it may be due to a pronounced cam shape to the body of the talus.[404] Everyone has a unique talar shape, and for some people, it is this shape that predisposes them to bone-on-bone contact even at very low angles of dorsiflexion. Again, yoga is not going to change that. You can stretch your calves all you want, or blame your tight Achilles tendon, but bone-on-bone compression is not going to go away.

Sometimes, the bone-on-bone compression is caused by *osteophytes*: bone spurs. These usually grow as a result of continued contact between two bones. As the bones repeatedly bang into each other, the surface of one starts to grow. These bumps (called osteophytes) may become large enough to limit movement. This is frequently observed in dancers and athletes. However, sometimes a growth in one area creates a corresponding divot in the opposite bone! One study of soccer players found that tibial osteophytes created a corresponding divot in the talus, which allowed full range of dorsiflexion to be maintained.[405]

A final cause of limitation to ankle dorsiflexion is subluxation of the bones. Subluxation is a movement of one or more bones so that they are misaligned.[406] Misaligned bones will not articulate normally, so range of motion is reduced. In the ankle, especially after a bad sprain, the fibula may become misaligned with either the tibia or the talus. This subluxation can limit the range of motion available. Recall that the proximal (top) end of the fibula needs to move freely to allow the ankle to move freely. If the fibula is subluxed forward (anteriorly) and downward (inferiorly) at the proximal or the distal tibial joint, normal dorsiflexion of the talus in the mortise will be limited.[407] However, the most common example of subluxation is that of the talus sitting forward after an ankle sprain. Most of the ankle sprains seen clinically present with limitation in the posterior glides of the talus, even with less severe ankle sprains. When the talus sits forward at the talocrural joint, this causes limitation in dorsiflexion due to the boney block of the talus hitting the tibia. This is something that can limit people even a long time after an ankle sprain, if they have not had it treated and specifically mobilized or manipulated. Chronic ankle sprains and instability can lead to the talus slipping into this anterior position without the person even rolling the ankle and can limit such activities as sitting cross-legged (with the foot in inversion and plantar flexion), due to the joint's instability.

Restrictions to Plantarflexion

Compression can and does arise in some people when they plantarflex the ankle. In most of these cases, the individual may have extra bones or bony growth, which can create compression. For some people, especially dancers who lift up onto the balls of their feet frequently, compression may arise between the calcaneus and the tibia. Figure 2.237 shows a full plantarflexed foot, with 90° of extension at the metatarsophalangeal joints. Notice the point of compression in this instance. We see a small extra bone that most people do not have: the os trigonum. It is getting caught in between the calcaneus and the tibia. In this case, a dancer rising up to *demi-pointe* may still be able to plantarflex the foot fully, but the continued compression of the os trigonum could cause pain and pathology.[408]

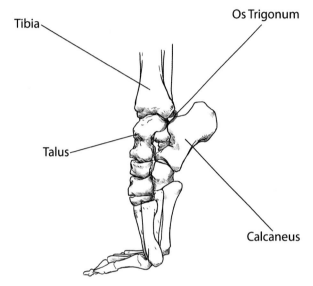

Tibia

Os Trigonum

Talus

Calcaneus

FIGURE 2.237 Plantarflexed foot, showing compression of the os trigonum (in red) between the tibia and the calcaneus.

Other causes of compression that can limit plantarflexion include osteophytes, ossicles or a Stieda process, which is an extended growth of the talus bone (see figure 2.227). These conditions may or may not cause painful posterior ankle impingement syndrome, but this syndrome does occur quite frequently in athletes and dancers due to their frequent need to fully plantarflex the foot with dynamic, transient stress applied.

Fortunately, in yoga, we rarely have to plantarflex so much and under such dynamic stress. Plantarflexion may be adopted, but we hold the position for a period of time, unlike an athlete who may need to make the movement only briefly—for example, a soccer player kicking the ball will forcefully but briefly plantarflex the foot.

Restrictions to Pronation

As shown in table 2.17, the ranges of abduction and adduction are similar, but the range for inversion is almost twice that as for eversion; it is easier to turn the sole inward than outward. One reason for that is the fibula. The distal (lower) end of the fibula prevents the talus from everting too much.

This is a bone-on-bone restriction, and its location is shown in red in figure 2.233c.

Restrictions to Supination

In extreme cases, compression can arise between the tarsal bones and the medial tibia, but this will normally only happen after a severe sprain of the lateral ligaments. However, as always, there are some people who possess amazing ranges of supination without having had sprained or otherwise injured ankles. Look back at figure 2.234c (page 230) for the example of B.K.S. Iyengar in Kandasana, which requires a lot of supination. His ankles were neither broken nor damaged; this was just part of his natural range of motion.

VARIATIONS IN RANGES OF MOTION

The ultimate range of motion we have, once we have worked through our tensile resistance, is dictated by where and when compression will occur, but that varies considerably due to normal variations in human shapes and sizes.

Dorsiflexion of the Ankle

How much dorsiflexion we can obtain will depend upon a number of factors, such as whether the movement is active or passive, or whether the knee is flexed or extended, or whether we are extending or flexing the toes. These variables dictate how much tension will be created in the muscles, tendons, ligaments and fascia of the leg and foot. A person who is limited in their range of dorsiflexion to 10° or less has a condition termed *ankle joint equinus*. This can lead to a number of pathologies, such as genu recurvatum (knock-knees) and excessive subtalar pronation, as well as an altered walking gait. Limited ankle dorsiflexion is also a factor in poor balance and falls in elderly people. Equinus can be caused by shortness or contracture in the calf muscles or by other pathologies that create joint stiffness.[409] Fortunately, where tension is a cause of equinus, stretching programs are effective in increasing range of motion.[410] Another factor may dictate a more significant barrier to deeper dorsiflexion: compression, where the top of the foot (the talus) comes into contact with the leg (the tibia), or soft tissue (various tendons) becomes trapped between the two bones.

VARIATIONS IN DORSIFLEXION RANGE

There is a significant difference between the range of dorsiflexion when the knee is fully extended and when it is fully flexed. (Yoga students often notice this; the stretch they feel in their calves is much more noticeable in Down Dog [Adhomukhasvanasana] when the legs are straight than when the knees are bent.) This is due to the tensile resistance of the gastrocnemius. When the knee is extended and the ankle is dorsiflexed, the gastrocs is at its longest and under the most tension. However, when the knee is flexed by 20° or more, the gastrocnemius is no longer a player in limiting dorsiflexion.[411] At 20° of knee flexion, the amount of dorsiflexion healthy people can do ranges from 20° passively (open chain/non-weightbearing) to 39° under stress (closed chain/weightbearing). One standard deviation for these measurements is 9° and 7°, respectively. This means the range of dorsiflexion for 95% of healthy individuals, with the knee bent and while bearing weight, is 25–53° (see figure 2.238).

It is interesting to recall the amount of ankle dorsiflexion required to:[412]

- Kneel (toes tucked under/ankles dorsiflexed): 26–45°
- Sit cross-legged: 26–39°
- Squat with heels on the floor: 33–45°

These three movements and positions often are required in yoga classes. Clearly, someone with a 53° range of dorsiflexion will have no problem with any of them, but someone with less than 20° of dorsiflexion available will find some of them challenging. It is instructive to learn what stops these students from obtaining greater dorsiflexion. Is it tension or compression? Can it be changed, or have they reached the limit of what their ankles can do? As we have seen in answering our WSM? question, the impediments to movements can come either from tension in tissues that do not easily stretch to accommodate movement, or from compression, where some part of the body comes into contact with another part of the body and further movement

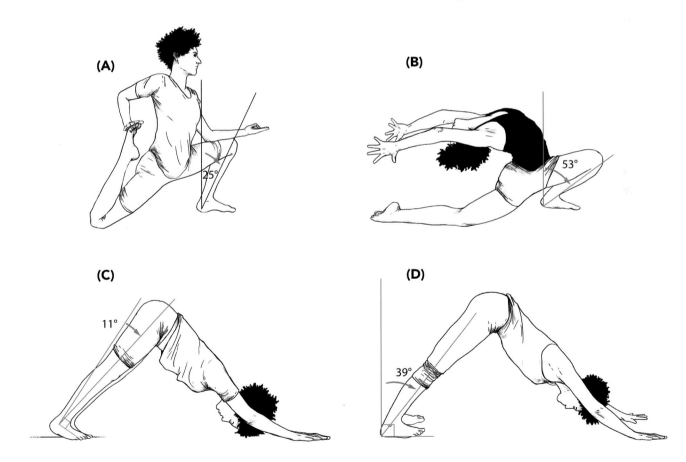

FIGURE 2.238 Ranges of dorsiflexion. With the knee flexed 20° or more, the normal range of active dorsiflexion goes from 25° (a) to 53° (b); with the knee fully extended, the normal range of active dorsiflexion is 11° (c) to 39° (d). When only 11° of dorsiflexion is available, most students will need to have their heels lifted off the floor in Down Dog if their legs are straight. Students with more dorsiflexion available can do a longer Down Dog and still keep their heels on the ground.

is not available. All these factors can come into play with dorsiflexion of the ankle. What is stopping you may be either tension or compression, and, as shown in figure 2.239, where you feel the resistance will give you the clue you need to determine the answer to your WSM? question.

Compression can arise from the talus coming into contact with the tibia, which is a hard, bone-on-bone form of compression, or from soft tissues becoming trapped between the two bones, which is the medium form of compression. Primates that climb trees generally require about 45° of dorsiflexion at the ankle, which is considerably more than the average human has available. One key cause of this enhanced range of motion in climbing primates such as

chimpanzees is the shape and width of their tibial plafond (see figure 2.221). Chimps' plafonds are trapezoid and wider at the front than human plafonds, which are more square. This means that the ankles of chimps can dorsiflex much more before the talus impinges upon the tibia. Human feet are not well adapted to climbing trees but are very good at walking and running.[413] If you happen to be someone with a wider or more trapezoid tibial plafond, you are likely to have a much greater range of ankle dorsiflexion (figure 2.238b) than an average person (figure 2.238a), not because you have stretched your calf muscles more but due to the variation in your ankle bones.

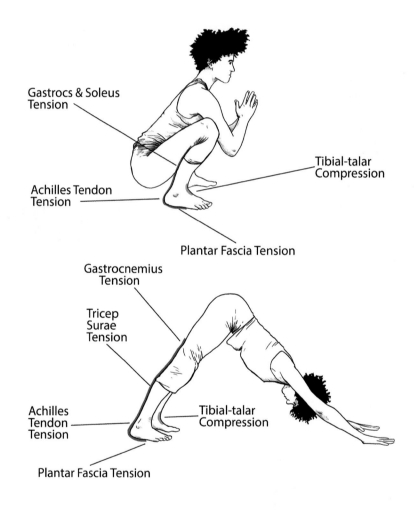

Gastrocs & Soleus Tension

Achilles Tendon Tension

Tibial-talar Compression

Plantar Fascia Tension

Gastrocnemius Tension

Tricep Surae Tension

Achilles Tendon Tension

Tibial-talar Compression

Plantar Fascia Tension

FIGURE 2.239 What stops you in dorsiflexion? Where do you feel resistance? The sensations may be due to muscular, tendinous, ligamentous or fascial tension (shown in blue), or bone-on-bone compression (shown in red).

IT'S IMPORTANT: Don't assume it's your ankles!

Here is a common question yoga students ask and the answer they commonly offer: "Why do my heels come up off the floor when I lower down into Squat (Malasana)? It must be my tight ankles." Yes, maybe it is your ankles, but as we have seen, squatting requires somewhere between 33° and 45° of dorsiflexion, and most people can get that much from their ankles when the knees are flexed. For 67% of the population, the range of dorsiflexion with knees flexed is 32° to 46°, nicely within the range needed for squatting.[414] So, why can't you get your heels to the ground in squats? Maybe you are the one person in six who can't dorsiflex their ankles enough to squat,[415] or maybe it is due to a lack of flexion available in your hips! For some people, restrictions in flexing the knees may be the limiting factor. It is not always about the ankles.

As shown in figure 2.240, when you descend into a squat, in order to counterbalance the weight of your derrière, which is hanging back over your heels, your knees need to come forward, or you will need to bring your arms out in front of your body, or you will lean your upper body over your feet more. The closer your knees can come to your chest, the closer your backside can come to the side-midline of the body when you squat, so the easier it is to find the counterbalance between the front and back body parts. However, if you are limited in your hip flexion, then your backside will be further back, away from the midline of the body as you descend into the squat. This added posterior distance of your posterior will require your knees to travel further forward for counterbalance; for many people, the only way to achieve that is to rise up onto the toes, lifting the heels, as shown in figure 2.240c. This is not because their ankles aren't flexible enough but because they can't flex their hips enough.

In reality, the amount of ankle dorsiflexion required to come into a squat is at the maximum when you are only halfway down! Figure 2.240 shows the ankle angles in both the full squat (d) and the halfway down to squat position (b). At halfway down, your knees need to be much further forward of the feet because your butt is much further backwards. Knees being further forward means a greater angle at the ankles is needed, or the heels have to lift.

One option for people who can't flex their hips enough to stay in a squat is to widen the distance between their feet and/or point their feet outward. When they do this, they increase the range of hip flexion available; it has nothing to do with adding more dorsiflexion in the ankles. With the legs abducted or with the femurs externally rotated further, there is less chance for the neck of the femur to impinge on the acetabulum or for the anterior superior iliac spine to come into compression with the top of the thighs. Through these adjustments, the back side of the body can track closer to the side-midline of the body as you descend into the squat, which means the knees do not have to come as far forward to counterbalance the body.

How do you know what is stopping you? Notice what you feel in your squat. Are you stopped from tracking your knees further forward due to tension in the back of your calves, or compression in the front of your ankles, or compression in the hips, or restrictions around the knee? If it is in your hips, try widening your feet; if it is in the back of your calves, work on lengthening the calf muscles; if it is compression in the front of the ankles, try using a wedge under your heels. Using a wedge or some other support is not cheating. Bone-on-bone compression is not going to change, so you might as well accept your reality and adjust accordingly.

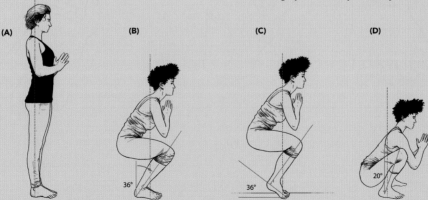

FIGURE 2.240 What stops me as I come into squats (Malasana)? The maximum dorsiflexion of the ankles is required in (b); (c) the heels may start to lift off the floor; (d) requires less dorsiflexion but maximum hip flexion.

IT'S COMPLICATED:
Where should the dorsiflexed foot point?

We have seen that the aesthetic requirement that the feet always point straight ahead in various standing postures—such as Mountain Pose (Tadasana), the front foot in Warrior Poses (Virabhadrasana) or lunges, or even in Down Dog (Adhomukhasvanasana)—is not a good alignment cue for every body. While it is easy for a teacher to see where the foot is pointing, changing the foot alignment has repercussions higher up. There are many factors we have already looked at that play a role in where the neutral foot will point: the degree of version of the acetabulum (lower version tends to point the foot more outward); the version of the neck of the femur (again, lower version angles will point the foot more outward); tibial torsion (the more torsion or twist to the tibia, the more the foot will point outwards); whether the knee is fully extended and locked or not (the tibia externally rotates coming into the locked position, and this can point the foot outward—and, if the knee is hyperextended, even more tibial rotation occurs);[416] the amount of tibial twist that is occurring if the knee is flexed; and the amount of rotation the femur is doing at the hip socket. All of these conditions can affect where the foot is pointing, and yet none of them have anything to do with the foot itself. Of course, the congruence of the bones in the ankle joint and the shape of these bones can also affect where the foot points.

The terms abduction and adduction, when applied to the foot, refer to movements away from or towards the second ray of the foot—i.e., the second toe. The second ray is considered the neutral line of the foot, thus, yoga teachers often will suggest students point their second toe straight ahead, or align their knee with the second toe. But this is an aesthetic request, not necessarily a functional one. Not every student is aligned in a natural neutral position when the second ray of the foot is pointing straight ahead! *Some* students are nicely aligned in this position, but most will not be, and for these students, rotating the foot to achieve this aesthetically pleasing position will require some sort of rotation of the leg (tibia) or thigh (femur), which may not be ideal.

The movement of the foot during dorsiflexion is another reason that the foot could be pointing anywhere but straight ahead and yet still be in its neutral position. To our list of conditions that affect where the foot will point we must add the shape of the ankle bones—both the shape of

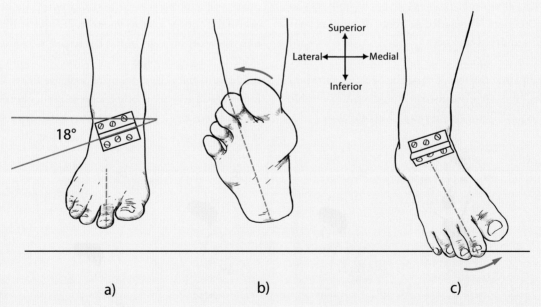

a)   b)   c)

FIGURE 2.241 The foot will exhibit medial or lateral movement as the ankle flexes (right foot); (a) the foot in neutral—notice how the second ray points straight ahead; with dorsiflexion (b), the foot abducts superiorly and laterally (outwardly); with plantarflexion (c), the foot adducts inferiorly and medially (inwardly). The greater the empirical axis angle, the more pronounced this effect will be.

the mortise formed by the tibia and fibula and the shape of the top of the talus (its trochlea). The rotation of the ankle follows its empirical axis, formed from the inferior tips of the fibula and tibia. The axis is angled both inferiorly and posteriorly from medial to lateral, as was shown in figure 2.223. The effect of the empirical axis being oblique can be seen in figure 2.241. Presented is a right foot. Notice how with dorsiflexion, the big toe of the foot abducts more laterally (outwardly) than when the foot is neutral. In the other direction, plantarflexion, the big toe of the foot adducts more medially (inwardly) than when the foot is neutral.[417] The greater the empirical axis angle, the more pronounced this effect will be.

We have seen that the range of human variation affects the empirical axis along which the ankle rotates. This reality means that for some people, when the ankle dorsiflexes, the foot naturally moves laterally and the second ray of the foot (the second toe) will naturally point more outward. Consequently, when the ankle dorsiflexes, it is natural for the foot to want to rotate laterally outward. This is just one more reason why the feet may want to abduct when we come into the deep flexion of the ankles required to do Squat Pose (Malasana). The same tendency may be observed in other postures that require a lot of dorsiflexion of the ankles: a low lunge with the knee over the toes, or in Down Dog. (See Note to Teachers: Aligning the feet in Down Dog, on page 246.)

Where should the foot point? That depends! It depends upon the shape and orientation of your acetabula, the torsion of your femurs and tibias, whether the knee is full extended or deeply flexed, upon the length of your fibula relative to your tibia and the amount of curvature in your talus, and upon how much you are flexing your ankles. There is no predefined "right" position for your feet—but there is an alignment that may be optimal for you, given your anatomical uniqueness. Your challenge is to find what works for you. To do that, you need to learn how to pay attention and observe what is going on when you are in certain postures and positions.

Plantarflexion of the Ankle

Plantarflexion results in the sole (the plantar portion) moving away from the front of the leg. We do this in many yoga postures: when we rise up on our toes to challenge our balance, or to lift the heels in Upward-Facing Bow (Urdvadhanurasana), the front foot in Triangle Pose (Trikonasana), in sitting or kneeling postures where the foot is pointed backwards, such as Hero Pose (Virasana), in postures where we grab and hold the back foot or big toe, such as King Dancer (Natarajasana), or when the legs are on the floor and straight backwards, as in Upward-Facing Dog (Urdhvamukhasvanasana). See figure 2.242 for a few examples of these postures, and notice the plantarflexion of the feet.

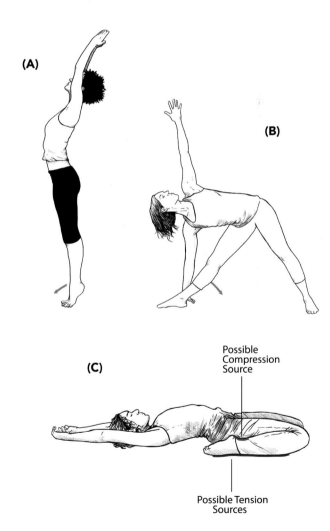

FIGURE 2.242 Some of the yoga postures that require plantarflexion: (a) standing stretch, (b) Triangle (Trikonasana) and (c) Hero Pose (Suptavirasana). Notice that compression may arise at the back of the heel, while tension may be felt on the top of the foot or in the front of the shin.

In most cases, our plantarflexion is passive: the foot comes into plantarflexion due to the shape of the pose, not due to strong action of the plantarflexion muscles. Passive postures include the Hero Pose. Sometimes, while in a posture that involves plantarflexion, we are encouraged to try to dorsiflex the foot; for example, in Upward-Facing Dog, or Cobra (Bhujangasana), or the back leg in lunges or Pigeon (Kapotasana), or the held foot in Bow Pose (Dhanurasana) or King Dancer, we may be requested to push the top of the foot into the floor or the hand. This action creates a co-contraction of the leg muscles and serve to stabilize the foot and back leg. Other times when active plantarflexion is required include rising onto the toes—then the plantarflexors must engage strongly. When we root the foot into the floor, which we may do for the front foot in Triangle Pose or in any of the Warrior Postures (Virabhadrasanas), we are plantarflexing. In these standing postures, we do not move the foot away from the leg but rather the leg away from the foot, but it is still plantarflexion.

VARIATIONS IN RANGE OF MOTION

An average, healthy person has the ability to plantarflex 50–60°. Most people require 8–46° of plantarflexion for normal living, so they have no problem with their daily functional need for plantarflexion. This range decreases slightly as we age and is a bit higher for women, but the differences are not very significant. Even men in the 45–69 age bracket have the ability to plantarflex 50°.[418] But these figures are for healthy individuals. There may be several reasons why someone cannot plantarflex their ankles very much, and these limitations can affect both their yoga practice and simple daily living. Pathology may prevent someone from achieving the plantarflexion range of motion daily life requires: disease, illness, accident, injury. Or there may be no pathology, and the limitations are just due to that person's natural genetic inheritance.

HOW MUCH PLANTARFLEXION DO WE NEED IN YOGA?

Figure 2.242 shows plantarflexion in a variety of yoga postures. We could say that "maximum"[419] plantarflexion is required for the sitting postures, such as Hero Pose (Virasana) or Lightening Bolt (Vajrasana) and their variations (Suptavirasana), where the top of the foot is flat on the floor. How much is this? Figure 2.243 shows us. Surprisingly, it is not 90°! The traditional (although not the most consistent) way to measure angles of foot movement is with a device called a *goniometer* (from the Greek for "angle" and "measure"). In figure 2.243, the goniometer shows that the angle of the ankle when the foot is fully pointed and the top of the foot is straight is about 70°.[420]

Most people are able to actively plantarflex their ankles 50–60°, so sitting on their heels with the tops of their feet flat on the floor may be challenging. That extra 10–20° of plantarflexion may not be available, but since the sitting postures are passive, there may be a little bit of extra plantarflexion available for most people to almost get there. If

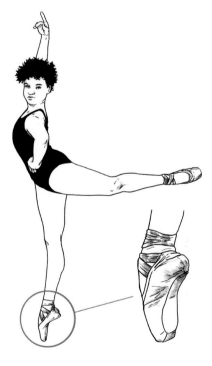

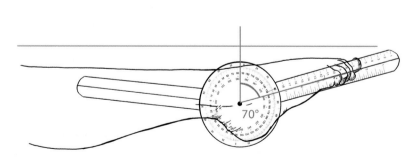

FIGURE 2.243 A fully plantarflexed foot requires only 70° of plantarflexion to get the top of the foot flat with the shin, as measured by a goniometer.

FIGURE 2.244 A dancer *en pointe*. Note how the foot is fully plantarflexed.

there is pain or discomfort in the tendons at the top of the foot, folded towels under the ankle may help make this pose more accessible. If resistance is felt in the top of the foot, this indicates that tension is restraining the movement, and it is possible, over time, to work out that tensile resistance and get the top of the foot flat on the floor. However, if the sensation is occurring in the rear of the foot, between the heel and the posterior tibia, we are now experiencing compression, and this impingement may not be resolvable through yoga. The student may have reached her ultimate limit of plantarflexion and may never be able to have the tops of her feet flat on the floor.

We say "may" in these cases because some causes of impingement at the back of the heel can be treatable or temporary. Inflammation may be causing local swelling in this area, and if that inflammation is removed, the impingement may also go away. If the impingement is caused by an ossicle, osteophyte or even an os trigonum or Stieda process, and if this is problematic for the student, these bony growths can be excised in surgery. Some athletes and dancers do need such interventions to resolve the pain of deep plantarflexion. But if there is no pain or injury, and deeper plantarflexion is blocked by the presence of one or more of these bones, it may be more yogic to simply accept that this is your body's limit.

In some elite dancers and athletes, the range of plantarflexion goes beyond the top of the foot being flat. Some people can deeply plantarflex at the transverse tarsal joints and the metatarsophalangeal joints in addition to the ankle joint. Figure 2.244 shows the foot of a dancer *en pointe*—standing on the tips of her toes. Notice how the top of her foot is beyond flat. We could say that she is hyper-plantarflexing the foot and ankle, because the line is past 180°. But notice how much of this plantarflexion is coming from her midfoot, not just her ankle.

This can happen also in Upward-Facing Dog (Urdhvamukhasvanasana), as shown in figure 2.245; some students can press the tops of their feet down so firmly while lifting their legs up that their foot hyper-plantarflexes like a ballerina, which may allow them be firmly rooted at the feet and raise their hips high off the floor.

Supination and Pronation of the Foot

Yoga teachers tend to ask students to minimize any observable pronation or supination of the feet. If the front foot in a lunge or Warrior Pose (Virabhadrasana) is pronating, the student will be asked to bring the knee back in line with the foot, thus supinating the foot. If the foot is supinating in Lotus Pose (Padmasana) or the back foot in Pigeon Pose (Kapotasana) is deemed to be *sickling* (which is a negative way to say "supinating"), the teacher will request that the student pronate the foot to bring it back to a neutral position. It almost seems that no amount of either supination or pronation is a good thing, and yet these movements are very natural and often very necessary. They do not always need to be corrected.

To be clear: there may be valid reasons for a student to correct a pronated or supinated foot. A pronated foot tends to shorten that leg, which in a standing posture could put strain on the knee or pull the hip laterally downward, into abduction. When pronated, the medial arch is diminished. A foot that is supinating may put more weight on the outside of the foot, lengthen the leg and laterally tilt the hip upward, into adduction. Pronation or supination of the foot can have ramifications further up the chain, but these movements by themselves are not inherently dangerous and do not automatically need fixing or addressing.

People who have larger ranges of pronation or supination of the feet than the norm do not have higher rates of injuries. A 2013 study of over 900 beginning runners (that's over 1,800 feet!) observed that 20% of the study population had supinated feet, 3% had highly supinated feet, 6% had pronated feet, 1% had highly pronated feet and 70% were "normal." The researchers found no correlation between the rate of injuries in normal feet and supinated feet, but interestingly, people with pronated feet actually had a lower

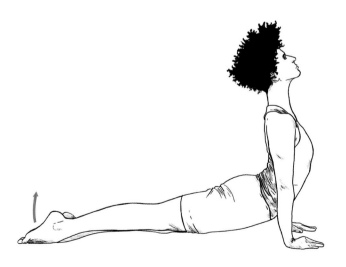

FIGURE 2.245 Upward-Facing Dog (Urdhvamukhasvanasana) also requires deep, active plantarflexion of the feet.

incidence of injury from running. The researchers concluded that the common belief that pronation automatically leads to higher injury rates is not true, although they admitted that for highly pronated feet, more study is needed.[421]

What does this imply for our yoga practice? Should we avoid pronation or supination? It all depends on what the student is experiencing. If there is a problem, if there is pain or some known underlying pathology, care should be taken and pain not tolerated. It is wise to back off when pain arises, unless the student is in the hands of a professional therapist who needs to work through some pain in order to mobilize a joint that has become stuck due to adhesions or scar tissue.

Figure 2.246 shows Lotus Pose, where a student is supinating his foot significantly. Most teachers will ask this student to straighten (pronate) the foot to avoid this degree of supination (or sickling). However, refer back again to figure 2.234c (page 230), which shows B.K.S. Iyengar in Kandasana. The feet are intentionally extremely supinated! In his book *Light on Yoga*, Mr. Iyengar says that this "cures stiffness in the hip, knee and ankle joints."[422] So, why is sickling the foot bad in Lotus Pose (or the back foot in Pigeon Pose [Kapotasana], or in many other postures), but perfectly okay, and even required, in Kandasana? Judge a pose not by

its looks, but by its effect. Figure 2.234b shows a variation of Butterfly (Baddhakonasana) in which the feet are again deliberately supinated to "open the book" and "have the soles face heaven." The point is: supination and pronation are normal movements of the foot, they are required for us to walk or run normally, and they are not necessarily bad things to do in our yoga practice.

OTHER CAUSES OF SUPINATION OR PRONATION

It is now no longer a surprise that where the foot is pointing is not always an indication of something occurring solely at the foot; its position may be due to alignment of the bones higher up the chain, at the knee or the hip. For example: the often observed sickled foot of the back leg of a student in a lunge or Pigeon Pose (Kapotasana) may be due to the student trying to avoid discomfort in the back knee. If the foot is perfectly centered, the kneecap may be painfully pushed into the floor, and to avoid that, the student may internally rotate the whole leg to allow the stress on the knee to slip to the outside, where it is more comfortable. This internal rotation at the hip may make the foot appear supinated, but it is actually the whole leg that has rotated, not the foot. Correcting the foot would not be helpful for this student; rather, padding the knee or pressing the top of the foot into the floor lightly may be sufficient to take pressure off the kneecap and keep the leg straight.

This is important for both teachers and students: before addressing the position of the feet, it is useful to look higher and see what is happening at the core of the body and work your way outwards towards the extremities, not vice versa.

CO-CONTRACTION WILL STABILIZE THE JOINT

Stiffness is always stabilizing. When a joint is relaxed and not bearing any stress, it can be safely moved through a far greater range of motion than when it is under stress or bearing weight. Open-chain, passive stress will result in greater ranges of movement than closed-chain, active stress. When a joint is bearing a load, we want to stabilize the joint, not try to get as much range of motion as possible. To stabilize the foot and ankle, stiffness is required, and we can achieve that through co-contraction of the muscles that move the ankle and foot. When the joints are not under stress, they can

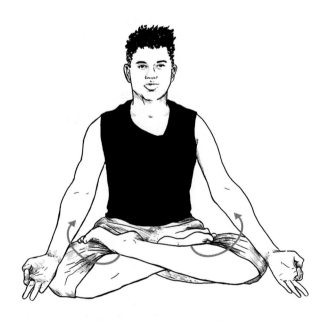

FIGURE 2.246 Supination in Lotus Pose (Padmasana). To reduce the amount of supination occurring, most teachers will advise that the student try to pronate the foot, as indicated by the red arrows.

passively move to their edges, which is what we do in Kandasana or Padmasana, or even with the back foot in lunges. However, when your feet passively pronate inward in a weightbearing, closed-chain posture such as Wide-Legged Standing Pose (Prasaritapadottanasana), it is a good idea to actively supinate the ankles to provide stability to this joint under stress. The same logic would apply to the back foot in standing postures like Triangle (Trikonasana) or the Warriors (Virabhadrasana): the tendency is to pronate the back foot, so active supination (moving the inner ankles away from the floor) will create a co-contraction of the muscles all around the ankle and midfoot, stiffening and thus supporting the joint.

The Four Movements of the Toes

We have simplified the movements of the foot and ankle, but the movements of the toes by comparison actually are quite simple. The toes can flex and extend, abduct and adduct. With the toes, the terms get changed a bit, but the basics still apply. Extension may be called dorsiflexion, while flexion may become plantarflexion. Abduction and adduction have a different plane of reference: they describe movements away from or towards the second toe. Toes are multi-jointed, and the movements of flexion and extension can happen where the metatarsals join the proximal phalanges (the *metatarsophalangeal* joint) or within the phalangeal joints.

LIMITATIONS TO EXTENSION (DORSIFLEXION) AND FLEXION (PLANTARFLEXION) OF THE TOES

Unfortunately, some people will never get 90° of freedom of extension, due to various causes of rigidity in the toe (called *hallux rigidus*), including osteophyte growths (bone spurs) on the dorsal (top) side of the metatarsal heads. Yoga will not help people with bone spurs increase their range of motion, but surgery might. So might alternative therapies—for *(continued on page 247)*

NOTE TO TEACHERS:
Sickling—plantarflexion with supination

The axis of the ankle, called the empirical axis, is oblique. As shown in figure 2.241, this means that when we plantarflex the foot, some adduction or supination of the foot naturally occurs. This is not a problem and does not necessarily need to be corrected. However, many yoga teachers do not like the look of a foot that in their view appears "sickled." They will suggest that the student "straighten" the foot by everting it. These teachers' intentions are valid: they wish to avoid torquing the knee by avoiding sickling the foot, but their prescription may not be effective. In some cases, the sickling that they are sick of is a natural outcome of the movement of the foot, and no stress is occurring in the knee.

Teachers may often notice the foot of the back leg in Pigeon Pose (Kapotasana), or Monkey Splits (Hanumanasana), or both feet in Upward-Facing Dog supinating slightly. This may be due entirely to the effects of plantarflexion, or a low amount of tibial torsion, or highly anteverted acetabula or femoral torsion. There may be many reasons why that back foot is supinated, and none of these reasons have anything to do with creating a torque in the knees. These positions of the foot may be quite normal and safe for the student. If sickling was always bad, well—look back at figure 2.234c for the example of B.K.S. Iyengar in Kandasana. Would you correct him? His feet are greatly sickled, but that is a requirement of this posture.

However, if you are concerned, feel free to ask the student what she is feeling in her knees. If there is discomfort or pain in the ankle, knee or hips, suggest she try straightening the foot and see whether that helps. But if she is nicely grounded already, firm and solid in her posture, and there is no pain when the foot is sickled, then why try to correct her natural alignment? Let her be. You may notice that when you do get your student to straighten her sickled foot, she can no longer plantarflex her foot fully, and the top of her ankle may come off the floor, losing some of her grounded sensation there. Which is more important: alignment or grounding? Remember your intention for the pose, and focus on function, not appearance.

NOTE TO TEACHERS: Aligning the feet in Down Dog

In your training to become a yoga teacher and probably for many years after that, you have heard the instructions to "keep your feet hip-distance apart and toes pointing straight ahead" when coming into Down Dog (Adhomukhasvanasana). You may have heard many variations on this theme: "Keep your feet parallel," "If you can see your heels, try turning them out slightly so you can't see them anymore," or even, from B.K.S. Iyengar, "Make sure your feet are in line with your hands and the same distance apart."[426] Throughout our exploration of the natural range of variation in the human body, we have seen that there are no alignment cues that work for every body, and for many bodies, the above cues will not be effective. To insist every student in your class must adhere to these dogmatic Dog instructions may do more harm than good for some. Even though the traditional, standardized alignment cues don't work for every body, there are personalized alignment cues that can and do work for individual bodies. One of the challenges of being a teacher is to help the student determine which alignment works for her body. This requires knowing what the *intention* of each pose is and paying close *attention* to what is happening while in the pose.

Before you offer Down Dog to a student, have a reason in your own mind as to what you want the student to feel: are you putting the student in Down Dog to build upper-body strength, lower-body length or a combination of both, to begin to stress the back of the calves, or the hamstrings, to

dorsiflex the feet in preparation for a squat? There are many valid reasons for using Down Dog; make sure your reason is also functionally valid.

But what is the right placement for the feet in every student's Down Dog? You will never know! So, help the student find her own answer. Give her some options, and let her decide what works best. Go ahead and offer the standard, traditional alignment cues—after all, you have to say something!—but ask her to notice how it feels for her body. Then offer some other options to compare with the standard approach, and direct her to notice how these positions feel.

For example, as shown in figure 2.247, start with the standard alignment cues, and direct the student's awareness to the feeling of stress in the legs, knees and ankles, but also in the pelvis, sacrum and lower back. Then offer the option of having the heels together and feet pointing outward. How does that feel? Some students may find that the heels are now firmly on the floor, whereas they were floating earlier. There may be greater rooting into the earth, but there may also be more compression in the sacrum. Is that good or bad? Compression is not necessarily bad, but painful compression is not good. Many students love this version of Down Dog! For some, it is not a good idea. Then try having the feet as wide apart as the mat, with the feet pointing inward. How does this feel? Most students will hate that version, but some will love it.

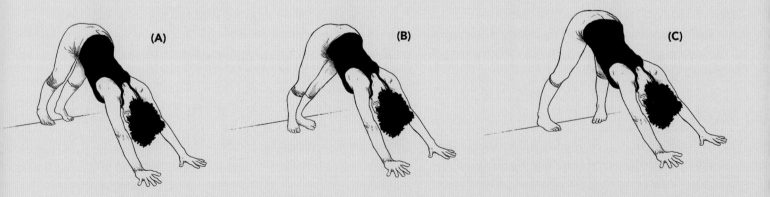

FIGURE 2.247 Down Dog (Adhomukhasvanasana) variations: (a) the Aesthetic Dog: feet hip-width apart and parallel; (b) the Narrow Dog, with heels together and feet externally pointed; (c) the Wide Dog, with feet as wide as the mat but internally pointed.

If you have time, play with all possibilities; there are nine orientations to experiment with, made up of three width variations (feet together, hip-width apart or as wide as the yoga mat) times three foot directions (parallel, externally pointed or internally pointed). You could play with all nine variations and ask the student to decide which one works best for her today. Of course, you would want to let her take some rest in between each exploration so fatigue is not a factor in deciding which one feels right.

The point is, no two dogs are exactly alike. A Saint Bernard is not jealous of a Chihuahua just because the Chihuahua is more flexible; there are other benefits to being a Saint Bernard (you get to carry whisky in the little barrel attached to your dog collar). Don't insist all the dogs in your class be of the same breed. Instead, let each student discover his inner canine.

example, stop wearing high heels, and start wearing shoes with wider toe boxes! Yoga may help people with other causes of hallux rigidus, but it really depends upon the source of the restriction.

Another, and surprising, cause of limitations to extending the toes is our skin! Tension in the fascia of the ball of the foot can be transferred to the surface skin of the proximal phalangeal joint, which can restrict extension.[423] Tightness in the flexors of the toes can also work against extension and vice versa: tension in the extensor muscles can restrict flexion.

ABDUCTION AND ADDUCTION
Abduction and adduction occur primarily at the metatarsophalangeal joint. Within the more distal interphalangeal joints, the movements allowed are flexion and extension, not abduction or adduction. Here we find that flexion is generally greater than extension, even though at the metatarsophalangeal joint extension is greater than flexion. Extension at the interphalangeal joints is limited by the passive resistance of the toe flexor muscles, plantar fascia and ligaments, and joint capsules.

INCREASING RANGE OF MOTION
Academically, the most interesting joint relating to the toes is the metatarsophalangeal joint, and the most interesting movement is extension (dorsiflexion), as shown by the fact that academics have produced virtually no studies on metatarsophalangeal flexion![424] This holds true for yoga teachers too; they are most interested in extension of the toes, although some teachers do like to ask for some abduction as well. Spreading your toes is a nice idea, especially before coming into a standing balance posture. One particularly effective posture for developing abduction of the toes is called The Zipper, as shown in figure 2.248. The Zipper can be done while students are in Butterfly Pose (Baddhakonasana). Toe Squats, shown in figure 2.249 and especially as they are practiced in yin yoga, are an effective way to passively increase extension range of motion of the toes, as well as develop ankle dorsiflexion.[425]

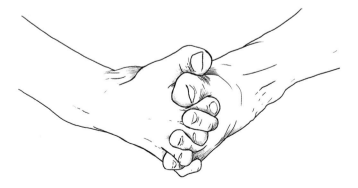

FIGURE 2.248 The Zipper, a great way to increase abduction.

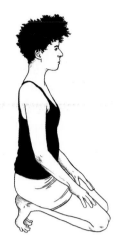

FIGURE 2.249 Toe Squat, a great way to increase extension.

There are yoga teachers who love to have their students work their toes—and why not! Normally, toes are the furthest thing from our minds, both literally and figuratively, but strong, flexible, healthy toes are valuable for growing old gracefully. Instead of imprisoning your toes in dead animals' skins all day long, then wondering why you have lost a lot of your balance as you grow older, yoga can free the feet and let the toes move. Figure 2.250 shows two toe movements that can be added to most seated, straight-legged postures. Extend the big toe while flexing the other toes (that should be easy), and then flex the big toe while extending the others—point the big toe while drawing the other four back (that may be hard, at first). Other good exercises include using your feet as hands and picking up things with your toes; picking up socks off the floor is a great starting practice, but then go for more challenging objects, such as golf balls (good luck with that!).

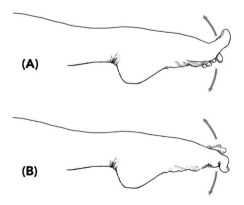

FIGURE 2.250 Toe exercises: (a) extend the big toe while flexing the other toes; (b) then flex the big toe while extending the others.

Ankle–Foot Segment Summary

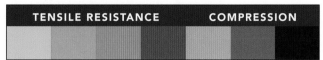

We can employ the WSM? spectrum to summarize what may stop you from greater ranges of motion in your feet and ankles. Table 2.20 shows the WSM? spectrum applied to each of the main movements possible in the ankle and foot. As we start from the left end of the spectrum, progress in working through tension is relatively easy, but as we get closer to the right, it becomes progressively harder (it is difficult to stretch ligaments), and at the far right, the game is over: no further progress in that direction for that pose will ever happen once one bone hits another. Asking WSM? helps to locate where you are along this spectrum, and thus you will know whether it is wise to try to go further. Remember, due to the reality of human variation, the shape and orientation of some people's bones mean that they will move very quickly to the right, while others will have a very large range of motion available to them before reaching their final edge.

Warning: This table does not indicate *why* the tension may have arisen. As we saw in Volume 1, there are many causes for tension; it is not always due to short muscles. The tension may be due to emotions, nervous system interactions, your state of hydration or pathologies. Scar tissue or inflammation can cause tension, and compression can arise from a torn labrum. The limitations suggested in the table are not static facts but indicators of possibilities. The table is for general guidance, not specific evaluation. Everyone has to answer for themselves, "What is stopping me?"

The ankle (talocrural joint) moves in dorsiflexion and plantarflexion. The foot can move in pronation and supination at several joints, but mostly at the subtalar joint and the transverse tarsal joint. The toes can flex, extend, abduct and adduct. What causes these motions has been described in the section on the muscles of the ankle-joint segment. The major factors that stop, hinder, prevent or reduce these movements are summarized in table 2.20.

TABLE 2.20 The WSM? spectrum for the ankle-joint segment.

MOVEMENT OF THE ANKLE AND FOOT	TENSILE RESISTANCE			COMPRESSION	
	MYOFASCIAL MERIDIANS* THAT RESIST MOVEMENT	MUSCLES THAT RESIST MOVEMENT	LIGAMENTS THAT RESIST MOVEMENT	SOURCE OF MEDIUM COMPRESSION	SOURCE OF HARD COMPRESSION
Ankle dorsiflexion	plantar fascia, superficial back line	**primarily**: gastrocnemius when knee is extended; soleus when knee is flexed over 20° **secondarily**: tibialis posterior plantaris, peroneus longus and brevis, flexor digitorum longus, flexor hallucis longus	deltoid ligament (the tibiotalar fibers), calcaneofibular ligament, posterior talofibular ligament	extensors tendons caught between talus and tibia, inflammation of tissues caught between talus and tibia	talus abutting the tibial mortise, talus abutting the distal ends of the fibula and/or tibia, osteophytes trapped between talus and tibia
Ankle plantarflexion	superficial front line	dorsiflexors: tibialis anterior, extensor digitorum longus, extensor hallucis longus, peroneus tertius	deltoid ligament (tibionavicular fibers), anterior talofibular ligament		calcaneus abutting the tibia, talus (Stieda process) abutting the tibia, osteophytes or os trigonum caught between the calcaneus and tibia
Foot pronation	deep front line	invertors: tibialis anterior, tibialis posterior	deltoid collateral ligaments: tibionavicular ligament, tibiocalcaneal ligament, tibiotalar ligament, medial talocrural joint capsule		talus against the distal fibula
Foot supination	lateral lines	evertors: peroneus longus, peroneus brevis, peroneus tertius	calcaneofibular ligament, tarsal interosseous ligaments, talocalcaneal ligament, lateral talocrural joint capsule		talus against the distal tibia

THE ANKLE-FOOT SEGMENT

MOVEMENT OF THE ANKLE AND FOOT	TENSILE RESISTANCE			COMPRESSION	
	MYOFASCIAL MERIDIANS* THAT RESIST MOVEMENT	MUSCLES THAT RESIST MOVEMENT	LIGAMENTS THAT RESIST MOVEMENT	SOURCE OF MEDIUM COMPRESSION	SOURCE OF HARD COMPRESSION
Toe extension (dorsiflexion)	fascia of the ball of the foot	flexors: flexor digitorum longus, flexor hallucis longus, flexor hallucis brevis, flexor digitorum brevis, the lumbricals, the interossei, quadratus plantae			osteophytes (bone spurs)
Toe flexion (plantarflexion)		extensor digitorum longus, extensor hallucis longus, extensor digitorum brevis			impingement of the distal phalanges upon the proximal phalanges

* See Volume 1, pages 71–74, for a description of the myofascial meridians.

Volume 2 Summary

There are many answers to the question "What stops me?" The causes can be arranged into a spectrum, with two major divisions: either we are stopped by tension in our tissues that prevents us from going any further, or we are stopped by compression arising from the body hitting itself. We have been investigating the sources of tension and compression in the action of the lower body joints and noting how the range of human variations can affect our natural range of motions.

In the hip joint, tension can arise (i) in the fascia around the hip as well as fascia quite far away, (ii) in the muscles that articulate the hip and (iii) in the ligaments that bind the femur into the hip socket. Compression can arise in all of its three forms: soft, tissue-on-tissue compression, which may limit flexion; medium, when tissue is squeezed between bones, which may also limit flexion, abduction and adduction; and hard, bone-on-bone compression, which may limit any of the possible movements in the hip sockets, with the possible exception of extension. The wide range of variation in the shape and orientation of the femur and pelvis can have a profound effect on a yoga student's ultimate range of mobility. For most students, it will take time, perhaps years, to loosen up the tight tissues that present tensile resistance to greater mobility, but eventually, limitations to most movements in the hip socket will come from compression.

The knee joint is structurally quite different from the hip: there is little opportunity for the bones to compress into each other, and most limitations to the range of movements at the knee are due to tensile resistance of the soft tissues. The knee primarily flexes and extends; however, when the knee is bent, a limited amount of rotation is available. Once again, human variations will dictate just how much movement is ultimately possible. Variations in the stiffness and length of the binding ligaments, as well as the shape of the surfaces of the tibia, femur and patella determine mobility.

The ankle and foot joints are quite complex and allow for a confusing array of movements. The ankle basically dorsiflexes and plantarflexes, and the range of movement here is initially constrained by fascia, muscles and ligaments; but ultimately, the compression of the talus against the tibia restricts dorsiflexion, while the calcaneus abutting the tibia can limit plantarflexion. Supination and pronation of the foot are more complicated movements, but here, too, their limitations are ultimately due to bone-on-bone contact.

Just as our body has a vast range of shapes, sizes and abilities, yoga has a vast range of teachings and teachers. Not surprisingly, not all teachings are consistent from one tradition to another. For example, hatha yoga can be defined as all the physical forms of yoga practiced today in the West; however, hatha yoga is also the term often applied to a particular gentle form of physical yoga practice, distinct from power yoga, hot yoga, Ashtanga yoga and so on. So, what does "hatha" really mean? It depends upon the teacher. Many teachers offer a deeper insight into the word "hatha," explaining that it is made up of two syllables: "ha" and "tha." "Ha" means sun and "tha" means moon, and together they symbolize the union of opposites, which is one of the goals of hatha yoga.[427] However, other senior teachers claim that "ha" means moon and "tha" means sun.[428] You would expect that yoga teachers could at least agree on whether "ha" means sun or moon!

Teachers also vary in the alignment cues they offer to students. One teacher may suggest an alignment for the feet, claiming this positioning is critically important, only to have another teacher warn against such an alignment as it may cause injury. As confusing as it is to get diametrically opposite instructions from two respected teachers, it is more confounding when the same teacher gives contradictory instructions, depending upon the posture being explained. We have seen some examples: in extension of the femur in the hip socket, a teacher may warn against externally rotating the back leg while in Monkey Splits Pose (Hanumanasana), and yet the same teacher will require the student to do exactly that for the back leg in Warrior 1 Pose (Virabhadrasana I). Why is external rotation bad in some hip extensions but required in others? Similarly, we have seen a common alignment cue in Warrior 2 Pose (Virabhadrasana II) demanding that the knee must be over the ankle and never past the foot, and yet in Chair Pose (Utkatasana), it is required to bring the knee in front of the toes.

There are two possible sources for contradictory alignment cues offered in asana practice: the first is related to the history of alignment teaching in the West, as explained in the Foreword by Paul Grilley—aesthetics. Unfortunately, much of what passes for alignment instruction is based upon what looks good, not what is functionally healthy. It is true: it does look good to have the back leg internally rotated at the hip socket in Monkey Splits and to have the knee lined up over the ankle in Warrior 1. If everyone looks the same way in every pose, our sense of aesthetics is rewarded, and a yoga teacher can be congratulated on her adherence to a dogmatic teaching principle. However, from a functional point of view, how a student looks in a yoga posture is irrelevant: what is important is what the student is feeling in the pose.

The second possible source for alignment cues is a teacher's own personal inquiry. In this instance, a teacher while doing Monkey Splits in a certain way may have discovered that the sensations she gets in the pose are stronger and safer if she internally rotates her back leg. For her, doing so may have reduced an uncomfortable stress on her adductor muscles, thus lowering the risk of injury. Unfortunately, not being aware of the uniqueness of her body, she offers this cue to all her students, thinking that if she benefits from the alignment offered, so will they. Her intention is commendable, her personal experience undeniable, but unfortunately, her students are not her, and what works for her may not work for them.

Alignment cues are necessary, but they should never become dogma. They are guidelines, and the important part of the physical practice is the "checking-in" the student must do to make sure that the alignment she is testing is working for her. Is it giving an appropriate amount of stress to the targeted areas? If not—if there is too much stress and pain, or too little stress—then a new alignment may be necessary. And that new alignment may not be aesthetically pleasing at all. Alignment cues based solely on aesthetics, focusing on changing the shape of the pose to conform to some ideal look, will not work for every body. A functional approach, however, will develop personalized alignment cues that will work for that student's body. Only by knowing what your body can do will you be able to develop your own yoga practice, one that is both safe and effective.

After all, it's your body. Why not do your yoga?

APPENDIX A
List of Anatomical Directions and Movements

These tables relate to the planes of movement. They list directions associated with the axial body (the core) and the appendicular body (the limbs), as well as various terms referring to directions of possible movements for the whole body.

AXIAL BODY

Anterior	Located on or pertaining to the front of the body
Axial	Pertaining to the head, neck and trunk of the body
Bilateral	Both sides
Caudad	Towards the tail or posterior
Central	Located at the center or interior of the body
Cephalad	Towards the head
Contralateral	On the opposite side of the body or structure
Coronal	Parallel to the coronal suture of the cranium
Cranial	Pertaining to the head
Deep	Below the surface of the body
External	Outer (sometimes lateral)
Frontal	Along the coronal plane, parallel to the coronal suture, dividing the front and back of the body
Horizontal	Along the transverse plane, dividing the upper and lower body
Inferior	Lower, below or located away from the head
Internal	Inner (sometimes medial)
Ipsilateral	On the same side of the body or structure
Lateral	To the side or located away from the midline of the body
Longitudinal	Along the long axis
Medial	Toward the median plane or the midline of the body

Median Plane	The sagittal plane
Medius	Situated in the middle
Midsagittal	Sagittal plane that lies on the midline
Oblique	Diagonal
Occipital	Pertaining to the back of the cranium
Parasagittal plane	A side plane (sagittal) that is not through the middle of the body and thus divides the body into unequal left and right regions
Peripheral	Located away from the center
Posterior	Located on or pertaining to the back of the body
Sagittal	Parallel to the sagittal suture of the cranium, dividing the left and right sides of the body
Side	Parallel to the sagittal suture of the cranium, dividing the left and right sides of the body
Superficial	Located on or close to the surface of the body
Superior	Upper, above or located towards the head
Temporal	Pertaining to the lateral side of the cranium
Transverse	Along the plane that horizontally divides the upper and lower body
Unilateral	One-sided
Ventral	Towards the abdomen, center or lower surface
Vertical	Perpendicular to the horizon
Visceral	Deep

APPENDICULAR BODY

Appendicular	Pertaining to the appendages or limbs
Arm	The region of the body from the shoulder to the elbow
Distal	Away from the trunk of the body or the point of reference, or towards the end of a limb
Dorsal	Pertaining to the back of the foot or hand (the other side from the sole or the palm)

Fibular	Pertaining to the lateral side of the leg
Forearm	The region of the body from the elbow to the wrist
Leg	The region of the body from the knee to the ankle
Palmar	Pertaining to the palm
Plantar	Pertaining to the sole
Proximal	Closer to the trunk of the body or the point of reference
Radial	Pertaining to the lateral side of the forearm
Thigh	The region of the body from the hip to the knee
Tibial	Pertaining to the medial side of the leg
Ulnar	Pertaining to the medial side of the forearm
Valgus	Distal segment of a joint deviates laterally (e.g., knock-kneed)
Varus	Distal segment of a joint deviates medially (e.g., bow-legged)

BODY MOVEMENTS

Remember that movements can be combined and often are. These terms may also apply equally to the upper and lower appendicular skeleton.

Abduction	Movement of a limb away from the midline of the body, usually in the frontal (coronal) plane
Adduction	Movement of a limb towards the midline of the body, usually in the frontal (coronal) plane
Angulation	Changing the angle between the axis of articulating bones
Circumduction	Circular movement of a limb that combines abduction, flexion, adduction and extension
Counternutation	Nodding of the sacrum posteriorly and slightly upward relative to the top of the pelvis
Depression	Moving the scapula downward in the frontal (coronal) plane
Deviation	Radial deviation: moving the wrist so the thumb comes closer to the forearm Ulnar deviation: moving the wrist so the little finger comes closer to forearm
Dorsiflexion	Moving the ankle so the toes move towards the knee
Elevation	Moving the scapula upward in the frontal (coronal) plane
Eversion	Twisting the foot laterally, outward so that the sole faces to the side
Extension	Straightening a joint that increases the joint angle, commonly posteriorly in the side (sagittal) plane

Flexion	Bending at a joint that decreases the joint angle, commonly anteriorly in the side (sagittal) plane
Inversion	Twisting the foot medially, inward so that the sole faces to the midline of the body
Nutation	Nodding of the sacrum anteriorly and slightly downward relative to the top of the pelvis
Opposition	Moving the thumb and palm closer together
Plantarflexion	Moving the ankle so the toes move away from the knee
Pronation	Forearm: rotation of the forearm so the palm faces inward, backward or downward Foot: rotation of the foot so the sole faces laterally outward
Prone	Lying on the stomach
Protraction	Abduction of the scapula away from each other
Retraction	Adduction of the scapula towards each other
Rotation	Circular turning along the long axis
Supination	Forearm: rotation of the forearm so the palm faces outward, forward or upward Foot: rotation of the foot so the sole faces medially inward
Supine	Lying on the back
Translation	Sliding with no rotation or angulation

APPENDIX B
Variations in the Female Pelvis

Humans' natural walking ability is due in large part to the shape of our pelvis. Other great apes find it tiring to walk upright for any length of time. Their pelvises have large ilia situated posteriorly, facing backwards. Human pelvises have shorter ilia facing more laterally, to the side of the body. This important evolutionary adaption allowed humans to stabilize the upper body over one leg while walking, thanks to the position and actions of our small gluteal muscles.[429] Human pelvises, however, pay a price for this advantage: giving birth is much more complicated. The shape of the inlet plane of the pelvis for apes is quite ovoid, deeper front to back than from side to side (this shape is called *anthropoid*), which allows for their babies to come through the birth canal without changing the position of the head. Human babies, because of the different shape of the pelvis, have to change orientation as they pass through.

A horizontal line drawn across the greatest width of the greater pelvis (the upper bowl) is called the *transverse diameter*. In women, the transverse diameter is longer than the line from the sacrum to the pubis, called the *true conjugate*. This ovoid shape requires a baby's head to turn sideways when it begins to enter the birth canal. When the head reaches the lesser pelvis (the lower bowl), it has to turn again, this time facing backwards, so that the back of the head, which is the narrowest part of the skull, can fit through the space between the ischial tuberosities and the tailbone. (It is similar to the way that you can more easily put on a tight pullover shirt by starting from the back of your skull, rather than from the top.) However, not all women have the same shape to their pelvic inlet bowl. A study in the 1930s created a standard way to categorize the variety of types of bowls women have (see figure 2.300). While more recent studies have sought to simplify the original classifications, these four types are still used in textbooks.[430]

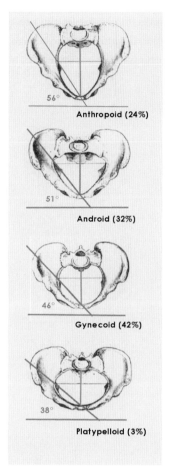

FIGURE 2.300 The four classical pelvic types, from Caldwell and Moloy (1933), based on their original illustration, with the angle of orientation of the side of the lesser (lower) pelvis bowl to the frontal plane. As the widest part of the lesser pelvis moves more forward, the orientation of the side of the pelvis is also more anterior, making external rotation in the hip socket more challenging. (Percentages show the frequency of occurrence in pelvises of Caucasian women.)

The four classifications named in the 1933 study were *gynecoid* (normal female form), *anthropoid* (ape-like), *android* (man-like) and *platypelloid* (flat), but there was a range of pelvises in between these four main types that varied by ethnic background and age. Girls' pelvic widths continue to widen as they get older, up to about age 25.[431] Approximately 42% of women have a gynecoid shape to their pelvis, and the number of incidences of problems giving birth are relatively low.[432] However, women who have narrower, android-shaped pelvises, occurring in 16–32% of women, find giving birth much more challenging and often require the use of forceps or Caesarean section.

With these images in mind, we can see how women's acetabula will generally be pointing more forward than men's. The sides of a gynecoid or platypelloid pelvis are orientated more anteriorly than the sides of an android or anthropoid pelvis. This helps us understand some findings that the acetabular angle of anteversion in women is, on average, 5° larger than for men.[433] We examine the consequences of this in detail in the section on Variations in External (Lateral) Rotation (see pages 130–134).

Curiously, the size of the ilia—those massive wings that spread up and out in the upper bowl—is unrelated to the size and shape of the inlet plane and the transverse diameter. A woman with very broad ilia, and thus very broad hips, may nonetheless have a very narrow inlet plane and thus may experience greater difficulty in delivering a baby than a woman with narrower ilia ("narrow hips") who happens to have a larger transverse diameter.[434]

APPENDIX C
Mechanical Advantage—Pulleys and Levers

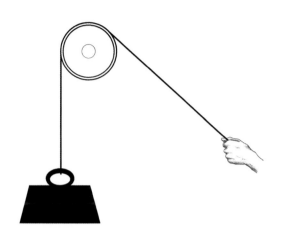

FIGURE 2.301 A simple pulley. Pulleys can change the direction in which a force is applied.

A vector is defined in physics as having both direction and magnitude. When a muscle contracts, it creates a force. A force can be depicted as a vector; it has a given strength (magnitude) and a direction in which it is applied (figure 2.302a). Physics has developed a useful concept of forces: we can view a force to be the summation of two other forces that form the sides of a rectangle, where the combination of the two component forces results in a net force along the diagonal of the rectangle (figure 2.302b). Thus, we can break a force into two forces working at right angles to each other. This little trick helps us understand how the pulleys we find in the body work. Pulleys are simple machines (figure 2.301) that can multiply a force if there is more than one pulley, or redirect the angle through which a force works (figure 2.302c). It is in this latter capacity that the various pulleys of our body function.

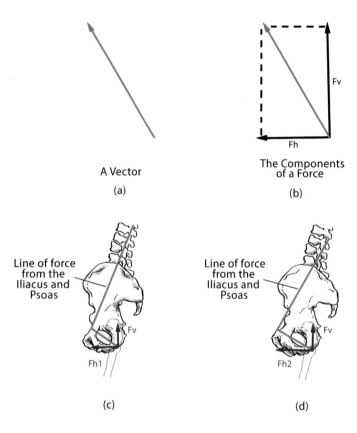

FIGURE 2.302 A force is a vector. Like a vector (a), a force has both magnitude (strength) and direction. It can be broken into components, as shown in (b). The horizontal force (Fh) provided by the psoas muscle contraction moves our femur around the hip socket, while its vertical force (Fv) helps to stabilize the joint by pulling the femur into the acetabulum. The larger the pulley of our pubis, the greater the horizontal force applied to the thigh. Notice how the Fh is larger in (d) than in (c) due to the more prominent pubis.

Figure 2.302 shows why the size of the pulley is important. The muscle or its tendon bends around the pulley and thus attaches to the bone at an angle. If the muscle fibers and its tendon did not go over the pulley, the muscle fibers would be in parallel to the bone, and when the muscle contracted, it would try to pull the bone directly into the joint. Articulation of our limbs requires a rotation *around* the joint, but this can only occur if a vector is applied at right angles to the bone. This force is shown as the horizontal component, Fh, in figure 2.302. The vertical component of the force of the iliacus and psoas muscles contracting, Fv, pulls the bone into the joint and does not contribute to movement, but it can contribute to stabilizing the joint. Fh, which operates at 90° (orthogonally) to Fv, serves to rotate the femur around the joint axis. When the pulley is bigger, Fh is stronger.

Unlike a pulley, a lever doesn't redirect force; instead, it multiplies forces. Everyone is familiar with teeter-totters and the fact that two people of unequal weight can find a balance if they vary the distance they are from the center of the beam. Someone who weighs half of the other person needs to be twice as far from the center to find the balance (see figure 2.303). This may sound like we are getting something for nothing, as a smaller person can create the same force as a larger person, but the tradeoff is in the distance each person has to travel to move to the balancing point. The lighter person will have to move twice as far as the heavier person. In the same way, where our muscles attach to our bones also creates differences in the effective force being applied to the bones. If the attachment point is further from the joint, the muscle will not have to work as hard to create a movement as it would were the attachment point closer to the joint. The tradeoff is that the distance the attachment moves is further, and thus it takes more time to articulate the joint through the same angle as it would if the attachment site were closer. We trade strength for speed.

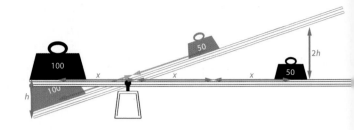

FIGURE 2.303 A lever. When we double the distance (*x*), we need only half the force to balance twice the weight, but the lever arm has to move twice as far (*2h*) to accomplish this.

Several bones act as pulleys, redirecting our muscles' angles of forces. The most famous are the pubis, the kneecap and the heel, but our various retinacula also act as pulleys. All these bones allow the body to change the effective direction of muscular forces. The pubic ramus is the bony bridge at the front of the pelvis. The ramus is easily palpated by feeling the bone directly below your navel (see figure 2.15). This is the pelvic bone that is most easily and commonly fractured in auto accidents.[435] It is quite variable[436] in size and prominence, and this can affect how easily we can flex the thigh. If the pubis is more prominent, it will act like a pulley redirecting the flexion force. Some students naturally seem to be able to flex their hips powerfully; they can keep both legs in the air in Boat Pose (Navasana) without any seeming effort, thanks in part to their prominent pubis and lower-situated lesser trochanters.

Since some of the pulleys of the body are bones, they have a range of sizes. Larger pulleys are more effective at articulating limbs than smaller pulleys. Similarly, where our muscles attach to the bone is also not constant. How distal the lesser trochanter is, how distal the tibial tuberosity, how far down the arm the deltoid muscle reaches before attaching to the humerus—these all determine how easily, but inversely how slowly, we can move the hip, leg or arm.

The same physics are at work around the heel: the plantarflexor muscles become the Achilles tendon, which in turn becomes the aponeurosis of the foot (the plantar fascia). This is all one continuous line of force. The posterior, inferior portion of the heel (calcaneus) acts like a pulley. If the heel bone is longer, the lever arm is longer, and thus the calf muscles need less force to plantarflex the foot. In people with longer heels, the calves are more effective at lifting the heels off the ground. The common metaphor to explain this is a wheelbarrow, as shown in figure 2.304. A wheelbarrow is a second-class lever. The handles of the wheelbarrow are equivalent to the heel bone, the hands lifting the wheelbarrow are equivalent to our calf muscles, and the wheel of the wheelbarrow is our toes, which stay on the ground. With longer handles, less work is needed to lift the wheelbarrow—the body.

The length of the calcaneus varies. One study found that the best sprinters had shorter heel bones. If longer heels mean the calf muscles don't need as much strength to plantarflex the foot, why do sprinters do better when the heels are shorter? The reason is time: the longer the lever, the greater the distance the calf muscles have to contract[437] and the more time it takes to move the object. With shorter levers, the reaction time is faster. In sprinting, initial speed is important. However, it is easier to stay standing up on your toes if your heel is longer. Whether it is better to have longer heels or shorter heels depends upon one's intentions; shorter heels are better for speed, longer heels for strength.

It is worth considering the influence of our bones and their unique shapes when we start to compare our strength and abilities with other people's. Their ability to move into and hold a pose may have less to do with how strong their muscles are and more to do with their unique anatomical structure.

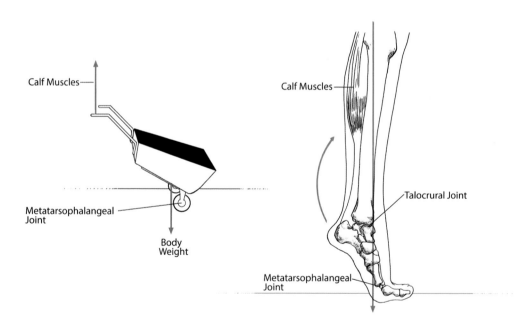

FIGURE 2.304 The pulley of the heel acts like the handles of a wheelbarrow to help us stand on our toes.

APPENDIX D
Flexion-Caused Impingement at the Hip Joint

Hip flexion may cause impingement of the superior labrum on the superior anterior neck of the femur when a rare combination of variations occurs. If (i) the acetabular abduction angle is very low, (ii) the acetabular version is very low, (iii) the femoral torsion is low, (iv) the neck angle is low and (v) the neck of the femur is thick and angled superiorly and anteriorly, then impingement may happen. It is challenging to visualize how compression could arise in flexion, because the axis of rotation in flexion is neither along the neck of the femur nor perpendicular to the acetabulum. Figure 2.305

shows the orthogonal lines (at 90°) of the femoral neck and the acetabulum. Notice how the axis of rotation of the femoral head is not aligned with either. In the rare combination of variations cited above, rotating the pelvis or the femur can bring the superior rim of the acetabulum onto the superior anterior neck of the femur. However, even a little bit of external rotation will prevent this from happening; allow the leg to rotate a bit externally away from the midline and no impingement will occur.

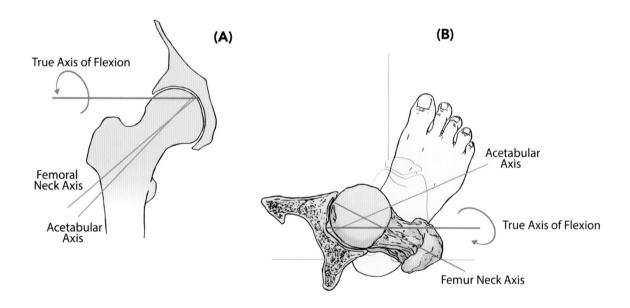

FIGURE 2.305 The axis of rotation in the hip joint: the angle of the femoral neck and a line perpendicular to the acetabulum are not the axis of rotation in flexion.

APPENDIX E
The Dangers and Benefits of Valgum or Varum Knee Orientation

Correlation is not causation. We must keep reminding ourselves of this fact. Many studies have correlated varum or valgum with osteoarthritis, varum being correlated more often than valgum.[438] One study found that over 60% of *healthy* people had either varum or valgum.[439] Thus, we cannot conclude that varum or valgum *causes* osteoarthritis. If they did, why do they not cause the condition in all healthy people? It is possible that arthritis causes varum or valgum. It is certainly fair to say, however, that if someone already has osteoarthritis in the medial condyles of the knee, varum could make it worse. Curiously, valgum may make the situation better! With a valgus orientation, compressive stress is shifted from the medial condyles to the lateral condyles. Most osteoarthritis occurs in the medial condyle, so a valgus shift of the stress to the lateral condyle may slow the progression of osteoarthritis.[440] Valgus could be healthy for some people with arthritis! For healthy knees, moderate amounts of varum and valgum do not seem to be a problem, at least as far as arthritis is concerned.

What about the ligaments? Injuries to the lateral collateral ligament are rare and are usually caused by transient, dynamic varus stresses occurring during movement or contact in sports.[441] This is unlikely to happen in a yoga class. Injuries to the medial collateral ligament can occur from a valgus force pushing the knee inward, but again these almost always occur during movement or from contact

injuries. It is highly unlikely that static valgus positioning (such as could occur in a Warrior pose, Virabhadrasana) on its own will damage the medial collateral ligament. When lateral ligaments are damaged, they fortunately have a good ability to repair themselves.[442] It is far more common for women to damage their knees from a dynamic valgus stress in sports than men, but the underlying cause for this gender difference is still being investigated. It is likely to be related to many factors, not just a valgus orientation of the knee;[443] it has been related to the effects of estrogen, the shape of the tibial plateau, the size of the ACL, generalized joint laxity, hyperextension of the knee, as well as poor biomechanical training.[444] Can valgus stress injure the ACL? Some studies say yes, yet other studies say no.[445] The jury is still out, but again, reported injuries are from dynamic, transient stresses, not from static stress. Valgum in static yoga postures is unlikely to cause ACL damage.

We are talking about moderate amounts of varum and valgum, and there certainly are individuals who have so much variation here that everyday activities are challenging. Such people often adopt compensatory behavioral patterns that result in long-term damage to the ankles, knees and hips. Large varus angles can lead a person to medially (internally) rotate the tibia and pronate the feet. For such individuals, maintaining balance can be a problem.[446]

APPENDIX F
The Movements of the Foot and Ankle

Normally, we like to describe movements of the body using three axes forming three planes: the frontal, horizontal and side planes. Unfortunately, this approach doesn't work very well for the foot and ankle because they do not move in just one of these planes. Instead, because the foot is angled with respect to the normal planes of the rest of the body, simple movements of the foot or ankle become very complicated when we try to describe them in the standard three planes. So, to keep things simple, we will look at the movements of the foot and ankle in their own unique, oblique orientations. Three basic pairs of terms for rotations are often used, as shown in figure 2.306: plantarflexion/dorsiflexion around the side axis; eversion/inversion in the frontal axis; and abduction/adduction in the horizontal axis. Again, these axes are related to the foot, not the whole body.

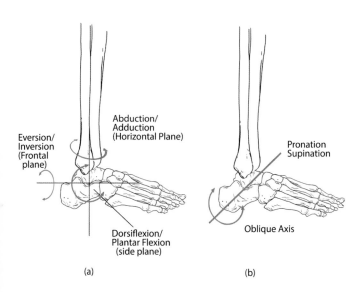

FIGURE 2.306 The directions defined in the three planes of the foot (a) and in the oblique axis (b).

Plantarflexion and Dorsiflexion of the Talocrural Joint (the Ankle)

Our feet may point out to the side and away from the purely sagittal (side) plane of the body for several reasons: retroversion of the acetabulum, very little anteversion of the femur, high tibial rotation, the amount of twist in the knee joint, and/or the amount of rotation in the hip joint. For any or all of these reasons, the foot points outward to varying degrees; consequently, movement at the ankle joint is not purely flexion or extension in the side plane of the body but includes movements in all three of the body's planes. However, for our purposes, we will define plantarflexion and dorsiflexion to be movement around an axis, called the empirical axis, which runs from the lateral malleolus to the medial malleolus. As shown in figure 2.307, this axis is not purely in any of the three planes we normally use to describe the body's movements. The empirical axis runs obliquely. The medial malleolus is higher (more superior) and more forward (anterior) than the lateral malleolus. You can feel this on your own body: check out where your inner and outer ankle bones are in relation to each other. Dorsiflexion, then, is a rotation around this axis that moves the top of the foot closer to the shin (in other places we would call this extension), and plantarflexion is rotation around the axis that moves the bottom (the plantar side) of the foot away from the shin (in other places we would simply call this flexion). These movements occur purely around the talocrural joint—the ankle joint.

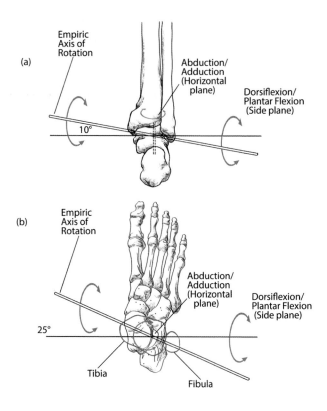

(a)

Empiric
Axis of
Rotation

Abduction/
Adduction
(Horizontal
plane)

Dorsiflexion/
Plantar Flexion
(Side plane)

10°

(b)

Empiric
Axis of
Rotation

Abduction/
Adduction
(Horizontal
plane)

Dorsiflexion/
Plantar Flexion
(Side plane)

25°

Tibia

Fibula

FIGURE 2.307 The axis of the talocrural joint of the right foot: (a) posterior view, (b) superior view.

But it is more complicated than that! Due to the shape of the talus, when the foot is plantarflexed, the joint is loose. Stability now comes not from the wedging of the bones together, as it does in extreme dorsiflexion, but from the ligaments binding the tibia to the fibula and from the tendons that run around the ankle. In many people, the ligaments and tendons are not tight enough to secure the ankle joint, so there is some "play" when the ankle is fully plantarflexed, which happens when you are on tiptoes or wearing high heels. Injuries to this joint occur most often when the foot is plantarflexed due to this reduced stability. Co-contracting the peroneal and tibialis muscles of the leg can stabilize a fully plantarflexed ankle because their tendons, which run on the lateral and medial sides of the ankle, will draw the distal ends of the tibia and femur more tightly together. Also, with plantarflexion there is some internal rotation of the talus, and with dorsiflexion there is some external rotation. (This is due to the shape of the talus: the lateral edge of the top of the talus' body, its trochlea, is longer than the medial edge, which causes the slight twisting during movement.)[447] Additionally, the fibula rotates slightly during dorsiflexion. Normally, we can think of the ankle as a pure hinge joint, but as we have seen, the reality is more complicated.

Supination and Pronation of the Foot

We have made the simplifying assumption that all other movements of the foot beyond plantarflexion and dorsiflexion are either supination (turning the sole inward) or pronation (turning the sole outward). However, the reality here is also much more complicated. Supination is a combination of three movements: inversion, plantarflexion and adduction. Pronation is a combination of eversion, dorsiflexion and abduction. Plus, supination and pronation can occur in different places. The hindfoot (the heel) can supinate or pronate with respect to the talus (which is what we normally refer to as supination or pronation), but the midfoot (the anterior tarsal bones) can pronate or supinate against the talus, and the forefoot can also move in these directions. It is quite common for hindfoot pronation to be accompanied by midfoot supination and vice versa. We need to understand these movements and where they occur to really appreciate how the foot moves. In general, unless we specify otherwise, supination and pronation refer to the movement of the heel under the ankle (the hindfoot movement).

There are usually 33 joints in the foot, and all these joints can allow some degree of movement, although most joints have very slight ranges of motion available. It is challenging to look at all these joints, and fortunately we don't have to. We need investigate only two. These are the subtalar joint of the talus and calcaneus (the hindfoot), and the transverse tarsal joint (the midfoot), which is actually comprised of several joints: the talus and the navicular joint, the calcaneus and the cuboid joint, and the cuboid articulation with the talus and cuneiform bones.

Starting with the subtalar joint: the talus and calcaneus usually have three sites of articulation (some people have two and some only one). Looking back at figure 2.228, we see an axis that runs through this joint. Rotation around this oblique axis can be divided into a combination of both inversion/eversion and abduction/adduction. The movement of the heel (calcaneus) under the ankle (talus) when the foot is not bearing any weight can either be from side to side— abduction and adduction, although some call this valgus and varus—or twisting (inversion and eversion). This is the open-chain situation. In a closed-chain, weightbearing situation, the heel remains stationary while the talus and all the leg bones above it move. The subtalar joint allows the foot to assume a variety of positions without affecting the posture of the ankle and leg, which is quite useful when walking on uneven terrain.

The Calcaneus and Talus Movements at the Subtalar Joint

In all cases of open-chain supination and pronation, it is easier to think of the talus as being the stationary bone around which all the others move. (Of course, the talus does move with respect to the leg, but those are the movements of dorsiflexion and plantarflexion.) When the foot is not bearing weight, when it is an open chain, such as when you rest your foot on the opposite thigh in Lotus Pose (Padmasana), the calcaneus moves along with the more distal segments of the foot. In figure 2.308, we see this situation: supination moves the calcaneus inwardly, and the distal foot moves in the same direction. In pronation, the same thing occurs but in the opposite direction.

However, when the foot bears weight, in a closed-chain position such as occurs in all standing yoga postures, the calcaneus and talus do not move in the same way, nor does the forefoot move with them. As shown in figure 2.309, when the forefoot is pinned by bearing weight, in supination the calcaneus inverts (moves inward), while the talus abducts and dorsiflexes (moves up and outward); in pronation, the calcaneus everts (moves outward), while the talus adducts and plantarflexes (moves down and inward). These movements have implications higher up the chain of bones. When we walk, and as the front leg swings forward, just before the heel strikes the ground, the leg is straight and extended at the knee, which is initially locked. If the knee stayed locked, that could cause a lot of the stress from the foot hitting the ground to travel up into the knee joint; however, as the heel strikes the ground, it everts and the foot pronates. This pronation does two things: it causes the tibia to slightly internally rotate, which "unlocks" the knee and allows it to begin flexing, and with pronation of the foot, the front leg shortens, which absorbs some of the stress of heel impact. Remember, also, that pronation loosens up the forefoot and allows it to accommodate the shape of the ground beneath it.

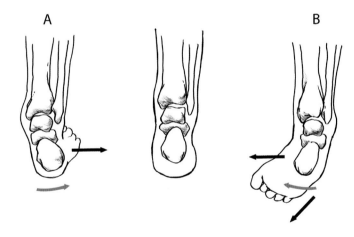

FIGURE 2.308 Open-chain subtalar movements of the right foot (posterior view). The calcaneus moves under the talus, which remains stationary; (a) shows pronation, (b) shows supination.

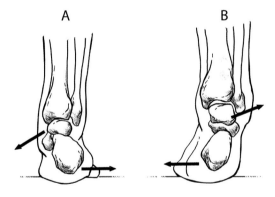

FIGURE 2.309 Closed-chain subtalar movements of the right foot (posterior view). Now the foot is fixed, so the leg and talus have to move over the calcaneus, which tilts in response; (a) shows pronation, (b) shows supination.

Inversion/Eversion and Abduction/Adduction

By classical definition, eversion and inversion are rotations around the axis that runs front to back (anterior to posterior). Similarly, abduction and adduction are rotations around the axis that runs from top to bottom (superior to inferior). Whether we call the movement abduction or adduction is decided by the direction of movement of the anterior portion of the limb (thus, moving the forefoot away from the midline of the body is termed abduction of the foot, even though the heel may actually be moving in the opposite direction, towards the midline of the body). As shown in figure 2.228, the axis of the subtalar joint does not run purely from front to back, or from top to bottom, but obliquely, so no pure eversion/inversion or abduction/adduction movements are possible; rather, a combination occur. Unfortunately, some anatomy texts choose to simplify this motion by equating eversion with pronation and inversion with supination, but as we just saw, these are not identical movements. Eversion is a *component* of pronation, not its synonym, and inversion is a *component* of supination.

The range of the inversion and eversion components of supination and pronation available at the subtalar joint is quite variable, and there is almost twice the range for inversion (~25°) as eversion (~12°).[448] Thus, the total range of inversion/eversion is ~37°, with one standard deviation being 8.5°. That means 2.5% of the population have a range of movement of 54° or more, while another 2.5% of the population have a very limited range of motion of 20° or less. The range of the abduction and adduction components of supination and pronation for the subtalar joint are quite similar: studies show around 31–47° of abduction and 27–42° of adduction, which is again a considerable variation.[449]

Movements at the Transverse Tarsal Joints

The transverse tarsal joint (also called the mid-tarsal joint or the Chopart joint) is where the hindfoot (calcaneus and talus) articulates with the midfoot (navicular and cuboid). It has two articulating sites: the talonavicular joint and the calcaneocuboid joint. As shown in figure 2.205, this joint, which is made up of four bones, creates a bit of an S-shaped curve. The talonavicular portion is a ball-in-socket interface, which allows significant rotation of the medial (inside) of the midfoot.[450] This means we can twist the midfoot independently of the hindfoot. The articulating surface of the calcaneocuboid section, however, has much less curvature, and when these two bones move, they act like wedges, locking the joint. The calcaneocuboid section is much more rigid, providing lateral support for the foot.

As shown in figure 2.310, there are two axes for the transverse tarsal joint: the longitudinal axis, at an angle of about 15° to the horizontal and about 9° to the ray of the second toe; and the oblique axis of about 52° to the horizontal and about 57° to the ray of the second toe.[451] (As always, these figures are just averages; your unique angles may be quite different, and that may affect your range of motion.) Rotation around the longitudinal axis is mostly eversion and inversion, but rotation around the oblique axis is a combination of abduction/dorsiflexion or adduction/plantarflexion.[452] Around the longitudinal axis, there is 20–25° of inversion available but only 10–15° of eversion.[453] In reality, the transverse tarsal joint moves as if it were one joint and is functionally uniaxial, not biaxial, as it might at first appear. Thus, the combination of eversion/abduction/dorsiflexion and inversion/adduction/plantarflexion again results in pronation and supination of the midfoot at this joint. Interestingly, due to the lack of range of motion of the calcaneocuboid joint, there is almost twice as much range of motion available in the midfoot for supination as for pronation. We can supinate here more than we can pronate.

We have just seen that supination and pronation can occur at the subtalar joint, the transverse tarsal joint or both. Together these make up most of the pronation and supination movements that we can do in the foot.[454] The transverse tarsal joint can amplify the movements that occur at the ankle joint and subtalar joint, which can be very useful if one loses some range of motion in either of these other two places due to injury or aging.[455] However, sometimes, especially in closed-chain, weightbearing situations, the hindfoot (subtalar joint) may pronate while the midfoot and forefoot (transverse tarsal joint) supinate, and vice versa, which again makes things complicated. The hindfoot and the midfoot do not always move together in the same directions.

Open- and Closed-Chain Movements

The talus is involved in all the joints we have discussed so far. This means that there is an intimacy between all these joints and their movements. It is rare for the transverse tarsal joint to articulate on its own: there is also movement in the subtalar joint. Most of what we call pronation and supination is a combination of movements at both the subtalar and the transverse tarsal joints. Thus, motion of the forefoot also contributes to pronation and supination. However, the situation becomes more complex when the foot is bearing weight (in the closed-chain position). Now, the forefoot may be pinned while talus and the leg above it move. When the forefoot and midfoot are pinned, the talus and calcaneus can move at the transverse tarsal joint. This is the situation that occurs during walking: sometimes the foot is bearing weight (the stance foot) and sometimes it is not (the swing foot).

When the foot is bearing weight and we supinate the whole foot, this means the forefoot adducts and plantarflexes while we abduct and dorsiflex the talus. Those movements are normally associated with pronation, but the talus is moving while the midfoot and forefoot are fixed. To understand this seeming paradox, let's consider only the movement of the talus bone in closed-chain supination. The talus is free to move; its anterior head moves inferiorly (which we can call talar plantarflexion) and medially (talar adduction). However, we do not normally look at a single bone when we describe movement; we look at the action of two or more bones around their joint, and we usually name the movement at the joint based on what the more distal bone is doing! In the closed-chain example, the talus, the more proximal bone, is free to move, and it goes down and medially, but the navicular is fixed and can't move. So the resulting joint movement is actually opposite to the talus' movement. Think of it this way: the anterior talus dips inferiorly, which is the same as the navicular rising

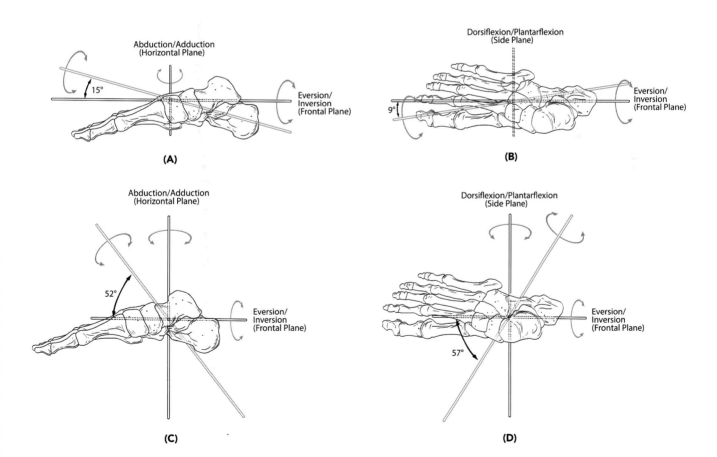

FIGURE 2.310 The transverse tarsal joint axes of movement (right foot): (a) medial view of longitudinal axis; (b) superior view of longitudinal axis; (c) medial view of oblique axis; (d) superior view of oblique axis.

superiorly, relative to the talus. At the joint level, this is called dorsiflexion of the talonavicular joint. Similarly, as the anterior talus moves medially, it is the same as the navicular moving laterally, and thus from the joint's point of view, this is abduction. When we have dorsiflexion and abduction of the transverse tarsal joint, it is called pronation. In the other direction, when forefoot and midfoot are pinned and we pronate the hindfoot, it is as if we were adducting and plantarflexing at the transverse tarsal joint, which is called supination.

Table 2.21 compares the movements of the calcaneus, talus, midfoot and forefoot in both open-chain and closed-chain positions.

Combining movements of the subtalar joint and the transverse tarsal joint can either free up or stiffen the forefoot. Figure 2.311 shows what happens with the two axes of the transverse tarsal joints when the hindfoot pronates or supinates. In the closed-chain, weightbearing situation, when the subtalar joint is in pronation, the axes of the transverse tarsal joint are parallel to each other, and the midfoot and forefoot are unlocked and quite flexible. This is important in walking; when we first strike the ground with our foot, the forefoot and midfoot need to be flexible enough to conform to the terrain.[456] However, in the final stage of walking, when the subtalar joint is supinating, the forefoot is pronating, the axes of the transverse tarsal joint converge, their bones wedge together, and the whole foot stiffens due to the compression of bone against bone.[457] This is important because the stiffened foot allows a rebounding of energy to help launch our next step.

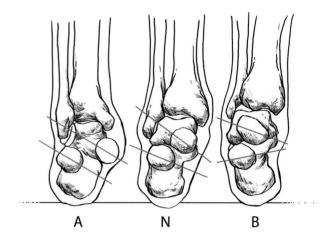

FIGURE 2.311 Comparing subtalar movement with transverse tarsal movement. Anterior view of right foot. The two lines show the axes of the two transverse tarsal joints; (a) shows pronation, (n) is neutral and (b) shows supination.

This can seem confusing: we can pronate the forefoot and end up supinating the hindfoot and vice versa. This is another reason we say, "It's complicated!" Indeed, even the experts do not all agree with the above idea that the divergent axes of the transverse tarsal joint are responsible for stiffening the foot when we push off from the ground during walking.[458] Biomechanical researchers are still trying to work this all out so we can completely understand what is going on. Fortunately, yoga teachers do not need to understand all these subtleties; we can get along quite nicely by simply referring to the four main movements of the ankle–foot segment: plantarflexion, dorsiflexion, pronation and supination.

TABLE 2.21 Open-chain versus closed-chain movements of the foot.

FOOT	PRONATION		SUPINATION	
	open chain (non-weightbearing: talus is fixed)	closed chain (weight-bearing: talus is not fixed)	open chain (non-weightbearing: talus is fixed)	closed chain (weight-bearing: talus is not fixed)
Subtalar joint	calcaneus everts	calcaneus everts	calcaneus inverts	calcaneus inverts
Transverse tarsal joint	talus is stable	talus adducts/plantar-flexes	talus is stable	talus abducts/dorsiflexes
Midfoot and forefoot	abducts/dorsiflexes	stable	adducts/plantarflexes	stable

Volume 2 Endnotes

1 See T.K.V. Desikachar and R.H. Cravens, *Health, Healing and Beyond: Yoga and the Living Tradition of Krishnamacharya* (New York: North Point Press, 2011), 41.

2 Cowface quiz answers: A—both legs are in adduction, flexion and external rotation at the hip joint; B—the right arm is in abduction, flexion and external rotation at the shoulder joint; C—the left arm is in adduction, extension and internal rotation at the shoulder joint. To be even more complete, the right scapula (B) is also in abduction and upward rotation, while the left scapula (C) is in adduction and downward rotation. (See American Council on Exercise, *Apley's Scratch Test for Shoulder Mobility*, retrieved from https://www.acefitness.org/certified-news/images/article/pdfs/ApleysScratchTest.pdf.)

Knowing that these are the movements required for this pose allows us to come into the posture in stages. For example, when you try to clasp your hands behind your back in Cowface pose, first extend your left arm out to the side, turn the palm down, then turn the palm towards the back of the room. If you have more room to move, keep (internally) rotating the arm until the palm faces the ceiling, but do this without moving your chest or shoulder forward. This is pure internal rotation of the arm. Next, move the arm backwards (extension) as far as you can before folding the elbow. Then, bending the elbow, bring the arm behind your back (adduction) and wiggle your hand as high up between your shoulder blades as possible. Positioning the arm first in internal rotation, then extension and finally adduction may allow you to reach higher up your back than you can by simply thrusting your arm behind your back.

For the right arm we do something similar: reach your right arm out to the side, turn the palm so it faces forward, (external rotation) and, if possible, rotate the palm towards the ceiling. Now, if possible, keep rotating until the palm faces the back of the room. Next, adduct the arm up alongside your head before flexing the elbow and reaching down your back for your other hand.

Understanding the limb movements required to achieve a posture allows us to come into the posture in the safest and most economical way and also may provide greater depth in the pose. As always, move with both intention and attention to avoid any possibility of injury.

3 See Anne M. Gilroy, Brian R. MacPherson, and Lawrence M. Ross, *Atlas of Anatomy*, corrected reprint (Harrogate, UK: Thieme, 2010), 388.

4 The movement of the sacrum is called *nutation*, which is from the Latin for nodding. To nod is to move up and down, which is what the sacrum does.

5 Femoral torsion is also called the *angle of anteversion*.

6 Another term for the femoral neck-shaft angle is the *angle of inclination*.

7 See C. Kisner and L.A. Colby, *Therapeutic Exercise: Foundations and Techniques,* 6th ed. (Philadelphia, PA: F.A. Davis, 2012), 710–1.

8 See N.B. Reese and W.D. Bandy, *Joint Range of Motion and Muscle Length Testing*, 2nd ed. (St. Louise, MO: Saunders, 2010), 296–7.

9 See B.G. Domb, D.E. Martin, and I.B. Botser, "Risk Factors for Ligamentum Teres Tears," *Arthroscopy* 29.1 (2013): 64–73. doi:10.1016/j.arthro.2012.07.009.

10 That the functions and limitations of various ligaments are debated is not surprising when we realize that everyone is different; if one study examines people who possess a particular range of length and rigidity in their ligaments, but another study examines people with different lengths and strengths, naturally they will not agree on the range of motion observed or the role of the tissues investigated.

11 See S.L. Delp, W.E. Hess, D.S. Hungerford, and L.C. Jones, "Variation of Rotation Moment Arms with Hip Flexion," *Journal of Biomechanics* 32 (1999): 493–501.

12 See M.C.G. Farias, B.D.R. Oliveira, T.D.S. Rocha, and V. Caiaffo, "Morphological and Morphometric Analysis of Psoas Minor Muscle in Cadavers," *Journal of Morphological Sciences* 29.4 (2012): 202–5.

13 See N.C. Moes, "Variation in Sitting Pressure Distribution and Location of the Points of Maximum Pressure with Rotation of the Pelvis, Gender and Body Characteristics," *Ergonomics* 50.4 (2007): 536–61.

14 See P.S. Igbigbi and A.M. Nanono-Igbigbi, "Determination of Sex and Race from the Subpubic Angle in Ugandan Subjects," *American Journal of Forensic Medicine and Pathology* 24.2 (2003): 168–72.

15 Sometimes this is called the *transverse angle of the acetabular inlet plane*.

16 Sometimes this is called the *sagittal aperture angle*.

17 Ideally, the version angle would be shown looking down on the pelvis; however, the ilium hides the acetabulum in that view, so the drawing on the right is meant to illustrate the displacement in the horizontal plane of the acetabulum, not its abduction angle. While not ideal, this view gives a sense of the acetabulum's forward position.

18 See Gilroy et al., *Atlas of Anatomy*, 379.

19 Study #1: from I.K. Sharp, "Acetabular Dysplasia: The Acetabular Angle," *Journal of Bone and Joint Surgery*, British Volume 43-B.2 (1961): 268–72. Study #2: from Y. Zheng, Y. Wang, Z. Zhu, T. Tang, K. Dai, and S. Qiu, "Differences in Acetabular Morphology Related to Side and Sex in a Chinese Population," *Journal of Anatomy* 220.3 (2012): 256–62; in

this study, I have only cited the range as being one standard deviation from the mean. Study #3: From P.E. Murtha, M.A. Hafez, B. Jaramaz, and A.M. DiGioia, 3rd, "Variations in Acetabular Anatomy with Reference to Total Hip Replacement," *Journal of Bone and Joint Surgery*, British Volume 90.3 (2008): 308–13, doi:10.1302/0301-620X.90B3.19548. Study #4: From A.C. Perreira, J.C. Hunter, T. Laird, and A.A. Jamali, "Multilevel Measurement of Acetabular Version Using 3-D CT-generated Models," *Clinical Orthopaedics and Related Research* 269.2 (2011): 552–61, doi:10.1007/s11999-010-1567-2.

20 See P. Udomkiat, L.D. Dorr, and Z. Wan, "Cementless Hemispheric Porous-coated Sockets Implanted with Press-fit Technique without Screws: Average Ten-year Follow-up," *Journal of Bone and Joint Surgery*, American Volume 84-A.75 (2002): 1195–200.

21 From Perreira et al., "Multilevel Measurement of Acetabular Version."

22 See Zheng et al., "Differences in Acetabular Morphology."

23 This is a summary of a number of different studies found in Perreira et al., "Multilevel Measurement of Acetabular Version." Included are only those findings that provided ranges.

24 See Perreira et al., "Multilevel Measurement of Acetabular Version."

25 See Domb et al., "Risk Factors for Ligamentum Teres Tears."

26 Ibid. Also see Murtha et al., "Variations in Acetabular Anatomy."

27 See Zheng et al., "Differences in Acetabular Morphology."

28 See Sharp, "Acetabular Dysplasia."

29 This could lead to more femoral acetabular impingement and thus more arthritis at the anterior labrum. Stu McGill, in a personal communication with me, noted that a deeper hip socket is far more common in people with a European heritage, especially those of Celtic background, who suffer much higher rates of femoracetabular impingement and hip replacement.

30 The labrum has also been called the *glenoidal labrum* and the *cotyloid ligament*.

31 See Y. Pinoit, O. May, J. Girard, P. Laffargue, T. Ala Eddine, and H. Migaud, "Low Accuracy of the Anterior Pelvic Plane to Guide the Position of the Cup with Imageless Computer Assistance: Variation of Position in 106 Patients," *Revue de Chirurgie Orthopédique et Réparatrice de l'Appareil Moteur* 93.5 (2007): 455–60.

32 See D. Lim et al., "Variations of the Anterior Frontal Pelvic Plane and Patient Positioning in Total Hip Arthroplasty (THA)," *Proceedings of the 52nd Annual Meeting of the Orthopaedic Research Society* (2006), paper 0453, http://www.ors.org/Transactions/52/0453.pdf.

33 See I. Gilligan, S. Chandraphak, and P. Mahakkanukrauh, "Femoral Neck-shaft Angle in Humans: Variation Relating to Climate, Clothing, Lifestyle, Sex, Age and Side," *Journal of Anatomy* 223.2 (2013): 133–51, doi:10.1111/joa.12073.

34 A formula shows how the neck-shaft angle (NSA) increases after birth: NSA = 158.71 – (0.77 x age). See J.L. Jouve et al., "Anatomical Study of the Proximal Femur in the Fetus," *Journal of Pediatric Orthopaedics B* 14.2 (2005): 105–10.

35 See John Y. Anderson and Erik Trinkaus, "Patterns of Sexual, Bilateral and Interpopulational Variation in Human Femoral Neck-shaft Angles," *Journal of Anatomy* 192 (1998): 279–85.

36 The correlation between femur length and neck-shaft angle was found to be NSA = 80.06° + 0.13 (total femur length); see S.M. Gujar, S. Vikani, J. Parmar, and K.V. Bondre, "A Correlation between Femoral Neck-shaft Angle to Femoral Neck Length," *International Journal of Biomedical and Advance Research* 4.5 (2013), doi:10.7439/ijbar.v4i5.354.

37 See Gilroy et al., *Atlas of Anatomy*, 367, which cites 126°, and Henry Gray

38 See Gilligan et al., "Femoral Neck-shaft Angle in Humans."

39 See J.C. Clohisy, R.M. Nunley, J.C. Carlisle, and P.L. Schoenecker, "Incidence and Characteristics of Femoral Deformities in the Dysplastic Hip," *Clinical Orthopaedics and Related Research* 467.1 (2009): 128–34.

40 One reason for believing coxa vara to be problematic is because the center of the head of the femur does not line up with the center point of the acetabulum. This is normally depicted diagrammatically with a neck-shaft angle showing coxa vara but with an average acetabulum. As we have seen, though, acetabula also vary considerably, so there can be cases where a coxa vara femur fits perfectly into an acetabulum that has a greater angle of abduction.

41 Graphic reproduction with the kind permission of John Anderson, from Anderson and Trinkaus, "Patterns of Sexual, Bilateral and Interpopulational Variation."

42 "A patient with excessive femoral neck anteversion will usually demonstrate an apparent excess of hip internal rotation and an apparent limitation of hip external rotation"; Fiona G. Neely, "Biomechanical Risk Factors for Exercise-Related Lower Limb Injuries," *Sports Medicine* 26.6 (1998): 395–413.

43 See O. Reikerås, I. Bjerkreim, and A. Kolbenstvedt, "Anteversion of the Acetabulum and Femoral Neck in Normals and in Patients with Osteoarthritis of the Hip," *Acta Orthopaedica Scandinavica* 54.1 (1983): 18–23.

44 See A. Høiseth, O. Reikerås, and E. Fønstelien, "Radiography and Computed Tomography in Cadavers and In Vivo," *Acta Orthopaedica Scandinavica* 60.1 (1989): 93–6.

45 See G. Gulan, D. Matovinović, B. Nemec, D. Rubinić, and J. Ravlić-Gulan, "Femoral Neck Anteversion: Values, Develop-

ment, Measurement, Common Problems," *Collegium Antropologicum* 24.2 (2000): 521–7.

46 "[In-toeing gait] is twice as common in girls as in boys"; see Gulan et al., "Femoral Neck Anteversion."

47 See Gulan et al., "Femoral Neck Anteversion."

48 See both Reikerås et al., "Anteversion of the Acetabulum," and A.V. Maheshwari, M.P. Zlowodzki, G. Siram, and A.K. Jain, "Femoral Neck Anteversion, Acetabular Anteversion and Combined Anteversion in the Normal Indian Adult Population: A Computed Tomographic Study," *Indian Journal of Orthopaedics* 44.3 (2010): 277–82.

49 See *Wheeless' Textbook of Orthopaedics* by Duke University Medical Center's Division of Orthopaedic Surgery, http://www.wheelessonline.com/ortho/12494.

50 See Maheshwari et al., "Femoral Neck Anteversion."

51 See Gulan et al., "Femoral Neck Anteversion."

52 Ibid., 523: "in our investigations (in press) we found negative correlation between lateral rotation and femoral anteversion."

53 The correlation is given as neck-shaft angle = 95.28° + 1.20 (length of neck); see Gujar et al., "A Correlation between Femoral Neck-shaft Angle to Femoral Neck Length."

54 See E.B. de Sousa et al., "Morphometric Study of the Proximal Femur Extremity in Brazilians," *International Journal of Morphology* 28.3 (2010): 835–40.

55 See K. Chin, M.C. Evans, J. Cornish, T. Cundy, and I.R. Reid, "Differences in Hip Axis and Femoral Neck Length in Premenopausal Women of Polynesian, Asian and European Origin," *Osteoporosis International* 7.4 (1997): 344–7.

56 See M.S. Patton, R.A. Duthie, and A.G. Sutherland, "Proximal Femoral Geometry and Hip Fractures," *Acta Orthopaedica Belgica* 72.1 (2006): 51–4.

57 See K.E. Poole et al., "Changing Structure of the Femoral Neck Across the Adult Female Lifespan," *Journal of Bone and Mineral Research* 25.3 (2010): 482–91.

58 See N. Narra, R. Nikander, J. Viik, J. Hyttinen, and H. Sievänen, "Femoral Neck Cross-Sectional Geometry and Exercise Loading," *Clinical Physiology and Functional Imaging* 33.4 (2013): 258–66, doi:10.1111/cpf.12022. See also L.C.V. Harrison et al., "MRI Texture Analysis of Femoral Neck: Detection of Exercise Load-associated Differences in Trabecular Bone," *Journal of Magnetic Resonance Imaging* 34.6 (2011): 1359–66, doi:10.1002/jmri.22751.

59 See John Michelotti and John Clark, "Femoral Neck Length and Hip Fracture Risk," *Journal of Bone and Mineral Research* 14.10 (1999): 1714–20.

60 See H. Xu, Y. Zhou, Q. Liu, Q. Tang, and J. Yin, "Femoral Morphologic Differences in Subtypes of High Developmental Dislocation of the Hip," *Clinical Orthopaedics and Related Research* 468.12 (2010): 3371–6.

61 See S.J. Preece et al., "Variation in Pelvic Morphology May Prevent the Identification of Anterior Pelvic Tilt," *Journal of Manual and Manipulative Therapy* 16.2 (2008): 113–7.

62 See J.F. Jarrell et al., "Consensus Guidelines for the Management of Chronic Pelvic Pain," *Journal of Obstetrics and Gynaecology Canada* (September 2005): 869–87, http://sogc.org/wp-content/uploads/2013/01/164E-CPG2-September2005.pdf. The authors recommended assessing the symmetry of the PSIS and ASIS. If one side's PSIS or ASIS is higher than the other, they conclude that there must be a tilt in the pelvis, probably due to unequal leg length or due to a pelvic twist (see page 872). This assessment ignores the reality that, for most people, the two sides of the pelvis are not symmetric, and this does not always imply a pathology.

63 See Preece et al. "Variation in Pelvic Morphology."

64 *Yogabody: Anatomy, Kinesiology, and Asana* (Berkeley, CA: Rodmell Press, 2009), 48.

65 See Leslie Aiello (ed.), *An Introduction to Human Evolutionary Anatomy* (Waltham, MA: Academic Press, 2006), 463.

66 See W. Bolanowski, A. Smiszkiewicz-Skwarska, M. Polguj, and K.S. Jedrzejewski, "The Occurrence of the Third Trochanter and Its Correlation to Certain Anthropometric Parameters of the Human Femur," *Folia Morphologica* 64.3 (2005): 168–75.

67 See E. Loth, "Odmiany mammalogeniczne w budowie człowieka," and E. Murawski, "Przyczyna występowania krętarza trzeciego u człowieka," cited in Bolanowski et al., "The Occurrence of the Third Trochanter."

68 Data from K.E. Roach and T.P. Miles, "Normal Hip and Knee Active Range of Motion: The Relationship to Age," *Physical Therapy* 71 (1991): 656–65, and for adduction from D.C. Boone and S.P. Azen, "Normal Range of Motion of Joints in Male Subjects," *Journal of Bone and Joint Surgery* 61 (1979): 756–9.

69 See Reese and Bandy, *Joint Range of Motion*, 31–2.

70 Ibid., 299.

71 From Kisner and Colby, *Therapeutic Exercise, 712.*

72 This is not the place of maximum joint congruence, however, which we normally do find in the close-packed position. For the hip joint, that comes at 90° of flexion, with a little bit of abduction and external rotation. This is why it is so comfortable for most people (but not all!) to sit with their legs slightly abducted and feet turned outward, as shown in figure 2.45; see Donald A. Neumann, ed., *Kinesiology of the Musculoskeletal System: Foundations for Rehabilitation*, 2nd ed. (St. Louis, MO: Mosby, 2010), 400.

73 See Kisner and Colby, *Therapeutic Exercise*, 711.

74 See M. Haversath et al., "The Distribution of Nociceptive Innervation in the Painful Hip: A Histological Investigation," *Bone and Joint Journal* 95-B.6 (2013): 770–6, doi:10.1302/0301-620X.95B6.30262.

75 From Gray et al., *Gray's Anatomy,* 1442–3.

76 See Zheng et al., "Differences in Acetabular Morphology."

77 See J. Cobb, K. Logishetty, K. Davda, and F. Iranpour, "Cams and Pincer Impingement Are Distinct, Not Mixed: The Acetabular Pathomorphology of Femoroacetabular Impingement," *Clinical Orthopaedics and Related Research* 468.8 (2010): 2143–51.

78 "A supernumerary [extra] muscle was noted in 33 (33.0%) out of the 100 thighs. In each of these thighs, it arose from the upper part of the inferior ramus of the pubis and ran obliquely downwards and laterally. It was inserted into the anterior surface of the insertion aponeurosis of the adductor minimus (17/33 thighs, 51.5%), the upper part of the pectineal line (9/33 thighs, 27.3%), or the posterior side of the base of the lesser trochanter (7/33 thighs, 21.2%)"; from E. Nakamura, S. Masumi S, M. Miura, S. Kato, and R. Miyauchi, "A Supernumerary Muscle between the Adductors Brevis and Minimus in Humans," *Okajimas Folia Anatomica Japonica* 69.2–3 (1992): 89–98.

79 See John Y. Anderson and Erik Trinkaus, "Patterns of Sexual, Bilateral and Interpopulational Variation in Human Femoral Neck-shaft Angles," *Journal of Anatomy* 192 (1998): 279–285. doi:10.1046/j.1469-7580.1998.19220279.x.

80 One study of 22 females found a mean anteversion of 24.1°, with a range from 14.0° to 33.3°. The same parameters for 20 males were 19.3°, with a range from 8.5° to 32.3°. See Murtha et al., "Variations in Acetabular Anatomy."

81 See H.D. Atkinson, K.S. Johal, C. Willis-Owen, S. Zadow, and R.D. Oakeshott, "Differences in Hip Morphology between the Sexes in Patients Undergoing Hip Resurfacing," *Journal of Orthopaedic Surgery and Research* 5 (2010): 76, doi:10.1186/1749-799X-5-76.

82 Indeed, there are studies that have found some people to have negative torsion (called retroversion) of –5° to –15°! See *Wheeless' Textbook of Orthopaedics* by Duke University Medical Center's Division of Orthopaedic Surgery, http://www.wheelessonline.com/ortho/12494, and Atkinson et al., "Differences in Hip Morphology." For our purposes, we do not need to cite such extreme variations to show that there are significant impacts on the range of femoral torsion.

83 See Gulan et al., "Femoral Neck Anteversion."

84 See A. Høiseth A, O. Reikerås, and E. Fønstelien, "Lack of Correlation between Femoral Neck Anteversion and Acetabular Orientation: Radiography and Computed Tomography in Cadavers and In Vivo," *Acta Orthopaedica Scandinavica* 60.1 (1989): 93–6.

85 "Few dancers make the cut with external rotation less than 60 degrees" (Steven J. Karageanes [ed.], *Principles of Manual Sports Medicine* [Philadelphia: Lippincott Williams & Wilkins, 2005], 497).

86 See E. Lieberman, *The Story of the Human Body: Evolution, Health and Disease* (New York: Pantheon, 2013), 85.

87 See Neumann, ed., "Axial Skeleton," 400.

88 From Kisner and Colby, *Therapeutic Exercise,* 712.

89 See Gray et al., *Gray's Anatomy,* 1442–3.

90 See D. Lim et al., "Variations of the Anterior Frontal Pelvic Plane."

91 See Gilroy et al., *Atlas of Anatomy,* 426.

92 The ligamentum teres is tense in semi-flexion, adduction and internal rotation. It is relaxed in abduction. See G. Michaels and A.L. Matles, "The Role of the Ligamentum Teres in Congenital Dislocation of the Hip," *Clinical Orthopaedics and Related Research* 71 (1970): 199–201.

93 See Delp et al., "Variation of Rotation Moment Arms with Hip Flexion," 410 and 415.

94 Ibid.

95 See A.S. Arnold, A.V. Komattu, and S.L. Delp, "Internal Rotation Gait: A Compensatory Mechanism to Restore Abduction Capacity Decreased by Bone Deformity," *Developmental Medicine and Child Neurology* 39.1 (1997): 40–4.

96 Indeed, restricted internal rotation has been used as a diagnostic tool for detecting osteoarthritis; see S. Reichenbach et al., "An Examination Chair to Measure Internal Rotation of the Hip in Routine Settings: A Validation Study," *Osteoarthritis and Cartilage* 18 (2010): 365–371.

97 See Delp et al. "Variation of Rotation Moment Arms with Hip Flexion."

98 Dr. Derek Ochiai, quoted by Joshua Hodges in *Kicking and the Hips,* retrieved from www.theshotokanway.com/kickingandthehips.html.

99 See Iyengar, *Light on Yoga,* 125.

100 See Reinhold Ganz, Michael Leunig, Katharina Leunig-Ganz, and William H. Harris, "The Etiology of Osteoarthritis of the Hip: An Integrated Mechanical Concept," *Clinical Orthopaedics and Related Research* 466 (2008): 264–72.

101 See Ganz et al., "The Etiology of Osteoarthritis of the Hip."

102 See M. Leunig et al., "Prevalence of Cam and Pincer-Type Deformities on Hip MRI in an Asymptomatic Young Swiss Female Population: A Cross-Sectional Study," *Osteoarthritis and Cartilage* 21.4 (2013): 544–50.

103 See S. Reichenbach et al., "Prevalence of Cam-Type Deformity on Hip Magnetic Resonance Imaging in Young Males: A Cross-Sectional Study," *Arthritis Care and Research* 62.9

(2010): 1319–27, and Leunig et al., "Prevalence of Cam and Pincer-Type Deformities."

104 See S. Reichenbach et al., "Prevalence of Cam-Type Deformity."

105 See Cobb et al., "Cams and Pincer Impingement."

106 This is known as mixed FAIS.

107 See Ganz et al., "The Etiology of Osteoarthritis of the Hip."

108 See Roach and Miles, "Normal Hip and Knee Active Range of Motion."

109 See Neumann, ed., "Axial Skeleton," 400.

110 See Leslie Kaminoff, *Yoga Anatomy* (Champaign, IL: Human Kinetics, 2007), 104–7.

111 See John Goodfellow and John O'Connor, "The Mechanics of the Knee and Prosthesis Design," *Journal of Bone and Joint Surgery* 60-B.3 (1978): 358–69.

112 See Gray et al., *Gray's Anatomy*, 1471.

113 See Neumann, ed., *Kinesiology of the Musculoskeletal System*, 439.

114 See Neumann, ed., *Kinesiology of the Musculoskeletal System*, 436.

115 See A.A. Faraj and P. Deacon, "Bipartite Sesamoids as a Cause of Disability in an Athlete," *European Journal of Orthopaedic Surgery and Traumatology* 11 (2001): 63–5.

116 See Carla Stecco and Antonio Stecco, *Fascia: The Tensional Network of the Human Body* (London: Elsevier, 2012), 32–3.

117 See Gray et al., *Gray's Anatomy*, 1480.

118 See Barry P. Boden, Joseph S. Torg, Sarah B. Knowles, and Timothy E. Hewett, "Video Analysis of Anterior Cruciate Ligament Injury Abnormalities in Hip and Ankle Kinematics," *American Journal of Sports Medicine* 37 (2009): 252, available at http://ajs.sagepub.com/content/37/2/252.

119 See B.P. Boden, F.T. Sheehan, J.S. Torg, and T.E. Hewett, "Noncontact Anterior Cruciate Ligament Injuries: Mechanisms and Risk Factors," *Journal of the America Academy of Orthopaedic Surgeons* 18.9 (2010): 520.

120 See T.E. Hewett, G.D. Myer, and K.R. Ford, "Anterior Cruciate Ligament Injuries in Female Athletes: Part 1, Mechanisms and Risk Factors," *American Journal of Sports Medicine* 34 (2006): 299–311.

121 See K.M. Sutton and J.M. Bullock "Anterior Cruciate Ligament Rupture: Differences Between Males and Females," *Journal of the American Academy of Orthopaedic Surgeons* 21.1 (2012): 41.

122 See K. Shelbourne, T. Davis, and T. Kootwyk, "The Relationship between Intercondylar Notch Width of the Femur and the Incidence of Anterior Cruciate Ligament Tears," *American Journal of Sports Medicine* 26 (1998): 402–8.

123 See Boden et al., "Video Analysis," 252.

124 See Neumann, ed., *Kinesiology of the Musculoskeletal System*, 451.

125 See C.M. Gupte, A. Smith, I.D. McDermott, A.M. Bull, R.D. Thomas, and A.A. Amis, "Meniscofemoral Ligaments Revisited. Anatomical Study, Age Correlation and Clinical Implications," *Journal of Bone and Joint Surgery*, British volume 84.6 (2002): 846–51.

126 See Neumann, ed., *Kinesiology of the Musculoskeletal System*, 451–3.

127 See Gray et al., *Gray's Anatomy*, 1481.

128 Ibid., 1479–81.

129 See Gilroy et al., *Atlas of Anatomy*, 401.

130 See Gray et al., *Gray's Anatomy*, 110.

131 See K.Y. Zhang, A.E. Kedgley, C.R. Donoghue, D. Rueckert, and A.M. Bull, "The Relationship between Lateral Meniscus Shape and Joint Contact Parameters in the Knee: A Study Using Data from the Osteoarthritis Initiative," *Arthritis Research and Therapy* 16 (2014): R27, doi:10.1186/ar4455.

132 See A.J. Fox, A. Bedi, and S.A. Rodeo, "The Basic Science of Human Knee Menisci: Structure, Composition, and Function," *Sports Health* 4.4 (2012): 340–51, doi:10.1177/1941738111429419.

133 Ibid.

134 See Bernie Clark, "Yin Yoga for the Knees," *Yin Yoga Newsletter* (July 2011), retrieved from http://www.yinyoga.com/newsletter7_yinyoga_knees.php.

135 See B.B. Mandal, S.H. Park, E.S. Gil, and D.L. Kaplan, "Stem Cell-Based Meniscus Tissue Engineering," *Tissue Engineering. Part A* 17.21–2 (2011: 2749–61.

136 See Gray et al., *Gray's Anatomy*, 1477.

137 See P.K. Levangie and C.C. Norkin, "The Knee," in Levangie and Norkin, eds., *Joint Structure and Function: A Comprehensive Analysis*, 5th ed., Philadelphia, PA: F.A. Davis Company, 2001, 399–443.

138 See V. Vedi et al., "Meniscal Movement: An In-Vivo Study Using Dynamic MRI," *Journal of Bone and Joint Surgery*, British volume 81.1 (1999): 37–41.

139 See Neumann, ed., *Kinesiology of the Musculoskeletal System*, page 442.

140 See Andrew Biel, *Trail Guide to the Body: A Hands-On Guide to Location Muscles, Bones and More*, 4th ed. (Boulder, CO: Books of Discovery, 2010), 375.

141 See S.R.R. Nascimento et al., "Morphometric Analysis of the Angle of the Femoral Trochlea," *Journal of Morphological Sciences* 28.4 (2011): 250–4.

142 M. Davies-Tuck et al., "Femoral Sulcus Angle and Increased Patella Facet Cartilage Volume in an Osteoarthritic Population," *Osteoarthritis Cartilage* 16.1 (2008): 131–5.

143 See Shelbourne et al., "The Relationship between Intercondylar Notch Width."

144 See Gray et al., *Gray's Anatomy,* 1491.

145 Garland et al.'s *Atlas of Anatomy* implies that a 23° torsion is "normal"; see page 373. However, Bengt-Gdran Clementz found the average to be slightly over 30°: "Tibial Torsion Measured in Normal Adults," *Acta Orthopaedica Scandinavica* 59.4 (1988): 441–2.

146 See R.P. Jakob, M. Haertel, and E. Stüssi, "Tibial Torsion Calculated by Computerised Tomography and Compared to Other Methods of Measurement," *Journal of Bone and Joint Surgery*, British volume, 62-B.2 (1980): 238–42.

147 See Pamela Sass and Ghinwa Hassan, "Lower Extremity Abnormalities in Children," *American Family Physician* 68.3 (2003): 461–8.

148 See Matsuda et al., "Posterior Tibial Slope in the Normal and Varus Knee," *American Journal of Knee Surgery* 12.3 (1999): 165–8.

149 See J. Robert Giffin et al., "Importance of Tibial Slope for Stability of the Posterior Cruciate Ligament–Deficient Knee," *American Journal of Sports Medicine* 35.9 (2007): 1443–9; and H. Marouane, "Steeper Posterior Tibial Slope Markedly Increases ACL Force in Both Active Gait and Passive Knee Joint Under Compression," *Journal of Biomechanics* 47.6 (2014): 1353–9.

150 See Faraj and Deacon, "Bipartite Sesamoids."

151 Drawings based upon those in H. Saupe, "Primare knochenmark seilerung der Kniescheibe," *Deutsche Zeitschrift für Chirurgie* 258 (1943): 386.

152 From Patellofemoral Foundation, "Patellar Morphology," in *Patellofemoral Foundation Online Education*, retrieved from www.patellofemoral.org/pfoe/c1/pat.

153 The number of sesamoid bones we have varies by individual, but one estimate suggests we are home to about 46! Not all of these show up in the anatomy textbooks, so we are rarely aware of them, but we will see them again when we look at the hands and feet. See V.K. Sarin, G.M. Erickson, N.J. Giori, A.G. Bergman, and D.R. Carter, "Coincident Development of Sesamoid Bones and Clues to Their Evolution," *Anatomical Record* 257.5 (1999): 174–80.

154 Exactly how often fabellae arise is unclear. Estimates range from 10–30% of the population, and this number tends to increase as we age. See J. G. Silva et al., "Morphological Analysis of the Fabella in Brazilians," *International Journal of Morphology* 28.1 (2010): 105–10.

155 See J.T. Zipple, R.L. Hammer, and P.V. Loubert, "Treatment of Fabella Syndrome With Manual Therapy: A Case Report," *Journal of Orthopaedic and Sports Physical Therapy* 33.1 (2003): 33–9.

156 Ibid.

157 See Kisner and Colby, *Therapeutic Exercise,* 767.

158 See A.C. Merchant et al., "The Female Knee: Anatomic Variations and the Female-Specific Total Knee Design," *Clinical Orthopaedics and Related Research* 466.12 (2008): 3059–65.

159 From P. Agliettis, J.N. Insall, and G. Gerulli, "Patellar Pain and Incongruence. I: Measurements of Incongruence," *Clinical Orthopaedics and Related Research* 176 (1983): 217–24.

160 See Neumann, ed., *Kinesiology of the Musculoskeletal System,* 438.

161 Ibid.

162 See "Q Angle of the Knee," in *Wheeless' Textbook of Orthopaedics*, retrieved from http://www.wheelessonline.com/ortho/q_angle_of_the_knee.

163 See C.H. Heath and L.T. Staheli, "Normal Limits of Knee Angle in White Children—Genu Varum and Genu Valgum," *Journal of Paediatric Orthopaedics* 13.2 (1993): 259–62.

164 See Leena Sharma, "The Role of Varus and Valgus Alignment in Knee Osteoarthritis," *Arthritis and Rheumatism* 56.4 (2007): 1044–7, doi:10.1002/art.22514.

165 See T.O. Smith, N.J. Hunt, and S.T. Donell, "The Reliability and Validity of the Q-angle: A Systematic Review," *Knee Surgery, Sports Traumatology, Arthroscopy* 16.12 (2008): 1068–79.

166 See E.M. Wojtys and L.J. Huston, "Functional Knee Braces: The 25-Year Controversy," in K.M. Chan, F. Fu, and N. Maffulli (eds.), *Controversies in Orthopaedic Sports Medicine* (Hong Kong: Williams & Wilkins, 2000).

167 It can be confusing to see *abduction* used to describe the knees moving together in valgus. The term is referring to the movement of the lower leg, not the knees per se. Think of the ankles: as the ankles move apart (abduct), the knees move together. The opposite occurs in adduction of the legs. To avoid such confusion, we will use the terms valgus instead of abduction and varus instead of adduction.

168 See Reese and Bandy, *Joint Range of Motion and Muscle Length Testing,* 473.

169 See Roach and Miles, "Normal Hip and Knee Active Range of Motion" and, for adduction, Boone and Azen, "Normal Range of Motion of Joints in Male Subjects."

170 From the author's own measurements on random pictures of students in Vajrasana and Virasana.

171 See Reese and Bandy, *Joint Range of Motion and Muscle Length Testing,* 333–4.

172 See M.S. De Carlo and K.E. Sell, "Normative Data for Range of Motion and Single-Leg Hop in High School Athletes," *Journal of Sport Rehabilitation* 6.3 (1997): 246–55.

173 See Reese and Bandy, *Joint Range of Motion and Muscle Length Testing*, 333.

174 See Garland et al., *Atlas of Anatomy*, 399.

175 See Thomas Myers, *Anatomy Trains: Myofascial Meridians for Manual and Movement Therapists*, 3rd ed. (New York: Elsevier, 2014), 111.

176 Ibid., 79–84.

177 Ibid., 191–4.

178 Ibid., 133.

179 Ibid., 206.

180 See Kisner and Colby, *Therapeutic Exercise*, 769.

181 Ibid.

182 Ibid.

183 See Goodfellow and O'Connor, "The Mechanics of the Knee and Prosthesis Design."

184 See Myers, *Anatomy Trains*, 85.

185 See Goodfellow and O'Connor, "The Mechanics of the Knee and Prosthesis Design."

186 See Neumann, ed., *Kinesiology of the Musculoskeletal System*, 451.

187 See S.E. Park et al., "The Change in Length of the Medial and Lateral Collateral Ligaments during In Vivo Knee Flexion," *Knee* 12.5 (2005): 377–82.

188 Ibid.

189 See Boden et al., "Noncontact Anterior Cruciate Ligament Injuries."

190 See Goodfellow and O'Connor, "The Mechanics of the Knee and Prosthesis Design."

191 Ibid.

192 Ibid.

193 See O. Missenard, D. Moettet, and S. Perrey, "The Role of Cocontraction in the Impairment of Movement Accuracy with Fatigue," *Experimental Brain Research* 185.1 (2008): 151–6.

194 See Stuart McGill, "Spine Flexion Exercise: Myths, Truths and Issues Affecting Health and Performance," retrieved from http://www.backfitpro.com/documents/Spine-flexion-myths-truths-and-issues.pdf.

195 "In a hatha yoga pose, to engage 'muscular' energy is to firm the muscles, 'hugging' them to the bones"; from Doug Keller, *Anusara Yoga: Hatha Yoga in the Anusara Style*, 3rd ed. (South Riding, VA: DoYoga Productions, 2005), 21. Available at http://www.doyoga.com/book.pdf.

196 See Bernie Clark, *The Complete Guide to Yin Yoga: The Philosophy and Practice of Yin Yoga* (Ashland, OR: White Cloud Press, 2012).

197 See Zipple et al., "Treatment of Fabella Syndrome."

198 See Reese and Bandy, *Joint Range of Motion and Muscle Length Testing*, 473.

199 See J.P. Pollard, W.L. Porter, and M.S. Redfern, "Forces and Moments on the Knee During Kneeling and Squatting," *Journal of Applied Biomechanics* 27.3 (2011): 233–41.

200 See Iyengar, *Light on Yoga*, 72.

201 See Desikachar and Cravens, *Health, Healing and Beyond*, 80.

202 See Mark Singleton, *Yoga Body: The Origins of Modern Postural Practice* (New York: Oxford University Press, 2010), 154.

203 "Recommendations for half or quarter squats to avoid degenerative changes in the knee joint [from deep squats] may be counterproductive. If the cartilage tissue of the odd facet is inadequately stressed then it receives insufficient nourishment that leads to consequent degeneration and atrophy"; from H. Hartmann, K. Wirth, and M. Klusemann, "Analysis of the Load on the Knee Joint and Vertebral Column with Changes in Squatting Depth and Weight Load," *Sport Medicine* 43 (2013): 993–1008.

204 From Iyengar, *Light on Yoga*, 72.

205 See R.F. Escamilla et al., "Effects of Technique Variations on Knee Biomechanics During the Squat and Leg Press," *Medicine and Science in Sports and Exercise* 33.9 (2001): 1552–66.

206 See G. McGinty, J.J. Irrgang, and D. Pezzullo, "Biomechanical Considerations for Rehabilitation of the Knee," *Clinical Biomechanics* 15 (2000): 160–6.

207 See Escamilla et al., "Effects of Technique Variations."

208 The area of contact between the patella and the femur was reported to be 2.6 +/– 0.4 cm^2 at 20° knee angle (KA), 3.1 +/– 0.3 cm^2 at 30° KA, 3.9 +/– 0.6 cm^2 at 60° KA, 4.1 +/– 1.2 cm^2 at 90° KA, and 4.6 +/– 0.7 cm^2 at 120° KA. See Escamilla et al., "Effects of Technique Variations."

209 The maximum amount of stress on the ACL in a lunge is reported to be about 50 newtons. However, the ACL's tolerance of stress ranges from 658 newtons for people over 60 to 2,160 newtons for people between 22 and 35 years of age. Clearly the amount of stress on the ACL in lunges is trivial. See Escamilla et al., "Cruciate Ligament Forces Between Short-Step and Long-Step Forward Lunge," *Medicine and Science in Sports and Exercise* 42.10 (2010): 1932–42.

210 Escamilla et al. found that all variations of squat were appropriate for rehabilitation patients who were trying to minimize ACL stress. See Escamilla et al., "Effects of Technique Variations."

211 See Escamilla et al., "Effects of Technique Variations."

212 The researchers claim that knee flexion angles beyond 80° may not be an issue for healthy athletes as long as they do not use heavy weights a lot. See Escamilla et al., "Effects of Technique Variations."

213 From Pattabhi Jois, *Yoga Mala*, 2nd ed. *(New York*: Eddie Stern/Patanjali Yoga Shala, 2000), 79.

214 The researchers found that preventing the knees from coming forward creates more leaning of the upper body, creating more flexion of the spine, leading to increased shear forces on the intervertebral discs. They concluded that directions to restrict the knees coming forward should be avoided. See Escamilla et al., "Effects of Technique Variations."

215 From Iyengar, *Light on Yoga*, 88.

216 Ibid.

217 From Jois, *Yoga Mala*, 54.

218 "[H]igher torque values in the knee joint [are] developed via a more upright posture" (from Hartmann et al., "Analysis of the Load on the Knee Joint").

219 "The influence of soft tissue contact between the back of the thigh and the calf plays a prominent role in reducing the knee-joint forces" (ibid.).

220 See R. Ramesh, O. Von Arx, T. Azzopardi, and P.J. Schranz, "The Risk of Anterior Cruciate Ligament Rupture with Generalised Joint Laxity," *Journal of Bone and Joint Surgery* 87-B.6 (2005): 800–3.

221 See Escamilla et al., "Effects of Technique Variations."

222 See Escamilla et al., "Cruciate Ligament Forces."

223 See K.L. Markolf, J.F. Gorek, J.M. Kabo, and M.S. Shapiro, "Direct Measurement of Resultant Forces in the Anterior Cruciate Ligament. An In Vitro Study Performed with a New Experimental Technique," *Journal of Bone and Joint Surgery*, American volume 72.4 (1990): 557–67.

224 See Clark, *The Complete Guide to Yin Yoga*, 108–11.

225 Drawing inspired by Neumann, ed., *Kinesiology of the Musculoskeletal System*, 561–2.

226 See De Carlo and Sell, "Normative Data."

227 See J.K. Loudon, H.L. Goist, and K.L. Loudon, "Genu Recurvatum Syndrome," *Journal of Orthopaedic and Sports Physical Therapy* 27.5 (1998): 361–7.

228 The literature varies on when to classify the hyperextended knee as genu recurvatum, with standards ranging from 0° to 10° of hyperextension.

229 See Ramesh et al., "The Risk of Anterior Cruciate Ligament Rupture."

230 See Lieberman, *The Story of the Human Body*, 42.

231 The range of hyperextension required for walking on level ground is 2–7°; see Reese and Bandy, *Joint Range of Motion and Muscle Length Testing*, 333.

232 See De Carlo and Sell, "Normative Data."

233 See K.D. Shelbourne, D.V. Patel, and D.J. Martini, "Classification and Management of Arthrofibrosis of the Knee Following ACL Reconstruction," *American Journal of Sports Medicine* 24 (1996): 857–62; K.D. Shelbourne and R.V. Trumper, "Preventing Anterior Knee Pain Following ACL Reconstruction," *American Journal of Sports Medicine* 25 (1997): 41–7.

234 See Ramesh et al., "The Risk of Anterior Cruciate Ligament Rupture."

235 See Yohei Shimokochi and Sandra J. Shultz, "Mechanisms of Noncontact Anterior Cruciate Ligament Injury," *Journal of Athletic Training* 43.4 (2008): 396–408.

236 See Hewett et al., "Anterior Cruciate Ligament Injuries in Female Athletes," and Boden et al., "Noncontact Anterior Cruciate Ligament Injuries."

237 See T.E. Hewett, K.R. Ford, B.J. Hoogenboom, and B.G. Myer, "Understanding and Preventing ACL Injuries: Current Biomechanical and Epidemiologic Considerations—Update 2010," *North American Journal of Sports Physical Therapy* 5.4 (2010): 234–51.

238 See Shimokochi and Shultz, "Mechanisms of Noncontact Anterior Cruciate Ligament Injury."

239 See T.E. Hewett, S.J. Shultz, and L.Y. Griffin (eds.), *Understanding and Preventing Noncontact ACL Injuries* (Champaign, IL: Human Kinetics, 2007), 25.

240 Drawings are based upon Iyengar, *Light on Yoga*, plate 591 from page 421 and plate 19 from page 75.

241 See Loudon et al., "Genu Recurvatum Syndrome."

242 See Escamilla et al., "Effects of Technique Variations."

243 See S.L. Woo, J.M. Hollis, D.J. Adams, R.M. Lyon, and S. Takai, "Tensile Properties of the Human Femur-Anterior Cruciate Ligament-Tibia Complex. The Effects of Specimen Age and Orientation," *American Journal of Sports Medicine* 19.3 (1991): 217–25.

244 See Escamilla et al., "Effects of Technique Variations."

245 See Markolf et al., "Direct Measurement of Resultant Forces."

246 See Loudon et al., "Genu Recurvatum Syndrome."

247 Given the statistics cited earlier on the average amount of hyperextension for men (5.5°, with one standard deviation of 2.5°), the 95% "norm" is 10.5° or less for men (compared with 12.1° or less for women).

248 The strength of the ACL does decline dramatically with age; see Woo et al., "Tensile Properties."

249 "Histological studies have indicated that applying some tension on healing ligaments will enhance the remodeling stage of healing. . . . [B]oth the ligament and the ligament attachment sites had greater tensile strength when they were subjected to tensile loads during healing. The absence of strain on ligaments, even those that have not been injured, has been shown to have harmful effects"; from G. Kelley Fitzgerald, "Open Versus Closed Kinetic Chain Exercise: Issues in Rehabilitation After Anterior Cruciate Ligament Reconstructive Surgery," *Physical Therapy* 77 (1997): 1747–54.

250 See Lan Chen, Paul D. Kim, Christopher S. Ahmad, and William N. Levine, "Medial Collateral Ligament Injuries of the Knee: Current Treatment Concepts," *Current Reviews in Musculoskeletal Medicine* 1.2 (2008): 108–13.

251 See S.E. Park et al., "The Change in Length of the Medial and Lateral Collateral Ligaments during In Vivo Knee Flexion."

252 See Shimokochi and Shultz, "Mechanisms of Noncontact Anterior Cruciate Ligament Injury."

253 See Sharma, "The Role of Varus and Valgus Alignment in Knee Osteoarthritis."

254 Ibid.

255 See Sharma et al., "Varus and Valgus Alignment and Incident and Progressive Knee Osteoarthritis," *Annals of the Rheumatic Diseases* 69.11 (2010): 1940–5, doi:10.1136/ard.2010.129742.

256 See Kenneth A. Krackow, *The Measurement and Analysis of Axial Deformity at the Knee* (Mahwah, NJ: Home Stryker Center, 2008), retrieved from http://www.smbs.buffalo.edu/ortho/axialdeformity.pdf.

257 See G.M. Brouwer et al., "Association between Valgus and Varus Alignment and the Development and Progression of Radiographic Osteoarthritis of the Knee," *Arthritis and Rheumatism* 56.4 (2007): 1204–11.

258 See Sharma et al., "Varus and Valgus Alignment."

259 The way we move our lower limbs during jumping was found to be independent of the physical attributes of the lower body, and thus it is the *way* we move that causes injury, not the shape of our bones; see Yasuharu Nagano et al., "Influence of Lower Limb Clinical Physical Measurements of Female Athletes on Knee Motion During Continuous Jump Testing," *The Open Sports Medicine Journal* 4 (2010): 134–9, doi:10.2174/1874387001004010134.

260 See Youri Thijs, Damien Van Tiggelen, Tine Willems, Dirk De Clercq, and Erik Witvrouw, "Relationship between Hip Strength and Frontal Plane Posture of the Knee during a Forward Lunge," *British Journal of Sports Medicine* 41 (2007): 723–7, doi:10.1136/bjsm.2007.037374.

261 See Stuart McGill, *Low Back Disorders: Evidence-Based Prevention and Rehabilitation*, 2nd ed. (Champaign, IL: Human Kinetics, 2007), and Maria Mountain, "Hockey Goalies: Spare Your Knees with These Two Exercises," *Hockey Training Pro*, retrieved from http://hockeytrainingpro.com/wordpress/2013/03/hockey-goalies-spare-your-knees-with-these-two-exercises.

262 See Chris Beardsley, "What Causes Knee Valgus?" (blog post, December 28, 2012), retrieved from www.strengthandconditioningresearch.com/2012/12/28/what-causes-knee-valgus.

263 See Jean-March Guichet, *Bone Deformities*, retrieved from www.leg-limb-stature-lengthening-taller-height-increase-cosmetic.eu/us/indications%20bone%20deformities.php.

264 See Gilroy et al., *Atlas of Anatomy*, 399.

265 *The Hatha Yoga Pradipika*, I-49 (English translation by Pancham Sinh, 3rd ed. [New Delhi: Oriental Books Reprint Corporation, 1980]).

266 Ibid., I-47.

267 See Reese and Bandy, *Joint Range of Motion and Muscle Length Testing*, 473.

268 Ibid.

269 See B.Y. Hwang et al., "Risk Factors for Medial Meniscus Posterior Root Tear," *American Journal of Sports Medicine* 40.7 (2012): 1606–10.

270 See B. Tangtrakulwanich, V. Chongsuvivatwong, and A.F. Geater, "Habitual Floor Activities Increase Risk of Knee Osteoarthritis," *Clinical Orthopaedics and Related Research* 454 (2007): 147–54.

271 See Neumann, ed., *Kinesiology of the Musculoskeletal System*, 445.

272 See McGinty et al., "Biomechanical Considerations for Rehabilitation of the Knee."

273 The medial patellofemoral ligament at 20° of flexion contributes 60% of the total restraining force. The medial patellomeniscal ligament provides 13% and the lateral retinaculum 10%. See S.M. Desio, R.T. Burks, and K.N. Bachus, "Soft Tissue Restraints to Lateral Patellar Translation in the Human Knee," *American Journal of Sports Medicine* 26.1 (1998): 59–65.

274 See McGinty et al., "Biomechanical Considerations for Rehabilitation of the Knee."

275 See Fiona G. Neely, "Biomechanical Risk Factors for Exercise-Related Lower Limb Injuries," *Sports Medicine* 26.6 (1998): 395–413.

276 McGinty et al. believe that there is no evidence to support the idea that the VMO can be exclusively recruited and strengthening the quadriceps may be sufficient to reduce

patellofemoral pain. See McGinty et al., "Biomechanical Considerations for Rehabilitation of the Knee."

277 See A. Techntahl, A. Wluka, and F. Cicuttini, "Abnormal Biomechanics: A Precursor or Result of Knee Osteoarthritis?" *British Journal of Sports Medicine* 37 (2003): 289–90.

278 See Goodfellow and O'Connor, "The Mechanics of the Knee and Prosthesis Design."

279 See Myers, *Anatomy Trains*, 85.

280 Goodfellow and O'Connor, "The Mechanics of the Knee and Prosthesis Design."

281 Ibid.

282 Ibid.

283 Ibid.

284 Ibid.

285 Ibid.

286 Sometimes, the metatarsal bones articulate with their neighboring bone. Some individuals have a facet between the first metatarsal and the middle cuneiform bone.

287 See Kisner and Colby, *Therapeutic Exercise*, 851.

288 See J.P. Gerber, G.N. Williams, C.R. Scoville, R.A. Arciero, and D.C. Taylor, "Persistent Disability Associated with Ankle Sprains: A Prospective Examination of an Athletic Population," *Foot and Ankle International* 19.10 (1998): 653–60, doi:10.1177/107110079801901002.

289 See W. Schamberger, *The Malalignment Syndrome: Implications for Medicine and Sport,* 2nd ed. (London: Churchill Livingston, 2013), 231.

290 Ibid.

291 See "Pes Planus / Flat Foot," in *Wheeless' Textbook of Orthopaedics,* Duke University Medical Center's Division of Orthopaedic Surgery, retrieved from http://www.wheelessonline.com/ortho/pes_planus_flat_foot.

292 See V. Sachithanandam and B. Joseph, "The Influence of Footwear on the Prevalence of Flat Foot. A Survey of 1846 Skeletally Mature Persons," *Journal of Bone and Joint Surgery,* British volume, 77 (1995): 254–7.

293 See A. Aminian and B.J. Sangeorzan, "The Anatomy of Cavus Foot Deformity," *Foot and Ankle Clinics* 13.2 (2008): 191–8, doi:10.1016/j.fcl.2008.01.004.

294 See "Pes Cavus / Cavovarus: Charcot Marie Tooth," in *Wheeless' Textbook of Orthopaedics,* Duke University Medical Center's Division of Orthopaedic Surgery, retrieved from http://www.wheelessonline.com/ortho/pes_cavus_charcot_marie_tooth.

295 See Rasmus G. Nielsen, Michael S. Rathleff, Ole H. Simonsen, and Henning Langberg, "Determination of Normal Values for Navicular Drop During Walking: A New Model Correcting For Foot Length and Gender," *Journal of Foot and Ankle Research* 2 (2009): 12, doi:10.1186/1757-1146-2-12.

296 See Karen P. Cote, Michael E. Brunet, II, Bruce M. Gansneder, and Sandra J. Shultz, "Effects of Pronated and Supinated Foot Postures on Static and Dynamic Postural Stability," *Journal of Athletic Training* 40.1 (2005): 41–6.

297 See Gray et al., *Gray's Anatomy*, 1512.

298 This trochlea is sometimes called the *trochlea tali*, but tali is just the plural for talus, and it is redundant to talk about the talus' trochlea tali, so when the context is clear, I will just say trochlea.

299 The talus provides 70% of the anteroposterior ankle stability, half of the foot's inversion/eversion stability, and 30% of the foot's internal/external rotation stability. See Rosdi Daud et al., "Three-Dimensional Morphometric Study of the Trapezium Shape of the Trochlea Tali," *Journal of Foot and Ankle Surgery* 30 (2013): 1–6.

300 See Kisner and Colby, *Therapeutic Exercise*, 853.

301 See J. Norgrove Penny, "Kinematics of the Subtalar and Tarsal Joints: How the Manipulation Method of Ponseti Works," (n.d.), retrieved from http://globalclubfoot.org/wp-content/uploads/downloads/2011/10/Tarsal-Kinematics-copy.pdf.

302 V.T. Inman, *The Joint of the Ankle* (Baltimore: Williams & Wilkins, 1976).

303 See Neumann, ed., *Kinesiology of the Musculoskeletal System*, 482.

304 It was from the work of V.T. Inman that anatomists first developed the idea of the trochlea approximating the surface of a cone. However, more recent research has determined that the top surface of the talus can be viewed as a truncated, skewed conic saddle shape with a laterally oriented apex. In other words, it's complicated! (Quotation from Soren Siegler, Jason Toy, Damani Seale, and David Pedowitz, "New Observations on the Morphology of the Talar Dome and Its Relationship to Ankle Kinematics," *Clinical Biomechanics* 10 (2013), doi:10.1016/j.clinbiomech.2013.10.009.

305 See Gray et al., *Gray's Anatomy*, 1524.

306 Ibid.

307 See Gray et al., *Gray's Anatomy*, 1526.

308 See Carla Stecco and Antonio Stecco, "Deep Fascia of the Lower Limbs," in *Fascia: The Tensional Network of the Human Body,* edited by R. Schleip, T.W. Findley, L. Chaitow, and P.A. Huijing (London: Elsevier, 2012), 33.

309 See Gray et al., *Gray's Anatomy*, 1508.

310 See Ching-Kuei Huang, Harold B. Kitaoka, Kai-Nan An, and Edmund Y. S. Chao, "Biomechanical Evaluation of Longitudinal Arch Stability," *Foot and Ankle International* 14.6 (1993): 353–7.

311 See Scott Wearing, "Anatomy of the Plantar Fascia," in Schleip et al., eds., *Fascia: The Tensional Network of the Human Body*, 253.

312 See Wearing, "Anatomy of the Plantar Fascia," 254.

313 See Wearing, "Anatomy of the Plantar Fascia," 255.

314 See Stecco and Stecco, "Deep Fascia of the Lower Limb," 33.

315 See Gray et al., *Gray's Anatomy*, 1509.

316 See Myers, *Anatomy Trains*, 77.

317 See Wearing, "Anatomy of the Plantar Fascia," 255.

318 See H. Lemont, K.M. Ammirati, and N. Usen, "Plantar Fasciitis: A Degenerative Process (Fasciosis) Without Inflammation," *Journal of the American Podiatric Medical Association* 93 (2003): 234–7.

319 See Wearing, "Anatomy of the Plantar Fascia," 255.

320 See Andrew Biel, *Trail Guide to the Body: A Hands-on Guide to Locating Muscles, Bones and More*, 4th ed. (Boulder, CO: Books of Discovery, 2010), 371.

321 See E. Vanderhooft, "The Frequency of and Relationship between the Palmaris Longus and Plantaris Tendons," *American Journal of Orthopaedics* 25.1 (1996): 38–41.

322 See Biel, *Trail Guide to the Body*, 374.

323 See Daysi Ramirez et al., "Clinical Evaluation of Fibularis Tertius Muscle Prevalence," *International Journal of Morphology* 28.3 (2010): 759–64.

324 See Gray et al., *Gray's Anatomy*, 1536.

325 See Gray et al., *Gray's Anatomy*, 1537.

326 See Kirsten L. Schroeder, Benjamin W.C. Rosser, and Soo Y. Kim, "Fiber Type Composition of the Human Quadratus Plantae Muscle: A Comparison of the Lateral and Medial Heads," *Journal of Foot and Ankle Research* 7 (2014): 54, doi:10.1186/s13047-014-0054-5.

327 See *Gray's Anatomy*, page 1541.

328 See Wearing, "Anatomy of the Plantar Fascia," 253.

329 See D.B. Thordarson, H. Schmotzer, J. Chon, and J. Peters, "Dynamic Support of the Human Longitudinal Arch: A Biomechanical Evaluation," *Clinical Orthopaedics and Related Research* 316 (1995): 165–72.

330 See Luke A. Kelly, Andrew G. Cresswell, Sebastien Racinais, Rodney Whiteley, and Glen Lichtwark, "Intrinsic Foot Muscles Have the Capacity to Control Deformation of the Longitudinal Arch," *Journal of the Royal Society Interface* 11.93 (2014), doi:10.1098/rsif.2013.1188.

331 See G. Mariani and V. Patella, "Valutazione statistica dei parametri articolari della tibio-tarsica," *Chirurgia Organi* 63 (1977): 333–40; and M.H. Fessy, J.P. Carret, and J. Bejui,

"Morphometry of the Talocrural Joint," *Surgical and Radiological Anatomy* 19 (1997): 299–302.

332 See M. Misiani, J. Nderitu, M. Pamela, O. Moses, and G. Gichambira, "Sexual Dimorphism in the Morphometric Characteristics of the Tibial Plafond and Medial Malleolus," *Indian Journal of Basic and Applied Medical Research* 2.7 (2013): 760–3.

333 See Jeremy M. DeSilva, "Functional Morphology of the Ankle and the Likelihood of Climbing in Early Hominins," *Proceedings of the National Academy of Sciences* 106.16 (2009): 6567–72.

334 See Inman, *The Joints of the Ankle*, 19, 26, 27, 31, 37, 70–3.

335 See Neumann, ed., *Kinesiology of the Musculoskeletal System*, 480, and Gray et al., *Gray's Anatomy*, 1512.

336 See K.A. Kirby, "Methods for Determination of Positional Variations in the Subtalar Joint Axis," *Journal of the American Podiatric Medical Association* 77.5 (1987): 228–34.

337 See Daud et al., "Three-Dimensional Morphometric Study."

338 All figures are from Daud et al., "Three-Dimensional Morphometric Study."

339 See Ned Amendola et al., "CAM-Type Impingement in the Ankle," *Iowa Orthopaedic Journal* 32 (2012): 1–8.

340 See Amendola et al., "CAM-Type Impingement in the Ankle."

341 See M.S. Burman and P.W. Lapidus, "The Functional Disturbances Caused by Inconstant Bones and Sesamoids of the Foot," *Archives of Surgery* 22 (1931): 936–75.

342 See "Os Trigonum / Posterior Talar Impingement," in *Wheeless' Textbook of Orthopaedics*, Duke University Medical Center's Division of Orthopaedic Surgery, retrieved from http://www.wheelessonline.com/ortho/os_trigonum_posterior_talar_impingement.

343 See M.B. Davies, "The Os Trigonum Syndrome," *The Foot* 14.3 (2004): 119–23.

344 See John Rogers et al., "Posterior Ankle Impingement Syndrome: A Clinical Review with Reference to Horizontal Jump Athletes," *Acta Orthopaedica Belgica* 76.5 (2010): 572–9.

345 See Evangelos Perdikakis and Apostolos Karantanas, "Stieda Process Versus Haglund's Deformity: An Uncommon Presentation of Posterior Ankle Impingement," *European Journal of Medicine* 6.2 (2011): 190–2.

346 See Mayank Javia et al., "Morphological Study of Squatting Facets on the Neck of the Talus in Indian Population," *Journal of Research in Medical and Dental Science* 2.4 (2014): 38–41.

347 See I.H. Oygucu, M.A. Kurt, I. Ikiz, T. Erem, and D.C. Davies, "Squatting Facets on the Neck of the Talus and Extensions of the Trochlear Surface of the Talus in Late Byzantine Males," *Journal of Anatomy* 192, Part 2 (1998): 287–91.

348 See K. Islam et al., "Symmetry Analysis of Talus Bone: A Geometric Morphometric Approach," *Bone and Joint Research* 3.5 (2014): 139–45.

349 See N. Muthukumaravel, D. Ravichandran, and S. Melani Rajendran, "Human Calcaneal Facets for the Talus: Patterns and Clinical Implications," *Journal of Clinical and Diagnostic Research* 5.4 (2011): 791–4.

350 Ibid.

351 This, remember, is a simplification. There are 33 joints in the foot, and most of these have some wiggle room. It is simply beyond our scope to investigate them all.

352 See Kirby, "Methods for Determination."

353 Ibid.

354 Ibid.

355 Ibid.

356 *Anatomy Trains*, 82.

357 See E. Trinkaus, *A Functional Analysis of the Neanderthal Foot* (PhD diss., University of Pennsylvania, 1975).

358 See Stephen J. Piazza, "The Sprinter's Advantage: Thinking Outside the Blocks," *Lower Extremity Review* (July 2012), retrieved from http://lermagazine.com/cover_story/the-sprinters-advantage-thinking-outside-the-blocks.

359 See S.S. Lee and S.J. Piazza, "Built for Speed: Musculoskeletal Structure and Sprinting Ability," *Journal of Experimental Biology* 212, Part 22 (2009): 3700–7, doi:10.1242/jeb.031096.

360 See A. Nagano and T. Komura, "Longer Moment Arm Results in Smaller Joint Moment Development, Power and Work Outputs in Fast Motions," *Journal of Biomechanics* 36.11 (2003): 1675–81.

361 See Lee and Piazza, "Built for Speed."

362 See D.A. Raichlen, H. Armstrong, and D.E. Lieberman, "Calcaneus Length Determines Running Economy: Implications for Endurance Running Performance in Modern Humans and Neandertals," *Journal of Human Evolution* 60.3 (2011): 299–308.

363 See O.K. Nwawka et al., "Sesamoids and Accessory Ossicles of the Foot: Anatomical Variability and Related Pathology," *Insights into Imaging* 4.5 (2013): 581–93.

364 See Nwawka et al., "Sesamoids and Accessory Ossicles of the Foot."

365 See Darron M, Jones, Charles L. Saltzman, and George El-Khoury, "The Diagnosis of the Os Trigonum Syndrome with a Fluoroscopically Controlled Injection of Local Anesthetic," *Iowa Orthopaedic Journal* 19 (1999): 122–6.

366 Ibid.

367 See J.J. Peterson and L.W. Bancroft, "Os Peroneal Fracture with Associated Peroneus Longus Tendinopathy," *American Journal of Roentgenology* 177.1 (2001): 257–8.

368 See D.M. Stormont and H.A. Peterson, "The Relative Incidence of Tarsal Coalition," *Clinical Orthopaedics and Related Research* 181 (1983): 28–36.

369 See Gray et al., *Gray's Anatomy*, 1520.

370 Dorsiflexion measurements were made with the subject sitting, so the knees were flexed 90°; see the *Normal Joint Range of Motion Study*, by the Centers for Disease Control and Prevention, retrieved from www.cdc.gov/ncbddd/jointrom.

371 This average was with the foot bearing weight and the knee completely extended. The standard deviation was 7°; see Sebastian F. Baumbach et al., "The Influence of Knee Position on Ankle Dorsiflexion—A Biometric Study," *BMC Musculoskeletal Disorders* 15 (2014): 246, doi:10.1186/1471-2474-15-246.

372 See Reese and Bandy, *Joint Range of Motion and Muscle Length Testing*, 347. These values represent the lowest average less one SD to the highest average plus one SD.

373 There is a slight difference between squatting with the heels on the floor or raised up, but only about 1° on average; see Reese and Bandy, *Joint Range of Motion and Muscle Length Testing*, 347. One study found that a dorsiflexion angle of 38.5° with one SD of 5.9° was necessary to keep the heels down during a full squat; see A. Hemmerich, H. Brown, S. Smith, S.S. Marthandam, and U.P. Wyss, "Hip, Knee, and Ankle Kinematics of High Range of Motion Activities of Daily Living," *Journal of Orthopaedic Research* 24 (2006): 770–81.

374 See M.L. Root, W.P. Orion, and J.H. Weed, *Normal and Abnormal Function of the Foot* (Los Angeles: Clinical Biomechanics Corporation, 1977).

375 Part of the discrepancy is due to variations in how to measure dorsiflexion; see Reese and Bandy, *Joint Range of Motion and Muscle Length Testing*, 347.

376 See Baumbach et al., "The Influence of Knee Position."

377 See P.C. Begeman and P. Prasad, "Human Ankle Impact Response in Dorsiflexion," SAE Technical Paper 902308, 1990, doi:10.4271/902308. Also see C.S. Parenteau, D.C. Viano, and P.Y. Petit, "Biomechanical Properties of Human Cadaveric Ankle-Subtalar Joints in Quasistatic Loading," *Journal of Biomechanical Engineering* 120 (1998): 105–11.

378 From Centers for Disease Control and Prevention, *Normal Joint Range of Motion Study*.

379 Ibid.

380 See Reese and Bandy, *Joint Range of Motion and Muscle Length Testing*, page 347.

381 Ibid. These values represent the lowest average less one SD to the highest average plus one SD.

382 See Neumann, ed., *Kinesiology of the Musculoskeletal System*, 491.

383 Values are from S.K. Grimston, B.M. Nigg, D.A. Hanley, and J.R. Engsberg, "Differences in Ankle Joint Complex Range of Motion as a Function of Age," *Foot and Ankle* 14 (1993): 215–22.

384 Ibid.

385 A 1979 study found average inversion to be 36° +/– 4° and eversion to be 19° +/– 5° in the 25–39 age range; see D.C. Boone and S.P. Azen, "Normal Range of Motion of Joints in Male Subjects," *Journal of Bone and Joint Surgery*, American volume, 61 (1979): 756–9.

386 Doug Keller suggests that these exercises can slow down the progression of bunions, also called hallux valgus; see "9 Poses to Prevent Bunions & Relieve Bunion Pain," *Yoga International* (June 4, 2013), retrieved from https://yogainternational.com/article/view/9-poses-to-prevent-bunions-relieve-bunion-pain.

387 See Neumann, ed., *Kinesiology of the Musculoskeletal System*, 505.

388 "Maximal dorsiflexion during push off was found to be 60 degrees for feet walking without shoes, 45–50 degrees for feet walking in soft shoes, and 25–30 degrees for feet walking in a stiff shoe of the minus-heel type"; see F. Bojsen-Møller and L. Lamoreux, "Significance of Free Dorsiflexion of the Toes in Walking," *Acta Orthopaedica Scandinavica* 50.4 (1979): 471–9.

389 See Myers, *Anatomy Trains*, 206.

390 Ibid., 100–3.

391 See Myers, *Anatomy Trains*, 206–7.

392 Equinus refers to the foot drooping downward, like a horse's foot (*equus* is Latin for horse).

393 See A. Gatt and N. Chockalingham, "Assessment of Ankle Joint Dorsiflexion: An Overview," *Revista Internacional de Ciencias Podológicas* 6.1 (2012): 25–9.

394 See Baumbach et al., "The Influence of Knee Position on Ankle Dorsiflexion."

395 See Gatt and Chockalingham, "Assessment of Ankle Joint Dorsiflexion."

396 See H. Danaberg, "Manipulation of the Ankle as a Method for Treating Ankle and Foot Pain," *Journal of the American Podiatric Medical Association* 94.4 (2004): 395–9.

397 See Gatt and Chockalingham, "Assessment of Ankle Joint Dorsiflexion."

398 The authors of a study on limited ankle dorsiflexion found that decreased dorsiflexion while weight-bearing reduces one's ability to lower the body's center of mass, which causes subtalar-joint pronation and tibial internal rotation. A knee valgus position could result due to increased tibial internal rotation, creating an associated increase in femoral internal rotation.

These changes in the frontal and transverse plane motion of the hip and knee could lead to patellofemoral pain. See E. Macrum, D.R. Bell, M. Boling, M. Lewek, and D. Padua, "Effect of Limiting Ankle-Dorsiflexion Range of Motion on Lower Extremity Kinematics and Muscle-Activation Patterns During a Squat," *Journal of Sport Rehabilitation* 21 (2012): 144–50.

399 These studies have shown that God does not keep lists of those people who can't do yoga poses in the most aesthetically pleasing ways. God does not keep lists. But Santa does!

400 See F.H. Bassett, III, H.S. Gates, III, J.B. Billys, H.B. Morris, and P.K. Nikolaou, "Talar Impingement by the Anteroinferior Tibiofibular Ligament. A Cause of Chronic Pain in the Ankle After Inversion Sprain," *Journal of Bone and Joint Surgery*, American volume, 72.1 (1990): 55–9.

401 See Neumann, ed., *Kinesiology of the Musculoskeletal System*, 486.

402 See L.A. Lavery, D.G. Armstrong, and A.J. Boulton, "Ankle Equinus Deformity and Its Relationship to High Plantar Pressure in a Large Population with Diabetes Mellitus," *Journal of the American Podiatric Medical Association* 92.9 (2002): 479–82.

403 See Bassett et al., "Talar Impingement by the Anteroinferior Tibiofibular Ligament."

404 See Amendola et al., "CAM-Type Impingement in the Ankle."

405 See S.M. Raikin and P.H. Cooke, "Divot Sign: A New Observation in Anterior Impingement of the Ankle," *Foot and Ankle International* 20.8 (1999): 532–3.

406 According to James Meadows, subluxation is "a biomechanical problem with the joint jamming at one end of the range of movement and blocking movement away from that range"; see *Orthopedic Differential Diagnosis in Physical Therapy: A Case Study Approach* (New York: McGraw-Hill, 1999), 114–5.

407 See Craig R. Denegar and Sayers J. Miller, III, "Can Chronic Ankle Instability Be Prevented? Rethinking Management of Lateral Ankle Sprains," *Journal of Athletic Training* 37.4 (2002): 430–5.

408 Many studies have implicated the presence of an os trigonum in posterior ankle impingement syndrome, a condition where pain arises when the ankle is in plantarflexion. Up to ~15% of the population may have one! Just because you have one does not mean that you will have pain in plantarflexion, but it may be a cause of compression and thus limitation in how far you can plantarflex your ankle.

409 See Rebekah Young, Sheree Nix, Aaron Wholohan, Rachael Bradhurst, and Lloyd Reed, "Interventions for Increasing Ankle Joint Dorsiflexion: A Systematic Review and Meta-Analysis," *Journal of Foot and Ankle Research* 6 (2013): 46.

410 Young et al., "Interventions for Increasing Ankle Joint Dorsiflexion."

411 This average was with the foot bearing weight and the knee completely extended. The standard deviation was 7°; see Baumbach et al., "The Influence of Knee Position on Ankle Dorsiflexion."

412 These ranges were derived by taking the average worst and best case study and subtracting or adding one standard deviation; see Reese and Bandy, *Joint Range of Motion and Muscle Length Testing*, 347.

413 See DeSilva, "Functional Morphology of the Ankle."

414 See Baumbach et al., "The Influence of Knee Position."

415 Thirty-three percent of the population has a range of dorsiflexion outside the range of one standard deviation cited here, but half of these people have a greater range of motion and half of them have less; half of 33% is about one person in six.

416 See J. Karrholm, S. Brandsson, and M.A. Freeman, "Tibiofemoral Movement 4: Changes of Axial Tibial Rotation Caused by Forced Rotation at the Weight-Bearing Knee Studied by RSA," *Journal of Bone and Joint Surgery*, British volume, 82-B (2000): 1201–3.

417 See Michael J. Coughlin, Charles L. Saltzman, and Roger A. Mann, *Mann's Surgery of the Foot and Ankle* (New York: Elsevier Health Sciences, 2013).

418 Females at ages 2–8: 67.1; ages 9–19: 57.3; ages 20–44: 62.1; ages 45–69: 56.5. Males at ages 2–8: 55.8; ages 9–19: 52.8; ages 20–44: 54.6; ages 45–69: 49.4. From Centers for Disease Control and Prevention, *Normal Joint Range of Motion Study*.

419 For our purposes, it is sufficient to claim that when the top of the foot is flat, we have reached the maximum functional amount of plantarflexion, but there are certainly cases in athletics and in dance when the ankle can plantarflex more. This additional range of motion is not required in yoga.

420 See AIM Trial, University of Oxford, *Guide for Assessing Ankle Range of Movement for the AIM Trial: Range of Movement Guide*, retrieved from www.aimtrial.org/?page=download&file_id=29.

421 See Rasmus Oestergaard Nielsen et al., "Foot Pronation is Not Associated with Increased Injury Risk in Novice Runners Wearing a Neutral Shoe: A 1-Year Prospective Cohort Study," *British Journal of Sports Medicine* 48 (2014): 440–7, doi:10.1136/bjsports-2013-092202.

422 See *Light on Yoga*, 352.

423 See Bojsen-Møller and Lamoreux, "Significance of Free Dorsiflexion of the Toes in Walking."

424 See Reese and Bandy, *Joint Range of Motion and Muscle Length Testing*, 349.

425 See Bernie Clark, The Complete Guide to Yin Yoga (Ashland, OR: White Cloud Press, 2012), 113.

426 See *Yoga Journal's* instructions at www.yogajournal.com/article/beginners/adho-mukha-svanasana and www.yogajournal.com/article/beginners/downward-facing-dog-pose-2/, as well as those from DoYouYoga.com at www.doyouyoga.com/10-alignment-tips-to-improve-your-downward-dog. Also see B.K.S. Iyengar, *Yoga: The Path to Holistic Health* (New York: DK Publishing, 2001), 184.

427 See Georg Feuerstein, *The Shambhala Encyclopedia of Yoga* (Boston, MA: Shambhala Publications, 2000), 118.

428 See T.K.V. Desikachar, *The Heart of Yoga* (Rochester, VT: Inner Traditions International, 1999), 137, 239. Also, see Swami Sivananda, *Yoga Asanas* (Richikesh, India: Divine Life Society, 1931 and 1998), xiii.

429 See Daniel Lieberman, *The Story of the Human Body* (New York: Pantheon Books, 2013), 35.

430 See Oksana Kolesova and Jānis Vētra, "Female Pelvic Types and Age Differences in Their Distribution," *Papers on Anthropology* 21 (2012), 147–54, doi:10.12697/poa.2012.21.11.

431 See Kolesova and Vētra, "Female Pelvic Types."

432 For descriptions and prevalences of these shapes, see W.E. Caldwell and H.C. Moloy, "Anatomical Variations in the Female Pelvis: Their Classification and Obstetrical Significance," *Proceedings of the Royal Society of Medicine* 32.1 (1938): 1–30.

433 See Murtha et al. "Variations in Acetabular Anatomy with Reference to Total Hip Replacement." They found for 22 females that the mean anteversion was 24.1°, with a range of variation from 14.0° to 33.3°. The same parameters for the 20 males in the study were 19.3°, with a range between 8.5° and 32.3°. We might assume that this would mean women would find external rotation more difficult than men, but other variations tend to balance out this effect: women, on average, have shallower acetabula, which allows more range of movement.

434 See Blandine Calais-Germain, *The Female Pelvis: Anatomy and Exercises* (Seattle: Eastland Press, 2003), 20.

435 See Adam J. Engler, "The Contribution of Geometrical Properties to Pubic Rami Fractures in Lateral Impact," *Journal of Young Investigators* 4.1 (2001), retrieved from http://legacy.jyi.org/volumes/volume4/issue1/articles/engler.html.

436 See Theodore E. Keats and Mark W. Anderson, "The Pubis and Ischium," in *Atlas of Normal Roentgen Variants That May Simulate Disease*, 9th ed., 265–74 (New York: Elsevier, 2013).

437 See Neumann, ed., *Kinesiology of the Musculoskeletal System*, 517.

438 See Leena Sharma, "The Role of Varus and Valgus Alignment in Knee Osteoarthritis," *Arthritis and Rheumatism* 56.4 (2007): 1044–7, doi:10.1002/art.22514.

439 Ibid.

440 See Leena Sharma et al., "Varus and Valgus Alignment and Incident and Progressive Knee Osteoarthritis," *Annals*

of the Rheumatic Diseases 69.1 (2010): 1940–5, doi:10.1136/ ard.2010.129742.

441 See Kisner and Colby, *Therapeutic Exercise*, 804.

442 See P.A. Indelicato, "Isolated Medial Collateral Ligament Injuries in the Knee," *Journal of the American Academy of Orthopaedic Surgeons* 3.1 (1995): 9–14.

443 See Boden et al., "Noncontact Anterior Cruciate Ligament Injuries."

444 Such as the tendency to engage the quadriceps exclusively when landing from a jump rather than co-contracting the hamstrings, and allowing the knees to come together (valgus) rather than keeping them neutral.

445 See Boden et al., "Noncontact Anterior Cruciate Ligament Injuries."

446 See A. Samaei, A.H. Bakhtiary, F. Elham, and A. Rezasoltani, "Effects of Genu Varum Deformity on Postural Stability," *International Journal of Sports Medicine* 33.6 (2012): 469–73.

447 See Craig R. Denegar and Sayers J. Miller, III, "Can Chronic Ankle Instability Be Prevented? Rethinking Management of Lateral Ankle Sprains," *Journal of Athletic Training* 37.4 (2002): 430–5.

448 See Neely, "Biomechanical Risk Factors."

449 See Neumann, ed., *Kinesiology of the Musculoskeletal System*, 491.

450 Ibid., 492.

451 Ibid., 495.

452 Ibid.

453 Ibid., 496.

454 Ibid., 493.

455 See Carol A. Oatis, "Biomechanics of the Foot and Ankle Under Static Conditions," *Physical Therapy* 68.12 (1988): 1815–21.

456 See Neumann, ed., *Kinesiology of the Musculoskeletal System*, 507.

457 See Thomas G. McPoil and Harry G. Knecht, "Biomechanics of the Foot in Walking: A Functional Approach," *Journal of Orthopaedic and Sports Physical Therapy*, 7.2 (1985): 69–72).

458 N. Okita, S.A. Meyers, J.H. Challis, and N.A. Sharkey, "Midtarsal Joint Locking: New Perspectives on an Old Paradigm," *Journal of Orthopaedic Research* 32.1 (2014): 110–5.

Credits and Permissions

Morgan Jeske created all the illustrations not otherwise credited.

Alex Hennig created the cover art, book layout and graphic designs.

The following photos are by Joe Dully, reproduced with the kind permission of Paul Grilley, from www.PaulGrilley.com/bone-photo-gallery: page 56, figure 1.39; page 106, figure 2.29; page 109, figure 2.33; page 111, figure 2.36; page 218, figure 2.221; and back cover.

Several images in this book, itemized below, are from OpenStax, which requires the following general copyright statement: "Textbook content produced by OpenStax College is licensed under a Creative Commons Attribution License 3.0 or 4.0, depending upon the specific material. The OpenStax College name, OpenStax College logo, OpenStax College book covers, OpenStax CNX name, and OpenStax CNX logo are not subject to the Creative Commons license and may not be reproduced without the prior and express written consent of Rice University."

VOLUME 1

page 5: "Each person has different proportions…" is quoted, with the author's permission, from Stuart McGill, *Ultimate Back and Fitness Performance*, 5th ed. (Waterloo, Canada: Backfitpro, 2014). www.backfitpro.com.

page 6, figure 1.6: This image was inspired by the drawing in Frank Netter, *Atlas of Human Anatomy*, 3rd ed. (Teterboro, NJ: Icon Learning Systems, 2003), plate 275.

page 8, figure 1.5: Graph generated based on data in Jonathan D. Schoenfeld and John P.A. Ioannidis, "Is Everything We Eat Associated with Cancer? A Systematic Cookbook Review," *American Journal of Clinical Nutrition* 97.1 (January 2013): 127–34. doi:10.3945/ajcn.112.047142.

page 9: "normal individuals are found from…" is quoted, with the kind permission of John Anderson, from John Y. Anderson and Erik Trinkaus, "Patterns of Sexual, Bilateral and Interpopulational Variation in Human Femoral Neck-shaft Angles," *Journal of Anatomy* 192 (1998): 279–285. doi:10.1046/j.1469-7580.1998.19220279.x.

page 10, figure 1.10: Graphic reproduced, with the kind permission of John Anderson, from John Y. Anderson and Erik Trinkaus, "Patterns of Sexual, Bilateral and Interpopulational Variation in Human Femoral Neck-shaft Angles," *Journal of Anatomy* 192 (1998): 279–285. doi:10.1046/j.1469-7580.1998.19220279.x.

page 14: "Differences aren't deficits" is quoted from Kate Douglas, "Reaping the Whirlwind of Nazi Eugenics," *New Scientist*, July 14, 2014. Reproduced with permission. © 2014 Reed Business Information Ltd., England. All rights reserved. Distributed by Tribune Content Agency.

page 27: "Our antifragilities have conditions…" is quoted, with the author's permission, from Nassim Nicholas Taleb, *Antifragile: Things That Gain from Disorder* (New York: Random House, 2012), 58.

page 27: "loading is necessary for optimal tissue health…" is quoted, with the author's permission, from Stuart McGill, *Low Back Disorders: Evidence-Based Prevention and Rehabilitation*, 2nd ed. (Champaign, IL: Human Kinetics, 2007), 14.

page 32, figure 1.24: Image inspired by a drawing in James Oschman, *Energy Medicine in Therapeutics and Human Performance* (Edinburgh, UK: Elsevier, 2003), 46.

page 33, figure 1.25: Graphic reproduced with the kind permission of Loren Fishman and Ellen Saltonstall, from *Yoga for Osteoporosis* (New York: W.W. Norton, 2010), 76.

page 42, figure 1.29: Images from the DVD *Interior Architecture: Exploring the Architecture of the Human Body*, reproduced with the kind permission of Jean-Claude Guimberteau.

page 45, figure 1.32: Images reproduced, with the author's permission, from Jaap van der Wal, "The Architecture of the Connective Tissue in the Musculoskeletal System—An Often Overlooked Functional Parameter as to Proprioception in the Locomotor Apparatus," in *Fascia Research II: Basic Science and Implications for Conventional and Complementary Health Care*, ed. Thomas W. Findley and Robert Schleip (Munich: Elsevier, 2009).

page 50: "It can be argued that stress…" is quoted, with the author's permission, from Timothy McCall, *Yoga as Medicine: The Yogic Prescription for Health and Healing* (New York: Bantam Books, 2007), 4.

page 55: "Two individuals may have very…" is quoted from the article "Enzyme in Saliva Helps Regulate Blood Glucose," published by Monell Chemical Senses Center, available at http://www.monell.org/images/uploads/amylase_final.pdf. Used with permission.

page 55, figure 1.38: © June 3, 2013 OpenStax College. Download the image for free at http://cnx.org/contents/9306de62-3f52-46f8-ab1a-94263c480eda@3.

page 57: "Stiffness is always stabilizing" is quoted, with the author's permission, from Stuart McGill, *Low Back Disorders: Evidence-Based Prevention and Rehabilitation*, 2nd ed. (Champaign, IL: Human Kinetics, 2006), 118.

page 62: "The longest period of low…" is republished with the permission of the *Journal of Orthopaedic and Sports Physical Therapy*, from "Contracture and Stiff Joint Management with Dynasplint," George R. Hepburn, vol., 8, no. 4, 1987; permission conveyed through Copyright Clearance Center, Inc.

page 71 : "lines of pull, based on…" is quoted, with the publisher's permission, from Thomas Myers, *Anatomy Trains: Myofascial Meridians for Manual and Movement Therapists*, 3rd ed. (New York: Elsevier, 2014), 5.

page 74, figure 1.49: Drawings of the meridian lines were inspired by information in Thomas Myers, *Anatomy Trains: Myofascial Meridians for Manual and Movement Therapists*, 3rd ed. (New York: Elsevier, 2014), chapters 3 to 9.

page 84n115: "[A]ll fibrous collagenous connective tissues…" is quoted, with the authors' permission, from Robert Schleip and Divo Gitta Müller, *Fascial Dysfunction: Manual Therapy Approaches—Use It or Lose It* (Pencaitland, Scotland: Handspring Publishing, 2014), 127.

page 86n169: "a higher proportion of elastic response…" is republished with the permission of the *Journal of Orthopaedic and Sports Physical Therapy*, from "Contracture and Stiff Joint Management with Dynasplint," George R. Hepburn, vol., 8, no. 4, 1987; permission conveyed through Copyright Clearance Center, Inc.

VOLUME 2

page 103, figure 2.23: © August 26, 2013 OpenStax College. Download the image for free at http://cnx.org/contents/14fb4ad7-39a1-4eee-ab6e-3ef2482e3e22@6.10.

page 103, figure 2.24: Drawing inspired by material in Blandine Calais-Germain, *Anatomy of Movement* (Seattle, WA: Eastland Press, 1993).

page 104, figure 2.25: © September 28, 2015 OpenStax College. Download for free at http://cnx.org/contents/cbdfe00f-2ef8-4348-9111-9fd-4ba7a02c5@5.

page 110, figure 2.34: This graph is reproduced with the kind permission of John Anderson, from John Y. Anderson and Erik Trinkaus, "Patterns of Sexual, Bilateral and Interpopulational Variation in Human Femoral Neck-shaft Angles," *Journal of Anatomy* 192 (1998): 279–285. doi:10.1046/j.1469-7580.1998.19220279.x.

page 116: "feel for any tension in…" quoted, with the author's permission, from Judith Lasater, *Yogabody: Anatomy, Kinesiology, and Asana* (Berkeley, CA: Rodmell Press, 2009), 48.

page 147: "Listening to one's body is important…" is a quotation of Dr. Derek Ochiai, cited by Joshua Hodges in *Kicking and the Hips*, www.theshotokanway.com/kickingandthehips.html. Reproduced with the permission of Joshua Hodges.

pages 158–159, figures 2.100, 2,101 and 2.102: © September 28, 2015 OpenStax College. Download for free at http://cnx.org/contents/14fb4ad7-39a1-4eee-ab6e-3ef2482e3e22@7.30.

page 166, figure 2.109: Drawings inspired by those in H. Saupe, "Primare knochenmark seilerung der Kniescheibe," *Deutsche Zeitschrift für Chirurgie* 258 (1943): 386.

page 167, figure 2.111: © July 30, 2014 OpenStax College. Download for free at http://cnx.org/contents/14fb4ad7-39a1-4eee-ab6e-3ef2482e3e22@6.27.

page 174: "a universal law of human…" is quoted, with the author's permission, from Stuart McGill, "Spine Flexion Exercise: Myths, Truths and Issues Affecting Health and Performance," http://www.backfitpro.com/documents/Spine-flexion-myths-truths-and-issues.pdf.

page 176: "man behind some of the most…" is quoted, with the publisher's permission, from Mark Singleton, *Yoga Body: The Origins of Modern Postural Practice* (New York: Oxford University Press, 2010), 154.

page 184, figure 2.127: Drawing inspired by Donald A. Neumann, *Kinesiology of the Musculoskeletal System: Foundations for Rehabilitation*, 2nd ed. (St. Louis, MO: Mosby, 2010), 561–562.

page 187: "the absence of strain on ligaments…" is quoted, with the permission of the American Physical Therapy Association, from Kelley Fitzgerald, "Open Versus Closed Kinetic Chain Exercise: Issues in Rehabilitation After Anterior Cruciate Ligament Reconstructive Surgery," *Physical Therapy* 77 (1997): 1747–54.

pages 204–5, figures 2.205 and 206: © July 30, 2014 OpenStax College. Download for free from http://cnx.org/contents/FPtK1zmh@6.27:c4okI-KQJ@4/Bones-of-the-Lower-Limb

page 209, figure 2.209: Drawing inspired by an illustration in V.T. Inman, *The Joint of the Ankle* (Baltimore: Williams & Wilkins, 1976).

pages 214–16, figures 2.216–19: © July 30, 2014 OpenStax College. Download for free from http://cnx.org/contents/FPtK1zmh@6.27:y9_gDy74@3/Appendicular-Muscles-of-the-Pe

page 222, figure 2.225: Drawing inspired by an illustration in Rosdi Daud et al., "Three-Dimensional Morphometric Study of the Trapezium Shape of the Trochlea Tali," *Journal of Foot and Ankle Surgery* 30 (2013): 1–6.

page 224: "Since the relative position of…" is quoted, with the permission of the American Podiatric Medical Association, from K.A. Kirby, "Methods for Determination of Positional Variations in the Subtalar Joint Axis," *Journal of the American Podiatric Medical Association* 77.5 (1987): 228–34.

page 240, figure 2.241: Drawing based on an illustration in Michael J. Coughlin, Charles L. Saltzman, and Roger A. Mann, *Mann's Surgery of the Foot and Ankle* (New York: Elsevier Health Sciences, 2013).

page 269, figures 2.308 and 2.309: Drawings based on those in Thomas G. McPoil and Harry G. Knecht, "Biomechanics of the Foot in Walking: A Functional Approach," *Journal of Orthopaedic and Sports Physical Therapy*, 7.2 (1985): 69-72.

page 272, figure 2.311: Drawing based on those in Thomas G. McPoil and Harry G. Knecht, "Biomechanics of the Foot in Walking: A Functional Approach," *Journal of Orthopaedic and Sports Physical Therapy*, 7.2 (1985): 69-72.

page 276n85: "Few dancers make the cut…" is quoted, with the permission of Wolters Kluwer, from Steven J. Karageanes (ed.), *Principles of Manual Sports Medicine* (Philadelphia: Lippincott Williams & Wilkins, 2005), 497.

page 279n195: "In a hatha yoga pose…" is quoted, with the author's permission, from Doug Keller, *Anusara Yoga: Hatha Yoga in the Anusara Style*, 3rd ed. (South Riding, VA: DoYoga Productions, 2005), 21. Available at http://www.doyoga.com/book.pdf.

page 279n203: "Recommendations for half or quarter…" is quoted from H. Hartmann, K. Wirth, and M. Klusemann, "Analysis of the Load on the Knee Joint and Vertebral Column with Changes in Squatting Depth and Weight Load," *Sport Medicine* 43 (2013): 993–1008, with kind permission from Springer Science+Business Media.

page 280n218: "[H]igher torque values in the…" is quoted from H. Hartmann, K. Wirth, and M. Klusemann, "Analysis of the Load on the Knee Joint and Vertebral Column with Changes in Squatting Depth and Weight Load," *Sport Medicine* 43 (2013): 993–1008, with kind permission from Springer Science+Business Media.

page 280n219: "The influence of soft tissue…" is quoted from H. Hartmann, K. Wirth, and M. Klusemann, "Analysis of the Load on the Knee Joint and Vertebral Column with Changes in Squatting Depth and Weight Load," *Sport Medicine* 43 (2013): 993–1008, with kind permission from Springer Science+Business Media.

page 281n249: "Histological studies have indicated that…" is quoted, with the permission of the American Physical Therapy Association, from Kelley Fitzgerald, "Open Versus Closed Kinetic Chain Exercise: Issues in Rehabilitation After Anterior Cruciate Ligament Reconstructive Surgery," *Physical Therapy* 77 (1997): 1747–54.

Index

Page numbers followed by *f* and *t* indicate figures and tables, respectively. Numbers followed by "n" indicate endnotes.

collagen, 39

collateral ligaments, 162–163, 172, 172*f*

colon, 51

color blindness, 26

compression, 14, 14*f*, 18–19, 91

    definition of, 13, 18

    descriptors of, 22, 22*t*

    examples, 13, 13*f*, 18–19, 19*f*

    hard, 13, 18, 19*f*, 21*t*, 51

    kinds of, 51

    medium, 13, 19, 21*t*, 51

    painful, 20

    sensing, 19–22, 21*t*, 22*t*

    soft, 13, 13*f*, 18–19, 21*t*, 51

    sources of, 51–62, 56*f*

        in ankle–foot segment, 234–236

        in hip joint, 121–123

        in knee joint, 175

    value of, 25, 30, 150

    WSM? spectrum of, 13–14, 14*f*

compressive stress. *see* compression

condyloid joints, 77, 78*f*, 157

connective tissues, 35

contraction

    co-contraction, 174

    concentric, 36

    eccentric, 36

    isometric, 36

    sarcomere, 37

contracture, in joints, 61–62

coronal ligaments, 163

coronal plane, 92, 92*f*

coronal suture, 92, 92*f*

cortex, 52

cortical bone, 52–53

Cowface Pose (Gomukhasana), 94, 94*f*, 97*f*, 273n2

    adduction of hip joint in, 142–143, 143*f*

    external rotation of hip joint in, 134

coxa anteverta, 111

coxa retroverta, 111

coxa valga, 9, 110–111

coxa vara, 9, 110–111, 274n40

coxal bones, 100, 101*f*

credit card effects, 30

creep, 67

cruciate ligaments, 162, 170–171, 172*f*

crural fascia, 161

cuboid bones, 204–205, 204*f*, 208–209

cuneiform bones, 204–205, 204*f*, 208–209

D

Dahners, Laurence, 61

deep back arm line (DBAL), 72*t*, 74*f*

deep fascia, 41

deep front arm line (DFAL), 73*t*, 74*f*

deep front line (DFL), 73*t*, 74*f*, 231, 232

deep leg muscles, 215–216, 216*f*

deltoid collateral, 210

deltoid ligament, 210

descriptors of sensations, 22, 22*t*

Diamond Pose or Thunderbolt (Vajrasana), 58, 169, 175, 242

diarthroses, 77

diets, ideal, 58

differences, 14. *see also* variations

digestion of carbohydrates, 55

directions

    anatomical, 253*t*–255*t*

    in planes of movement, 92–93, 93*f*

discs, intervertebral, 59, 59*f*

distraction, 25

disuse osteoporosis, 25

Dobzhansky, Theodosius, 14

Down Dog (Adhomukhashvanasana), 30, 83n77, 214

    alignment of feet in, 240, 241, 246–247, 246*f*

    ankle dorsiflexion in, 226, 227*f*, 237, 237*f*

    co-contraction in, 174

    external rotation of arm in, 95

    restrictions to dorsiflexion in, 232

dynaments, 45, 45*f*

E

Eagle Pose (Garudasana), 111

    adduction of hip joint in, 141, 141*f*

    internal rotation of hip joint in, 95, 95*f*, 143, 146–147

ears, 41

eating, 29

edge

    emotional, 15–16

    physical, 15

    playing your edge, 15–16, 23, 129, 174

    psychological, 16

    spiritual, 16

Egyptian or Pyramid Pose (Parsvottanasana), 226

elastic response, 86n169

elastin, 39

ellipsoid joints, 77–78, 78*f*, 157

emotional edge, 15–16

empirical axis, 218–221, 221*f*

en pointe (ballet), 242*f*, 243

endomysium, 38

endosteum, 55

energy, muscular, 174

epimysium, 38

epiphyseal plates, 53

epithelia tissues, 35

equinus, 232, 236, 285n392

eversion, 270

exercising joints, 57

extension, 93–94, 93*f*, 94*f*

    biomechanics of, 79

    definition of, 255*t*

extensor digitorum brevis, 216, 216*f*

extensor digitorum longus, 215, 215*f*

extensor hallucs longus, 215, 215*f*

external rotation, 94–95, 95*f*

extracellular matrix (ECM), 32–33, 32*f*

eyes, 19, 29

eyesight, 26, 27

F

fabella, 166, 278n154

faces, 18

fan-shaped muscles, 69

farts, 51

fascia, 41–44, 42*f*

    and bone, 55, 55*f*

    crural, 161

    deep or profound, 41

    of foot, 212–213, 212*f*

    of knee, 161, 161*f*

    myofascia, 38–39, 39*f*

    myofascial meridians, 43, 71, 71*t*–73*t*, 74*f*

    nerve endings in, 46–47

    plantar, 212, 212*f*

    sources of tension from, 118, 170, 231–232

    superficial, 41, 42*f*

fascia lata, 161

fascicles, 38

fasciculus, 38

fascinados, 41

fascinistas, 41

fascists, 41

fat pads, 60

feet. *see* foot

female pelvis, 105, 105*f*

variations in, 257–258, 257*f*

femoral acetabular impingement syndrome (FAIS), 145–146, 149, 149*f*

femoral anteversion, 111, 112, 112*f*, 112*t*, 113

femoral neck, 53

compression against acetabular rim, 121–122, 122*f*

length of, 128, 128*f*

variations in, 113, 113*f*

femoral neck-shaft angle, 102, 110–111, 110*f*, 273n6

variations in, 9, 9*f*, 10, 10*f*, 110–111, 110*f*, 127, 127*f*

femoral retroversion, 111

femoral torsion, 111–113, 111*f*, 131, 131*f*, 273n5

femur, 100, 100*f*, 102, 102*f*, 159, 159*f*

abduction of hip joint by moving, 128–129, 128*f*

external rotation of, 131, 131*f*, 132*f*, 194*f*

variations in, 165

variations of, 110–114, 114–117, 155, 155*t*

fencing lunge, 178, 178*f*

fibroblasts, 25, 43–44

fibronectins, 33

fibrous joints, 77

fibularis tertius, 215, 215*f*

fight-or-flight response, 46

fingerprints, 59

first position (ballet), 133, 133*f*

flat foot (pes planus), 206

flexion, 93–94, 93*f*, 94*f*

biomechanics of, 79

definition of, 256*t*

side, 96, 96*f*

flexion-caused impingement at hip joint, 263

flexor digiti minimi brevis, 216*f*, 217, 218

flexor digitorum brevis, 216*f*, 217

flexor digitorum longus, 215, 216*f*

flexor hallucis brevis, 216*f*, 217

flexor hallucis longus, 215, 216*f*

foot, 28, 204–205. *see also* ankle–foot segment

abduction/adduction of, 270

alignment of, 240–241, 240*f*

in Down Dog, 246–247, 246*f*

with knee, 180, 195–197

with thigh, 196–197, 196*f*

arches of, 205–207, 205*f*

bones of, 204–205, 204*f*, 207–209

claw foot, 206

fascia of, 212–213, 212*f*

flat foot (pes planus), 206

forefoot, 201

hindfoot, 201

hollow foot (pes cavus), 206

interossei of, 218, 218*f*

intrinsic muscles of, 216–218, 216*f*

ligaments that resist movements of, 234*t*

midfoot, 201

movements of, 201, 202*f*, 267–272, 267*f*

open- and closed-chain, 271–272, 272*t*

restrictions to, 234*t*

variations in, 54

muscles of, 216–218, 216*f*, 219*t*

muscles that cause or resist movements of, 233*t*

pronation of, 92–93, 93*f*, 224*f*, 228–230, 229*f*, 230*f*, 268–269, 272*t*

causes of, 244

definition of, 256*t*

restrictions to, 233, 233*t*, 234*t*, 236

variations in, 243–244

retinacula of, 211–212, 211*f*, 212*t*

sling of, 220, 220*f*

supination of, 92–93, 93*f*, 224*f*, 228–229, 229*f*, 230*f*, 268–269

causes of, 244

definition of, 256*t*

plantarflexion with, 245

restrictions to, 233, 233*t*, 234, 234*t*, 236

variations in, 243–244

variations in, 54, 225

forefoot, 201

fractures, 75

fragility, 28, 29*f*

freeze reaction, 46

front functional line (FFL), 72*t*, 74*f*

frontal plane, 92, 92*f*

Fuller, Buckminster, 52

functional yoga, 22–23

fusiform muscles, 69, 69*f*

G

gaits, 40, 236

gastrocnemius, 164, 214

gastrocnemius contracture, 232

gender differences, 105, 105*f*

genes, 23

genu recurvatum, 186

genu valgum or varum, 5*f*, 167–168, 167*f*, 184–185, 184*f*, 185*f*, 188*f*, 189*f*, 192*f*

cause of, 188–189

correction of, 189–191, 190*f*, 191–192, 191*f*

dangers and benefits of, 265–266

how to reduce, 191–192, 191*f*

in Lotus Pose (Padmasana), 194–195, 194*f*

when to change, 189–191

ginglymoid joints, 78

glands, 47, 63

gliding joints, 78, 78*f*

glycosaminoglycans, 49, 49*f*, 51

Goddess Pose (Utkatakonasana)

abduction in, 96, 128–129

external rotation of arms in, 95, 95*f*

external rotation of hip joint in, 95, 95*f*, 133, 133*f*

horizontal abduction in, 97, 97*f*

Goldilocks Curve, 25, 25*f*

Goldilocks Philosophy, 26, 27, 30, 62

Goldilocks Position, 25

Golgi, Camillo, 84n125

Golgi tendon organs (GTO), 46, 47–48

greater trochanter, 114

compression against pelvis, 122, 122*f*

compression zone between ilium and, 128, 128*f*

Grilley, Paul, xv–xvi, 10, 92–93

ground substance, 49, 51

grounding, 206

GTO. *see* Golgi tendon organs

guts, 51

H

Half-Moon Pose (Ardhachandrasana)

hyperextension of knee in, 187, 187*f*

lateral flexion in, 96, 96*f*

hallux, 209

hallux rigidus, 245

hallux valgus (bunions), 218, 285n386

hamsprings, 135–136, 135*f*

hamstrings, 13, 13*f*, 48, 48*f*, 135, 136, 138*f*, 164, 170, 184, 184*f*

Happy Baby (Ananda Balasana), 137, 138

Hatha yoga, 3, 17

Head-to-Knee Pose (Janusirsasana)

flexion of hip joint in, 138, 139*f*

movements of toes in, 231, 231*f*

health, 25, 25*f*

heartbeat, 48

Hedley, Gil, 84n108

heel
    alignment with ankle, 224–225, 224*f*
    variations in, 224–225, 224*f*

helical lines, 72*t*, 74*f*

hematopoietic cells, 53

Hero Pose (Virasana), 112, 113, 163, 169
    ankle plantarflexion in, 241, 241*f*, 242
    flexion of knee in, 175, 175*f*
    internal rotation of hip joint in, 146, 146*f*, 148, 148*f*
    internal rotation of knee joint in, 192, 192*f*, 193

high ankle sprain, 204

hindfoot, 201

hinge joints, 78, 78*f*

hip bone. *see* ilium

hip joint, 99–156, 99*f*, 101*f*
    abduction of, 126–130, 126*f*, 128*f*, 130*f*, 154*t*
        with external rotation and extension, 151
        with flexion, 138–139, 138*f*, 139*f*, 153*t*
        horizontal, 129–130, 129*f*, 130*f*, 154*t*
        with internal rotation, 147–148
        limits to, 126, 126*f*, 128
        range of, 129, 130*f*
        variations in, 126–130, 128*f*
    adduction of, 139–143, 140*f*, 141*f*, 154*t*
        with flexion, 141–143, 141*f*, 143*f*, 154*t*
        with internal rotation, 146–147, 147*f*, 154*t*
    architecture of, 100
    axis of rotation, 263, 263*f*
    bones of, 100–102, 101*f*
    circumduction of, 124–125, 124*f*
    extension of, 150–151, 153*t*
    external (lateral) rotation of, 132*f*, 133*f*, 135*f*, 153*t*
        with extension and abduction, 151
        with flexion, 134, 134*f*, 154*t*
        with horizontal abduction, 133, 133*f*
        variations in, 130–134
    flexion-caused impingement at, 263
    flexion of, 135–139, 136*f*, 137*f*, 152*t*
        with abduction, 138–139, 138*f*, 139*f*, 153*t*
        with adduction, 141–143, 141*f*, 143*f*, 154*t*
        with external rotation, 134, 134*f*, 154*t*
        with internal rotation, 138, 145–146, 152*t*, 154*t*

        with internal rotation and abduction, 148
    horizontal abduction of, 129–130, 129*f*, 130*f*, 154*t*
    horizontal adduction of, 142
    internal (medial) rotation of, 143–148, 144*f*, 145*f*, 154*t*
        with abduction, 147–148
        with adduction, 146–147, 147*f*, 154*t*
        with flexion, 145–146, 152*t*, 154*t*
        with flexion and abduction, 148
    joint capsule of, 103, 103*f*
    leveling the hips, 114–116, 114*f*, 115*f*
    ligaments of, 103, 103*f*
    muscles of, 104, 104*f*
    muscles that cause and restrict movement of, 118, 119*t*
    range of abduction of, 129, 130*f*
    range of motion of
        estimating, 124
        normal, 117–118, 118*t*
        variations in, 124–151
    rotation of
        external (lateral), 130–134, 132*f*, 133*f*, 134*f*, 135*f*, 153*t*, 154*t*
        internal (medial), 143–148, 152*t*, 154*t*
    sources of compression in, 121–123
    sources of tension in, 118–119, 121*t*
    summary, 152–156, 251
    variations, 5*f*, 105–117, 274n29
    variations in abduction, 126–130, 128*f*
    variations in adduction, 139–143, 140*f*
    variations in circumduction, 124–125, 124*f*
    variations in extension, 150–151
    variations in external (lateral) rotation of, 130–134
    variations in flexion, 135–139
    variations in internal (medial) rotation of, 143–148
    variations in range of motion, 124–151
    and the WSM? spectrum, 152, 152*t*–155*t*
    in yoga postures, 117–151

hip openers, 194

hip socket. *see* acetabulum

Hispanics, 26

hockey goalies, 147, 147*f*

hollow foot (pes cavus), 206

Holmes, Bob, 33

horizontal abduction, 97, 97*f*, 129–130, 129*f*, 133, 155*t*

horizontal plane, 92, 92*f*

hyaline cartilage, 58

hyaluronan, 49

hyaluronic acid, 49, 51

hydraulic amplification, 44

hydraulics, 50

hygiene hypothesis, 28–29

hyperplasia, 84n105

hypertonia, 47

hypertrophy, 84n105

hypotonia, 47

I

ideal diets, 58

identical twins, 26

iliac crest, 100, 100*f*

iliofemoral ligament, 103, 103*f*
    effects of movement on, 119, 120*f*
    sources of tension from, 119, 121*t*

iliotibial band (IT band), 161

ilium, 100, 100*f*

immune system, 49–50, 63
    adaptive, 49
    development of, 28–29
    innate, 49
    key components, 49

impingement
    femoral acetabular impingement syndrome (FAIS), 145–146, 149, 149*f*
    flexion-caused, at hip joint, 263
    as form of compression, 107
    posterior ankle impingement syndrome (PAIS), 222, 285n408

individuality, 5. *see also* variations

injuries
    caused by yoga, 17
    stress when injured, 31

Inman, V.T., 282n304

innate immune system, 49

integrins, 32, 32*f*, 46

intercondylar eminence, 160, 160*f*

intercondylar fossa, 159, 159*f*

intercondylar groove, 159, 159*f*, 197

intercondylar notch, 159, 159*f*

internal rotation, 94–95, 95*f*

interossei, of foot, 218, 218*f*

intervertebral discs, 59, 59*f*, 77

intervertebral symphysis, 77

intestines, 51

inversion, 270

ipsilateral functional line (IFL), 72*t*, 74*f*

ischiofemoral ligament, 103, 103*f*

    effects of movement on, 119, 120*f*

    sources of tension from, 119, 121*t*

Iyengar, B.K.S., xvi, 176

    hyperextension of knee, 187, 187*f*

    options for beginners, 148

    version of Kandasana, 230*f*, 244, 245

    version of Utkatasana, 180

    version of Warrior Two (Virabhadrasana), 176, 176*f*

Iyengar Yoga, xv, xvi, 177, 177*f*

J

jaws, 28

joint segments, 89

joints, 57–62

    in ankle–foot segment, 201

    ankle joint, 203–204, 203*f*

    ball-and-socket, 77, 78*f*

    biomechanics of, 79–80, 80*f*

    cartilaginous, 77, 86n191

    condyloid, 77, 78*f*, 157

    contracture in, 61–62

    definition of, 57

    ellipsoid, 77–78, 78*f*, 157

    exercising, 57

    fibrous, 77

    ginglymoid, 78

    gliding, 78, 78*f*

    hanging out in, 195

    hinge, 78, 78*f*

    hip joint, 99–156, 99*f*, 101*f*

    knee joint, 60, 60*f*, 157–199

    of lower body, 99–156, 157–199, 201–250

    parts of, 60

    patellofemoral joint, 157

    pivot, 78, 78*f*

    rolling, 79, 79*f*, 80, 80*f*

    saddle, 78, 78*f*

    safely stressing, 57

    spheroidal, 77

    syndesmosis, 204

    synovial, 57, 77–78, 78*f*, 86n191

    tibiofibular joint, 157

    types of, 77–78, 78*f*

Jois, Pattabhi, xv, xvi, 177, 180

Jois, Sharat, 179, 179*f*

K

Kabat, Herman, 47–48

Kalama Sutta, 11

Kaminoff, Leslie, 3

Kandasana, 230*f*, 244–245

King Dancer (Natarajasana)

    ankle plantarflexion in, 241, 242

    extension of hip joint in, 150

    hyperextension of knee in, 187, 187*f*

knee joint, 60, 60*f*, 157–199

    adduction of, 194–195, 194*f*

    alignment of, 176–179, 195–197

    architecture of, 157–158

    biomechanics of, 80, 80*f*

    bones of, 157, 158*f*, 159–160, 166

    extension of, 180–183

    fascia of, 161, 161*f*

    flexion of

        normal, 169, 169*t*

        variations, 175–176

    hyperextension of, 180, 182–184, 182*f*, 183*f*, 186–187, 187*f*

        reducing, 183–184

    joinings, 157

    ligaments of, 158, 158*f*, 160–164, 162*f*

    locking in full extension, 195

    loose-packed position, 61

    movements of, 168–169, 168*f*

    muscles causing or resisting movement, 171*t*

    muscles of, 164

    range of motion

        normal, 169, 169*t*

        variations, 175–198

    rotation of, 192–195, 192*f*

        internal, 192, 192*f*

        in Lotus Pose (Padmasana), 194–195, 194*f*

        normal, 169

    screw-home mechanism, 195

    sideways movement of, 184–188

    sources of compression, 175

    sources of tension, 169–172, 173*t*

    summary, 199, 251

    thigh muscles that cross, 158, 159*f*

    valgum or varum orientation of, 188, 188*f*, 189*f*, 192*f*

        cause of, 188–189

        correction of, 189–191, 190*f*, 191–192, 191*f*

        dangers and benefits of, 265–266

        how to reduce, 191–192, 191*f*

        in Lotus Pose (Padmasana), 194–195, 194*f*

        when to change, 189–191

    variations, 165–168

    variations in range of motion, 175–198

    and the WSM? spectrum, 199, 199*t*

    in yoga postures, 168–198

knee-joint capsule, 163, 172

knee valgum or varum. *see* genu valgum or varum

Knees-to-Chest Pose (Apanasana), 137, 137*f*

knock-knees (genu valgus). *see* genu valgum or varum

Kripalu yoga, xvi

Krishnamacharya, Tirumalai, 89, 176, 177*f*

Kundalini yoga, 182

kyphosis, 59

L

labrum, 58, 77, 103, 108, 117, 121–122, 122*f*, 125, 132*f*, 134*f*, 145, 149, 149*f*, 263

language

    anatomical directions, 253*t*–255*t*

    for body movements, 255*t*–256*t*, 267

    descriptors of sensations, 22, 22*t*

    for directions in planes of movement, 92–93, 93*f*

    for foot and ankle movement, 267, 267*f*

    metric standards, 36

Lasater, Judith, 116

last straw effect, 26

lateral collateral ligament (LCL), 162–163, 162*f*, 172, 172*f*

lateral leg muscles, 215, 215*f*

lateral line (LL), 71*t*, 74*f*, 231, 232

lateral plantar flexors, 215, 215*f*

lateral rotation, 94

Law of Transformation of the Bone (Wolff's Law), 30

LCL. *see* lateral collateral ligament

leg muscles

    anterior, 215, 215*f*

    deep, 215–216, 216*f*

    lateral, 215, 215*f*

    posterior, 214–216, 214*f*

lesser trochanter, 54, 54*f*, 116–117, 116*f*

leveling the hips, 114–116, 114*f*

leveling the pelvis, 114–116, 114*f*, 115*f*

levers, 259–261, 260*f*

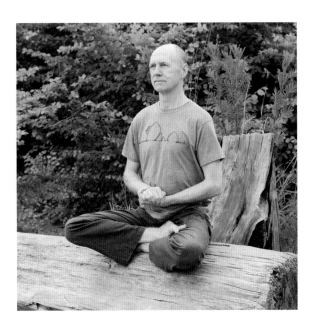

ABOUT THE AUTHOR

Bernie Clark has had a passion for science, health, sports and spirituality since childhood. He has a degree in science from the University of Waterloo and spent over 25 years as a senior executive in the high-tech/space industry. Bernie has been investigating the path of meditation for over three decades and began teaching yoga and meditation in 1998. He conducts yoga teacher trainings several times a year and aims to build bridges between the experiences of yoga and the understandings of modern science. He is creator of the www.YinYoga.com website. Bernie lives and teaches in Vancouver, Canada.

Other books by Bernie Clark:

YinSights: A Journey into the Philosophy and Practice of Yin Yoga

The Complete Guide to Yin Yoga: The Philosophy and Practice of Yin Yoga

From the Gita to the Grail: Exploring Yoga Stories and Western Myths

To stay current with Bernie Clark's teaching, workshops, videos, writings and books, subscribe to the Yin Yoga Insights newsletters at www.YinYoga.com.

Also by Bernie Clark

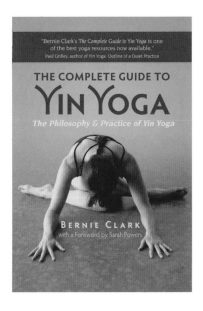

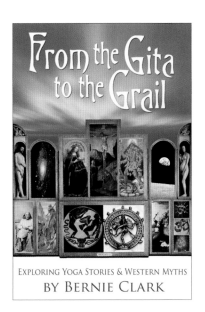

THE COMPLETE GUIDE TO YIN YOGA

The Philosophy & Practice of Yin Yoga

Bernie Clark's *The Complete Guide to Yin Yoga* provides an in-depth look at the philosophy and practice of Yin Yoga, with illustrated sections on how to practice it. All forms of yoga can provide physical, emotional and mental benefits, but Yin Yoga works at the deeper levels of the body/heart/mind: the connective tissues of the ligaments, fascia, joints and bones, and the energetic channels of the meridians, nerves and blood system. One big difference noticed by students of Yin Yoga is the long-held, passive nature of the postures, which gives time for a deeper journey to unfold, a journey into the meditative aspects of yoga, a bridge to living life mindfully.

Bernie presents comprehensive information on how to do the practice, including a deep look inside over two dozen Yin Yoga postures, showing the benefit of the pose, how to get into and out of the pose, contraindications and warnings for those who may have trouble with particular aspects of the posture, and other important information. The benefits are explored in three main sections: the physiological benefits, the energetic benefits and the mental/emotional benefits.

FROM THE GITA TO THE GRAIL

Exploring Yoga Stories & Western Myths

Learn what the myths of yoga mean to those of us who grew up in Western culture and with Western stories.

"In this insightful book, Bernie reminds us that we have a choice in how we live our lives; we can hold tight to our beliefs, allowing them to dictate our reality, or we can invite every story (or even encounter) to be a gateway into the poetic, multifaceted dimensions of truth, and the fluid nature of reality." —*Sarah Powers, author of* Insight Yoga *and founder of the Insight Yoga Institute*

"Bernie's book covers mythical territory any student of yoga should be aware of. Diving into both unfamiliar and familiar stories of creation and the path of the hero, Bernie's readable style is like the voice of an Elder. If you could record Joseph Campbell and Carl Jung's conversation over a game of chess, it might sound something like this." —*Daniel Clement, founder of Open Source Yoga*